böhlau

Tiere in der Geschichte | Animals in History

Band 2 | Volume 2

Herausgegeben von | Edited by
Christian Jaser, Mieke Roscher, Nadir Weber

Die Buchreihe *Tiere in der Geschichte* versammelt historische Studien zur Geschichte der Mensch-Tier-Beziehungen. Die Werke beleuchten die Rollen von Tieren in Gesellschaften von der Antike bis zur Gegenwart. Sie untersuchen die vielfältigen Interaktionsformen zwischen Menschen und anderen Lebewesen und analysieren wirkmächtige Unterscheidungen wie die zwischen Wildtieren auf der einen und Haus- und Nutztieren auf der anderen Seite im historischen Kontext. Auch die sich wandelnden kulturellen Repräsentationen von Tieren werden in den Blick genommen, zugleich spüren die Studien der Materialität der gelebten Beziehungen nach. Der geographische Fokus der Reihe liegt auf dem europäischen Kontinent und seinen Verflechtungen mit anderen Weltregionen. Die ausgewählten Titel bereichern die methodischen Entwicklungen im neuen Forschungsfeld der historischen Human-Animal Studies und leisten damit zugleich einen Beitrag zu aktuellen Debatten der Sozial-, Kultur-, Politik- oder Umweltgeschichte.

The *Animals in History* book series publishes historiographical studies on the history of human-animal relations. The monographs and anthologies shed light on the roles of animals in societies from antiquity to the present. They examine the various interactions between humans and other living beings and historicise powerful categories such as the distinctions between domesticated animals and wild animals or between pets and livestock. They also look at the changing cultural representations of animals and trace the materiality of interspecific relationships. The geographical focus of the series is on the European continent and its interconnections with other world regions. The selected titles enrich the methodological developments in the new research field of historical human-animal studies and contribute to current scholarly debates in social, cultural, political, or environmental history.

Die Herausgeber | The Editors

Axel C. Hüntelmann / Christian Jaser /
Mieke Roscher / Nadir Weber (eds.)

Animals and Epidemics

Interspecies Entanglements in Historical Perspective

BÖHLAU

Published with the financial support of the University of Klagenfurt and the Research Committee of the University of Lucerne.

Forschungskommission der Universität Luzern

Bibliographic information published by the Deutsche Nationalbibliothek:
The Deutsche Nationalbibliothek lists this publication in the Deutsche Nationalbibliografie; detailed bibliographic data available online: https://dnb.de.

Cover image: Professional rat catchers with a dog and dead rats during "cleansing operations" in the quarantine area in Sidney, 1900, Western Sidney Records Centre / Wikimedia Commons.
Typesetting: le-tex publishing services, Leipzig
Cover design: Guido Klütsch, Köln
Printed and bound: Hubert & Co, Göttingen
Printed in the EU

Vandenhoeck & Ruprecht Verlage | www.vandenhoeck-ruprecht-verlage.com

ISBN 978-3-412-52570-5 (print)
ISBN 978-3-412-52572-9 (digital)

Contents

Perspectives

Case Studies

The *Longue Durée*

Perspectives

Axel C. Hüntelmann, Christian Jaser, Mieke Roscher, Nadir Weber

Introduction

Animals and Epidemics in Historical Perspective

Epidemics seem to be everywhere. Within the last few decades alone, BSE was followed by SARS and avian influenza, swine influenza, Ebola, MERS, and Zika. The outbreak of another respiratory illness in Wuhan in late 2019 appeared to be then just another epidemic episode: regionally limited, largely ignored by the Western world, and no doubt soon to be forgotten. As we know now, things turned out differently. However, all of these epidemics had two things in common: animals played a central role in the outbreak as well as in the spread of the disease; and yet their importance has been largely overlooked by historians. This volume aims to correct and fill this research gap.

The Covid-19 pandemic, with its severe economic, social, and public health consequences all over the world has shown plainly how animals figure prominently as possible causes, disease carriers, or alternate hosts in scientific research and public debates.[1] The emergence and rapid spread of the virus has been attributed to a new, ecologically problematic, and intensified human-animal relationship characterized by human infringement on the habitats and retreat areas of so-called wild species, as well as by the global animal market.[2] As environmental historians have remarked, it is quite astonishing how "nonhuman animals have emerged as key figures and flashpoints in the drama of an all-too-human disease."[3]

At the same time, animals also appeared as *agents* in the narratives that accompanied the pandemic, from stories about the origins of the disease in isolated bat caves or at a public wet market to animals' "reclaiming" of places after humans had been forced into lockdown. Did the coronavirus even represent the "revenge of the pangolins" – the retribution of a highly endangered species against humankind?[4] Wherever in the

1 See, for example, Christos Lynteris (ed.), Framing Animals as Epidemic Villains. Histories of Non-Human Disease Vectors, Cham 2019; id., Human Extinction and the Pandemic Imagery, London 2019.

2 Christine K. Johnson et al., Global Shifts in Mammalian Population Trends Reveal Key Predictors of Virus Spillover Risk, in: Proceedings of the Royal Society B (2020), http://dx.doi.org/10.1098/rspb.2019.2736 (last accessed 4 June 2023).

3 Peter Alagona, All of Us, Animals, in: id. et al., Reflections: Environmental History in the Era of COVID-19, in: Environmental History 25 (2020) (Special Issue), 595–686, 597–600.

4 Wufei Yu, Coronavirus: Revenge of the Pangolins, in: New York Times, 5 March 2020, https://www.nytimes.com/2020/03/05/opinion/coronavirus-china-pangolins.html (12 June 2023); Matthias Glaubrecht, Die Rache des Pangolin. Wild gewordene Pandemien und der Schutz der Artenvielfalt, Berlin 2022. Among others, WHO experts later discussed the possible roles of bats and pangolins as carriers, and civets, cats, or mink as hosts. WHO-convened Global Study of Origins-CoV-2: China Part. Joint Report, 30 March

long chain of human-animal entanglements the prime cause for the current pandemic may lie, epidemics and pandemics serve as a linchpin in reflections on the current and historical state of human-animal relationships and on their respective roles as historical agents.

1. (Re)considering Animals in the History of Epidemics

The historical epidemics and pandemics, the plagues and pests that are discussed in this book are all defined by their animal momentum. A closer look, inspired by the research questions and concepts of historical animal studies,[5] shows that humans have ascribed non-human animals numerous roles in connection with such epidemics since antiquity. Animals have appeared as causative agents or early indicators, but also as victims and–through animal-based remedies, and later through vaccines – as potential saviours. This points to the extent to which humans and animals share not only a bodily nature and potential for action, but above all a vulnerability. It also shows that the history of human societies has always been a history of (biological and cultural) co-evolution with other animals.[6] Looking at the animals' roles in historical epidemics therefore not only helps us "to make sense of the traces of human-animal entanglements in proliferating news reports,"[7] but also allows us to analyse historical sources in a different way, revealing the history-shaping character of interspecies entanglements. By focusing on the *longue durée* of zoonotic constellations and the role of animals during epidemics, we aim to historicise and contextualize human-animal relations across epochal boundaries from a multi-perspective viewpoint that focuses on health crises and their impacts on human both and non-human animals.

In the long genealogy of historical diseases, a first glance at (perceived or real) zoonotic transmissions already illustrates how they can frame historical periodization. The Justinianic Plague of 542 and its endemic aftermath has been considered by many scholars of late antiquity as a cultural, religious, and social cesura rather than a merely demographic or economic one in the transitional phase between antiquity and the Middle Ages.[8] In a similar way, the plague epidemic at the end of the 1340s was already seen by

---

2021, https://www.who.int/health-topics/coronavirus/origins-of-the-virus (4 June 2023). See also the contribution by Matthias Glaubrecht in this volume.

5 For a recent overview of this field of research, see the Mieke Roscher/André Krebber/Brett Mizelle (eds.), Handbook of Historical Animal Studies, Berlin/Boston 2021.

6 See Edmund Russell, Coevolutionary History, in: The American Historical Review 119 (2014), 1514–1528.

7 Dolly Jørgensen, Tracking Animals in a Pandemic, in: Alagona et al., Reflections (note 3), 626–631, 626.

8 See the discussion between Lee Mordechai et al., The Justinianic Plague. An Inconsequential Pandemic?, in: PNAS 116 (2019), 25546–25554, and Mischa Meier, The "Justinianic Plague": An "Inconsequential Pandemic"? A Reply, in: Medizinhistorisches Journal 55/2 (2020), 172–199. See Kyle Harper, The Fate of Rome. Climate, Disease, and the End of an Empire, Princeton 2017; and id., Plagues upon the Earth.

contemporaries as an epochal shift and is still in many compendiums and handbooks on the era used as an index of the alleged "crisis" of the late Middle Ages. Insofar as these zoonotic pandemics, at least in their historical reflection, are ascribed to specific human-animal relations, non-human animals emerge as potent co-actors in the shaping of epochs and their construction. With this focus, the question to be asked by historians is how animals impacted time regimes and thus also structured historical thinking.

However, in previous historiography of epidemics' effects, human-animal relationships have rarely been considered. When they have, animals have mainly been discussed as features of the (natural) environment, rather than as part of the societies affected by the epidemics. Accordingly, epidemics are seen primarily as arguments for the far-reaching significance of environmental factors on the course of human history. Kyle Harper, for instance, has emphasized how climate change and the Justinianic Plague influenced the so-called fall of the Roman Empire, and the same is true of publications on plague in the Middle Ages.[9] Publications on the history of cholera have emphasized the impact of epidemics on social developments,[10] social turmoil,[11] or, in the case of smallpox, on warfare.[12]

Hence, even recent historical overviews of epidemics have understood these outbreaks primarily as interactions between microbiotic pathogens and humans, and then focused on their social and political impact. Volker Reinhardt's widely read study of the plague years 1347–1353, for instance, draws on similarities and differences to the Covid pandemic, yet its animal origins are just a side note.[13] Instead, the author focuses on the discriminating factor of epidemics among humans. Similarly, in a recently published "short history of the Covid pandemic", Malte Thießen, among others, discusses the social stigmatization of Asian people in Europe during the first weeks and months of the pandemic, drawing a connection to older tropes of Jews as scapegoats during plague

---

Disease and the Course of Human History, Princeton, NJ 2022; critical to Harper Karl-Heinz Leven, Mimesis, Miasma und Molekularmedizin.Die "Justinianische Pest" in der neueren Forschung, in: Marcel Bubert/André Krischer (eds.), Zwischen Gottesstrafe und Verschwörungstheorien. Deutungskonkurrenzen bei Epidemien von der Antike bis zur Gegenwart, Frankfurt am Main 2023, 60–91.

9 Harper, Fate of Rome (note 8); Jams Belich, The World the Plague Made. The Black Death and the Rise of Europe, Princeton 2022; Klaus Bergdolt, Der Schwarze Tod in Europa. Die Große Pest und das Ende des Mittelalters, Munich 2003; Mischa Meier, Die Pest. Die Geschichte eines Menschheitstraumas, Stuttgart 2005.

10 See Richard J. Evans, Death in Hamburg. Society and Politics in the Cholera Years, Oxford 1987; id., Epidemics and Revolutions. Cholera in the Nineteenth-Century Europe, in: Past and Present 120 (1988), 123–146; Christopher A. Hamlin, Cholera. The Biography, Oxford 2009.

11 See exemplarily Evans, Epidemics and Revolutions; or for cholera and other epidemics Samuel K. Cohn Jr., Epidemics. Hate and Compassion from the Plague of Athens to AIDS, Oxford 2018.

12 See for other epidemics, Stefan Winkle, Geißeln der Menschheit. Kulturgeschichte der Seuchen, Zurich 1997.

13 Volker Reinhardt, Die Macht der Seuche. Wie die Große Pest die Welt veränderte, Munich 2021, 11.

epidemics.[14] In contrast, animals, apart from the figurative scapegoat, are more or less absent in these accounts.[15] In Jacalyn Duffin's recent Covid-19 history, animals (and human-animal relationships) are present, but ephemeral,[16] just as they are in Frank M. Snowdon's (revised) overview on epidemics "from the black death to the present" or in Charles Kenny's "plague cycle".[17]

The marginal role that animals have played in the historiography of epidemics makes them all the more susceptible to stereotypical attributions, which have had far-reaching consequences right up to the recent past. The co-presence of animals – especially "pests" – in historical accounts on epidemics often appears primarily as a sanitary problem and danger, a one-sided view of the past that can, in turn, shape perceptions in the present. A striking example of this is the "global war" on rats in the first half of the twentieth century, driven by their then newly identified (potential) role as carriers of plague via the rat flea.[18] Although rats were not the direct causative agent, they were now closely associated with plague and became an iconic symbol for past and present diseases. For example, a poster displayed in Marseille in 1920 called for the total extermination of rats, referring to the plague outbreak two hundred years earlier (fig. 1).[19] Even today, on the semantic level, the term "pest" refers to both the plague and the vermin, especially the rat. This interpretation of rats as a potentially deadly threat

---

14 Malte Thießen, Auf Abstand. Eine kurze Geschichte der Coronapandemie, Frankfurt a. M. 2021.

15 Ibid.; Martin Subrow (ed.), Seuche und Gesellschaft, Leipzig 2022. See also Malte Thießen (ed.), Infiziertes Europa. Seuchen im langen 20. Jahrhundert, Munich 2014; or Heiner Fangerau and Alfons Labisch, Pest und Corona: Pandemien in Geschichte, Gegenwart und Zukunft, Freiburg 2020. In Thießen's history about immunization (vaccination), animals play also only a minor role: Malte Thießen, Immunisierte Gesellschaft. Impfen in Deutschland im 19. und 20. Jahrhundert, Göttingen 2017.

16 Revealingly, animals are listed separately (as bats, pangolins), but also summarized as "animals" in the index; see Jacalyn Duffin, Covid-19. A History, Montreal 2022.

17 Frank M. Snowden, Epidemics and Society. From the Black Death to the Present, New Haven 2019; a more social and economic history of plagues: Charles Kenny, The Plague Cycle. The Unending War Between Humanity and Infectious Disease, New York 2021. In addition to the above-mentioned, see for example Joseph P. Byrne/Jo N. Hays, Epidemics and Pandemics. From Ancient Plagues to Modern-Day Threats, 2 vols., Santa Barbara 2021. Although Mitchell L. Hammond, Epidemics and the Modern World, Toronto 2020, a more student-oriented introduction to the history of epidemics combining various topics like race, gender, space, and industrialization with epidemics, has a separate chapter on rinderpest, as epizootics and animals were exemplarily linked to imperialism and environmental history. A similar introduction, addressed to a broader readership, Rae-Ellen W./Allison Kavey, Viral Pandemics. From Smallpox to COVID 2019, London 2021, discusses in one chapter the transmission of pathogens from animals to humans.

18 This connection was made following the seminal discovery of *Yersinia pestis* by Paul-Louis Simond, La propagation de la peste, in: Annales de l'Institut Pasteur 12 (1898), 625–687. See Michael McCormick, Rats, Communications, and Plague. Toward an Ecological History, in: Journal of Interdisciplinary History 34/1 (2003), 1–25.

19 On the global fight against rats and other rodents, see the contributions by Jules Skotnes-Brown and Matheus Duarte Da Silva in this volume.

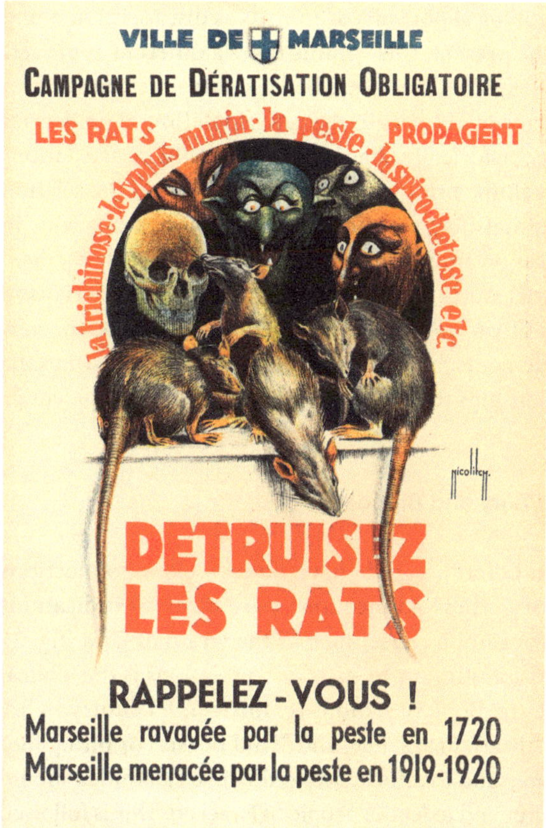
VILLE DE MARSEILLE
CAMPAGNE DE DÉRATISATION OBLIGATOIRE
LES RATS PROPAGENT
la trichinose · le typhus murin · la peste · la spirochetose etc.
DETRUISEZ LES RATS
RAPPELEZ-VOUS !
Marseille ravagée par la peste en 1720
Marseille menacée par la peste en 1919-1920

Fig. 1 Public poster by the city authorities of Marseilles calling for the extermination of rats. Colour lithograph by Obrad Nicolitch, Marseille, 1920. Due to the transmission of the plague bacillus by rat fleas, postulated a few decades earlier, rats were retrospectively blamed for the spread of numerous epidemics, including the devastating plague in Marseille in 1720. Through the grotesque faces in the background, the poster further links this negative image to anti-Asian and anti-Semitic stereotypes.

still shapes our image of them today – even though recent research has fundamentally challenged their role as plague reservoirs in the past.[20]

20 See Nils Stenseth et al., No Evidence for Persistent Natural Plague Reservoirs in Historical and Modern Europe, Proceedings of the National Academy of Sciences PNAS 119/51 (2022), https://doi.org/10.1073/pnas.2209816119 (11 May 2023).

To avoid such one-sided and stereotypical portraits of animals as disease carriers and pathogenic agents in the past and the present, this volume takes a different approach. Inspired by recent research in animal studies, the essays here examine the connections between semiotic signifying functions of animals in the representation of epidemics and the material practice of diverse, historically changing interspecific constellations of relationships.[21] In doing so, the volume brings together discussions on the relation between human epidemics and animal diseases that were previously dealt with in separate research discourses. It focuses on animals and the animals' historically ascribed agency as transmitters, hosts, patients, and – in the case of smallpox, diphtheria, and tuberculosis – as potential sources of vaccines, sera, or diagnostics. This opens new perspectives on interspecies entanglements, biopolitics, economics, ecologies, and the *longue durée* of human-animal relationships that impact and are impacted by epidemics.

2. Threats or Saviours? Animal Polity and Biopolitics

Since antiquity (and arguably even before), people have noticed close connections between human and animal diseases. These connections were taken as indications either of zoonotic infection or of a common cause, such as the wrath of God (fig. 2). An impressive and culturally powerful testimony to such interpretations is the biblical narrative of the plagues of Egypt in the Book of Exodus (c. thirteenth century BCE), in which animals appear in various roles. Frogs, lice, and "wild beasts" or biting flies (plagues 2 to 4), which affected people and livestock, foretold worse calamities should the Pharaoh fail to obey Yahweh's command to let the people of Israel go. This is followed by a devastating pestilence of livestock (5), immediately followed by terrible "festering boils", which again agonized both people and livestock. The plague of locusts (8), and finally, the death of all the firstborn – including "all the firstborn of the cattle" – mark the end of the story.[22] Animals are thus portrayed in multiple roles, as plague carriers (a possible link between the fourth and fifth plagues) and as victims of the diseases.[23]

Such archetypal narratives were perpetuated and illustrated in medieval Europe in both the Christian and Jewish traditions (fig. 3) and linked to the animal knowledge of classical natural history as well as to the animal images in contemporary bestiaries. Based on the Galenic miasma theory, sick animals were also considered to cause "bad air", which could lead to illness in humans. Both in the case of farm animal epidemics and in the great plague waves from the fourteenth century onwards, urban authorities

21 Mieke Roscher, New Political History and the Writing of Animal Lives, in: Hilda Kean/Philip Howell (eds.), The Routledge Handbook of Human-Animal History, London 2018, 53–75.

22 Exodus 7:14–12:36.

23 Daniel Hillel, The Natural History of the Bible. An Environmental Exploration of the Hebrew Scriptures, New York 2006.

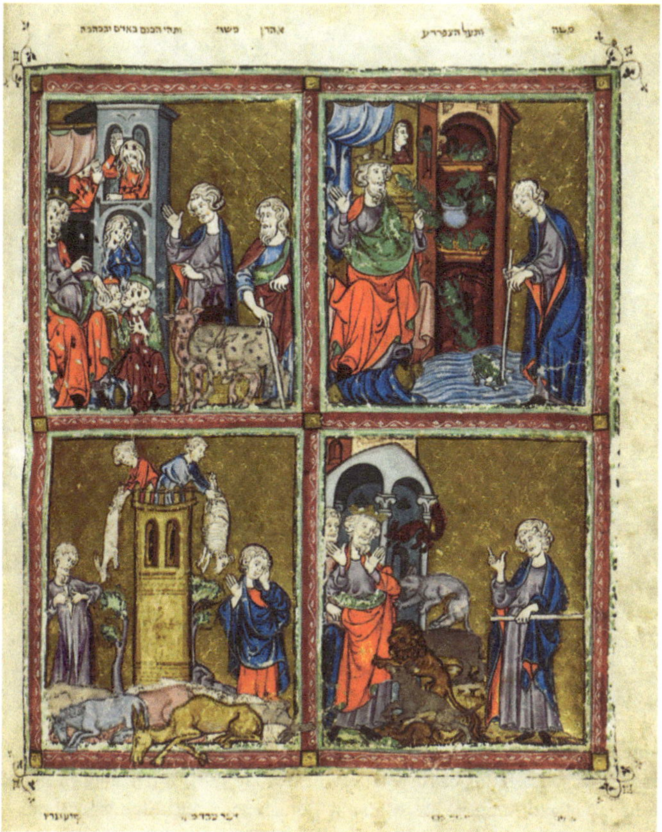

Fig. 2 Illustration of the Plagues of Egypt in the Jewish *Haggadah for Passover* (the "Golden Haggadah"), c. 1320–30. The representation shows four of ten plagues in which animals played prominent roles as disruptive factors (frogs), fellow sufferers of a fly plague, mourned victims of an animal epidemic, and as "wild beasts" attacking humans.

set about "cleansing" the streets of dirty, potentially infected animals.[24] Interestingly, these sanitary measures rarely applied to rats and other small animals, which were later to become the main targets of such efforts, but rather to poultry, dogs, and livestock. Through the fight against epidemics, non-human animals thus became a prominent object of governmental biopolitics, which in the course of the early modern period also increasingly extended to larger territories.[25]

---

24 See the contributions by Carole Rawcliffe, Willam Riguelle, and Dominik Hünniger in this volume.

25 In his seminal work on the history of governmentality and biopolitics, Michel Foucault identified the fight against epidemics as an important moment in the formation of spatial, life-related practices of sovereignty, but barely mentioned animals; see Michel Foucault, Security, Territory, Population. Lectures

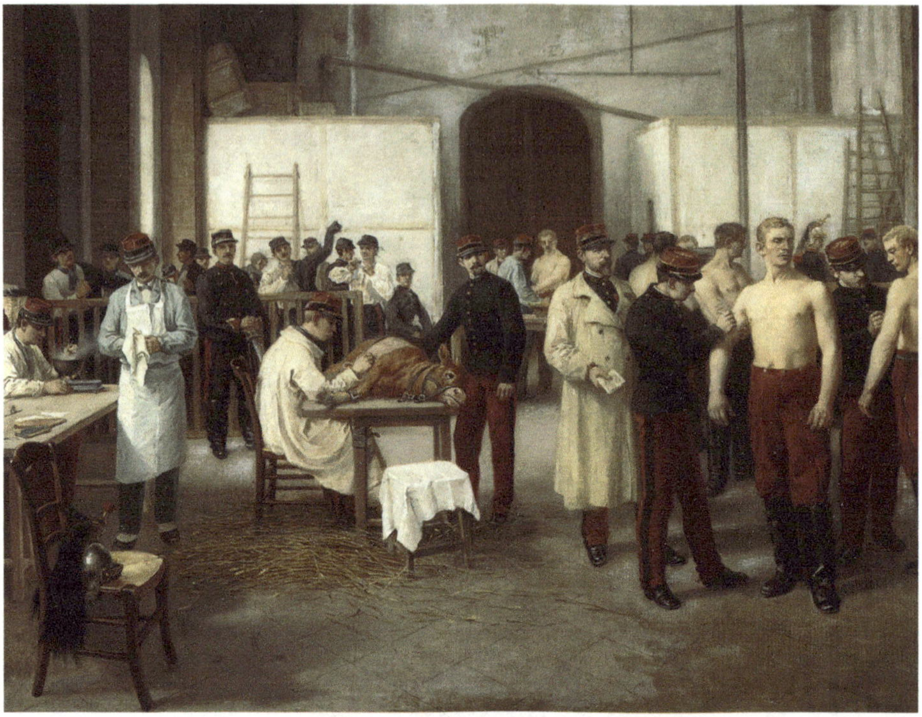

Fig. 3 Jan Smit, "God's Punishment on the Netherlands through the Cattle Plague", etching, 1745 (detail). This representation interprets the devastating cattle plague, which led to the death of about 135,000 animals between November 1744 and August 1745, as divine punishment, but at the same time shows the rural subjects' expectation that the authorities would provide them with sanitary measures, compensation, and other support.

The bacteriological turn in medicine in the late nineteenth century again contributed to shifts in the perception of certain animals as epidemic factors. Smaller animal species, such as mosquitos, rats, ticks, lice, flies, beetles, and bats, were now identified – in historical as well as bacteriological literature – as transmitters, sources of danger, and, more generally, antagonists to human interest and wellbeing. They were, in short, portrayed as "epidemic villains"[26] that would descend on humans, the "innocent victims forced

at the Collège de France, 1977–1978, Basingstoke 2008. On the role of animals in the premodern genealogy of biopolitics, see also the contributions in Nadir Weber (ed.), Hege und Herrschaft. Höfische Jagdtiere in der europäischen Vormoderne, Cologne 2023.

26 Christos Lynteris, Introduction: Infectious Animals and Epidemic Blame, in: id. (ed.), Framing Animals (note 1), 1–25, here 5. See Abigail Woods et al. (eds.), Animals and the Shaping of Modern Medicine. One Health and Its Histories, London 2018; Dawn Day Biehler, Pests in the City. Flies, Bedbugs, Cockroaches, and Rats, Washington D.C. 2013.

to fight back."[27] In this sense, non-human animals were cast in an active role in the dramatic composition of epidemics and their underlying knowledge and power structures.[28] Faced with an epidemic threat, authorities now implemented rigid measures against their infected human subjects (or those who were suspected to be infected), and especially against animals that were seen as potential carriers of the disease. Governmental authorities hoped that epidemics could be prevented, or at least controlled, with the help of medical policing and other progressive hygienic measures, from traditional practices of quarantine and isolation to fumigation and, beginning in the late nineteenth century, disinfection.[29]

In this context, animals that were considered infected or vectors for germs became targets of drastic extermination campaigns. As early as the 1860s, cattle from the continent suspected of carrying rinderpest were banned from the British Isles, and the slaughtering of herds was widely discussed, prefigurating the numerous large extermination campaigns against livestock in the second half of the twentieth century.[30] Around 1900, formerly harmless – or at worst annoying – insects such as flies and mosquitos transformed into a threat as they were considered carriers of typhoid fever and malaria.[31] But above all, it was again the rat, as a supposed vector for disease, that was hunted systematically. Killed by (semi-)professional rat-catchers and their animal assistants, as visual sources from early twentieth-century Australia illustrate (see the cover image), traps and poisons were now employed that could also affect humans. Such *othering* of potentially contagious animals revealed not only a diverse set of political and public health aspirations, conflicts, and debates, but also the potential for social and colonial denigration and for militant semantics of annihilation of the human enemy.[32]

At the same time, supposedly dangerous beings such as rats and mosquitos could also serve – although involuntarily – to provide a better understanding of the course and treatment for diseases.[33] In the artificial, more or less controlled environment of the research laboratory, they became co-agents in the fight against disease. Until this day, most countries require vaccines to be tested on animals before being approved for human use. Thus, all cures for infectious diseases have in one form or another "required the

27 Hao Chen, Nonhuman Animals in a Human Pandemic: Past and Present, in: Alagona et al., Reflections (note 3), 604–607, 606.

28 Kevin Bardosh, Unpacking the Politics of Zoonosis Research and Policy, in: id. (ed.), One Health Science. Politics and Zoonotic Disease in Africa, London, New York 2016, 1–20; Rohan Deb Roy, Malarial Subjects: Empire, Medicine and Nonhumans in British India, 1820–1909, Cambridge 2017.

29 Lynteris, Introduction (note 26), 9.

30 See the chapters by Lucinda Cole and Brett Mizelle in this volume.

31 See the chapter by Axel C. Hüntelmann in this volume.

32 Lynteris, Introduction (note 26), 5, 11. See also Christoph Gradmann, Bazillen, Krankheit und Krieg. Bakteriologie und politische Sprache im deutschen Kaiserreich, in: Berichte zur Wissenschaftsgeschichte 19 (1996), 81–94; and Susan Sontag, AIDS and its Metaphors, New York 1989.

33 See the chapter by Axel C. Hüntelmann in this volume.

use of animals, almost entirely mammals, ranging from mice to horses to apes."[34] Some animals were even used to produce effective means to fight the outbreak and spread of diseases. Beginning in the late eighteenth century, cows and calves served as the source of smallpox vaccines; one hundred years later, horses were used to "produce" sera against diphtheria and tetanus (fig. 4).[35] In the collective imagination, such animals, whose bodies served to save humans and other creatures from disease and death, were stylized as saviour figures, influenced by the Christian iconography of the innocent sacrificial lamb. In turn, however, the bodily connections that such vaccines and sera established between humans and other animals could also prompt irritation and defiance. Thus, in political and social debates on the nature of the disease, the cure, and possible side effects, cows and horses became icons of (satirical) illustrations (fig. 5) that condensed the fears and anxieties of people implicated in such mediated transspecies encounters.

3. Animal Patients: Bioeconomy, Livestock, and Veterinary Medicine

Since zoonoses affect both animals and humans, some animals were also seen as patients and treated in a similar manner as humans. Consequently, humans were not the only beneficiaries of biologicals of organic origin: anti-tetanus serum, obtained from horse blood, was also administered to horses suffering from tetanus, just as anti-erysipelas serum, obtained from pigs, was administered to those animals suffering from swine erysipelas (fig. 6). Usually, this care was motivated by economic reasons rather than compassion; even companion animals such as dogs, at the latest with the advent of defined breed standards in the late nineteenth century, were also considered an economic resource to be protected from disease and other dangers.[36]

As has been shown with avian flu, swine pest, and BSE, the outbreak of epizootics or zoonoses came with considerable economic consequences. On a micro-historical level, diseased animals could ruin a farm. Especially in premodern agrarian societies, the loss of livestock through disease could destroy the basis of existence of countless people. Animal diseases were thus considered a serious threat to public order, and have left numerous traces in historical sources since antiquity. Even for the otherwise poorly

34 Anita Guerrini, Animals, vaccines, and COVID-19, in: Endeavour 45/3 (2021), https://doi.org/10.1016/j.endeavour.2021.100779 (4 June 2024).

35 See Axel C. Hüntelmann, Diphtheriaserum and Serumtherapy. Development, Production and Regulation in fin de siècle Germany, in: Dynamis. Acta Hispanica ad Medicinae Scientiarumque Historiam Illustrandam 27 (2007), 107–131; id., Smallpox Vaccination in the German Empire. Vaccination between Biopolitics and Moral Economy, in: Asclepio. Revista de Historia de la Medicina y de la Ciencia (2020), no. 1, https://doi.org/10.3989/asclepio.2020.01 (12 June 2023).

36 Michael Worboys, et al., The Invention of the Modern Dog. Breed and Blood in Victorian Britain, Baltimore 2018; Sarah Franklin, Dolly Mixtures. The Remaking of Genealogy, Durham 2007.

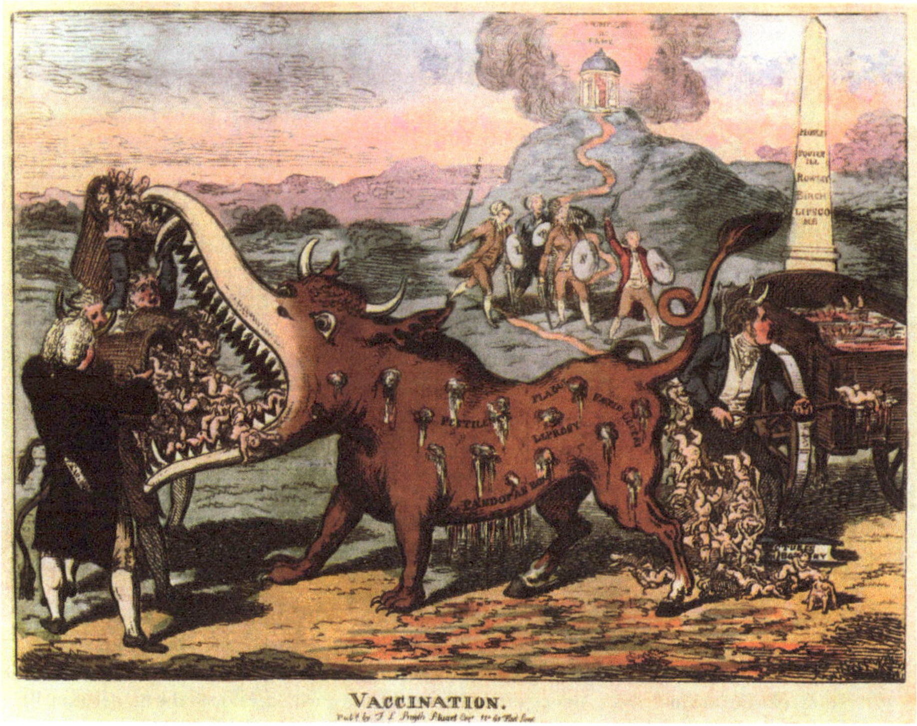

Fig. 4 Alfred Touchemolin, *Vaccination*, oil on canvas, c. 1895. The picture shows French soldiers being vaccinated against smallpox in the Val-de-Grâce hospital in Paris and directly relates the bodies of the calf from which the vaccine is taken to those of the soldiers.

documented centuries of the early Middle Ages, it is possible to reconstruct waves of animal plagues.[37] In the early modern period, the prevention of cattle epidemics was increasingly understood as a task of the "good police" of the authorities. When animal diseases appeared abroad, measures such as border closures and trade bans were introduced to prevent the import of dangerous diseases. To compensate for lost livestock populations, new breeds were brought in from other territories. In addition to the practical knowledge that livestock farmers had handed down over centuries for the care of their animals' diseases, and which was partly disseminated in agricultural household literature, a specialized medical discourse emerged in the eighteenth century that laid the foundations for veterinary medicine as an independent discipline.[38]

37 See the contribution by Timothy Newfield in this volume. For the perception of health and sickness of pigs in the early medieval West, see Jamie Kreiner, Legions of Pigs in the Early Medieval West, New Haven, London 2020, 35.

38 See the contribution by Dominik Hünniger in this volume.

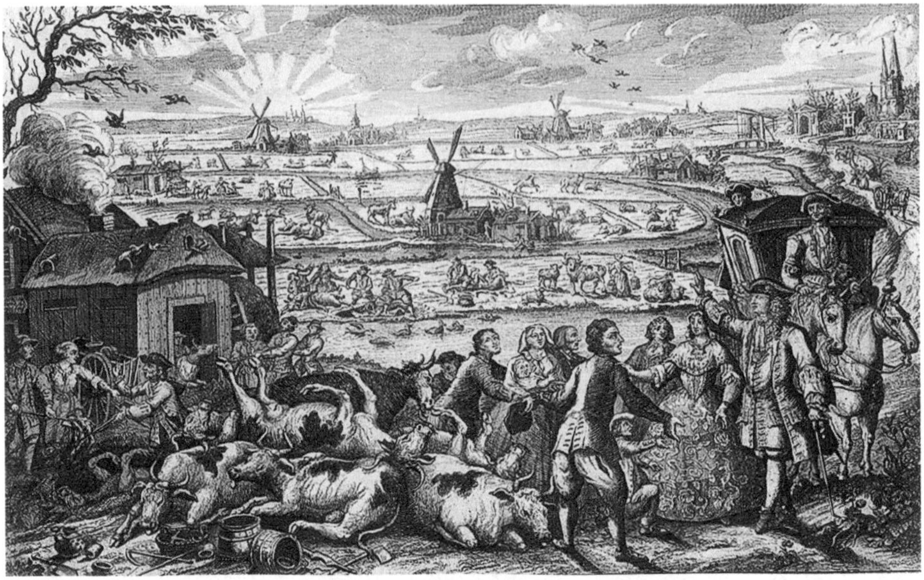

Fig. 5 "Vaccination", satirical coloured etching, published by John Ferdinand Smyth Stuart, c. 1802. In the context the large-scale vaccination campaign around 1800, this vaccine-critical representation portrays the death of numerous human children caused by a cow-like monster on which the names of various plagues are inscribed. Among others, Edward Jenner, who developed the modern smallpox vaccination method and was awarded a sum of 10,000 pounds by the British Parliament for the vaccination campaign, is shown in the background.

Despite increased knowledge of treatment options and the first vaccination programmes for livestock, animal diseases remained a serious problem in the nineteenth and twentieth centuries, spreading faster and further than ever before due to increasing globalization.[39] When a disease had no effective cure, the measures to protect one's own (or the national) livestock or precious breeds and to prevent the outbreak of an epizootic were often far more radical than with human epidemics. In Britain, for instance, the 1860s ban on trade of cattle from the continent and the slaughtering of imported cattle, mentioned above, had been discussed by the British Parliament as well as in the

39 See, for example, Lise Wilkinson, Animals and Disease. An Introduction to the History of Comparative Medicine, Cambridge 1992; Joanna Swabe, Animals, Disease and Human society. Human-Animal Relations and the Rise of Veterinary Medicine, London 1999; Susan R. Schrepfer and Philip Scranton (eds.), Industrializing Organisms. Introducing Evolutionary History, New York 2004; Harriet Ritvo, Noble Cows and Hybrid Zebras. Essays on Animals and History, Charlottesville 2010, chap. 6, 12; Karen Brown/Daniel Gilfoyle (eds.), Healing the Herds. Disease, Livestock Economies, and the Globalization of Veterinary Medicine, Athens 2010; Alex Blanchette, Porkopolis. American Animality, Standardized Life & the Factory Farm, Durham 2020.

Fig. 6 Cover of a brochure of the *Serum-Gesellschaft*, Berlin, c. 1900. Humans were not the only beneficiaries of biologicals of organic origin: anti-tetanus serum, obtained from horse blood, was also administered to horses suffering from tetanus, while anti-erysipelas serum, obtained from pigs, was administered to those animals suffering from swine erysipelas as this merchandising brochure shows.

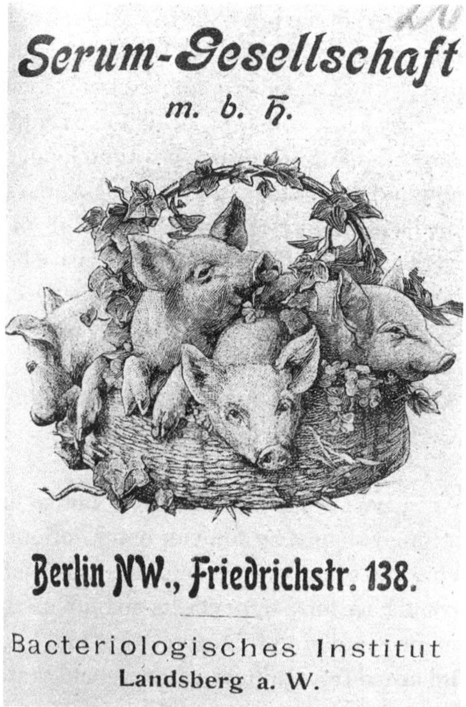

public sphere.[40] In the global twentieth century, epidemiologically based, often purely preventive mass slaughter could, furthermore, not only lead to the reorganization of entire economic sectors (and the people associated with them), but also to the extermination of individual animal populations, such as the *kochon kreyol* in Haiti.[41] Thus, the societal fallout – which also affected interspecific relations – could sometimes cause more damage than the epidemic itself.

This illustrates that, within the human-animal relationship, animal health and veterinary medicine are deeply intertwined with biopolitics and bioeconomy. These practices have led, and continues to lead, to often rapid and usually drastic measures, which spare neither property rights nor animals' lives in order to avoid greater damage to the animals, but above all to countries' international reputation and trade. Therefore, similar methods were still being applied in the 1990s, when the import of British beef and cattle was banned by the European Community and accompanied by a mass killing of cattle

40 See the contribution of Lucinda Cole in this volume. On the killing of imported dogs from the continent, see Neil Pemberton/Michael Worboys, Mad Dogs and Englishmen. Rabies in Britain, 1830–2000, Basingstoke 2007; for a similar discussion of cows in France in the twentieth century, see the chapter by Delphine Berdah in this volume.

41 See the contribution by Brett Mizelle in this volume.

suspected of having BSE. The extreme act of mass slaughter of suspected animals to prevent the outbreak of, or at least to control, an epizootic has since become common practice and was also employed against avian flu and swine pest.[42]

Thus, in the course of the past two centuries, the late medieval concept of quarantine was turned upside down. It was no longer the potentially diseased group (of animals and human animals) that had to be quarantined and excluded from the healthy, but the healthy who were to be isolated from the potential threat of "the others". Due to epidemic dangers, new boundaries have been and are constantly being drawn not only between humans and animals, but between different non-human animals.

4. Framing Discourses and Shared Vulnerabilities: Epidemics and Animal Knowledge

As we have already seen, human-animal interactions in the context of epidemics were strongly shaped by contemporary notions of living bodies, disease, and medicine. As episodes of crisis, epidemics were also catalysts of epistemic ruptures, which in turn could have long-term effects on human-animal relationships. For centuries, the dominant paradigm of interpretation had been Galen's aforementioned miasma theory, inherited from antiquity, which held that diseases were caused by a noxious form of "bad air" caused by animal perspiration, excrement, and corpses.[43] In this context, the concept of contagion (*contagium*, *contagio*) was widely adopted, emerging from a long-standing theological discourse on the habituation of bad character – referring to the notion of original sin (*contagium originale*) – and then applied rigorously to the plague epidemic of 1348/1349.[44]

In the early modern period, such Galenic interpretations remained effective, but were repeatedly reconfigured as fields of knowledge became differentiated. In particular, the categorization of animals changed amid new attempts at taxonomic systematization and empirical experiments, whose results were disseminated in letters and printed papers.[45]

42 Ibid.

43 See John Henderson, "Filth is the Mother of Corruption": Plague, the Poor and the Environment in Early Modern Florence, in: Lukas Engelmann/John Henderson/Christos Lynteris (eds.), Plague and the City, London 2019, 69–90; Carole Rawcliffe, "Great Stenches, Horrible Sights and Deadly Abominations": Butchery and the Battle Against Plague in Late Medieval English Towns, in: ibid., 18–38.

44 See Lawrence I. Conrad/Dominic Wujastyk (eds.), Contagion: Perspectives from Pre-Modern Societies, Abingdon, New York 2017; Christian Jaser, Ecclesia maledicens. Rituelle und zeremonielle Exkommunikationsformen im Mittelalter, Tübingen 2013, 334–347.

45 See Nicholas Jardine/Jim A. Secord/Emma C. Spary (eds.), Cultures of Natural History, Cambridge 1996; Erica Fudge (ed.), Renaissance Beasts. On Animals, Humans, and Other Wonderful Creatures, Champaign, Ill. 2004; Karl A. E. Enenkel/Paul J. Smith (eds.), Early Modern Zoology. The Construction of Animals in Science, Literature and Visual Arts, 2 vols. Leiden, Boston 2007; and more broadly, Bruce

The discovery of the circulation of the blood and studies of the nervous system revealed extensive physical similarities between humans and other animals. Even differentialist positions, such as those of René Descartes, accepted the common physical basis of humans and animals (the notorious body-machine, or *res extensa*) and emphasized the difference mainly on the cognitive level.[46] This made the first experiments with xenotransfusion between animals and humans possible in the seventeenth century and paved the way for the use of vaccines a century later.[47] Animals were now primarily distinguished according to categories of usefulness, which was reflected in a firmer distinction between "domestic" and "wild" animals. In this context, the new categories of "vermin" or "pests" as a cause for epidemics was established, based on the nexus between miasma theory and the close relationship with domesticated animals that should be protected.[48]

The bacteriological turn in the second half of the nineteenth century represented an epistemic revolution that ushered new animal (or biotic) actors onto the scene. Nevertheless, at the same time, the interpretation and control of epidemics remained linked to earlier notions of (moral, social, and physical) purity and impurity.[49] The discourses on (social) hygiene in the nineteenth century combined these notions with novel findings in the field of medicine, in particular the discovery of bacteria, viruses, and bacilli. With the externalization of illnesses and their deferral to micro entities, which could now be made apparent by the microscope, came new ascriptions: the intrusion of alien organism into the – often racialized – body was part of a political language of inclusion and exclusion.[50]

Boehrer (ed.), A Cultural History of Animals in the Renaissance, Oxford/New York 2007; Matthew Senior (ed.), A Cultural History of Animals in the Age of Enlightenment, Oxford/New York 2007.

46 See, for example, Erica Fudge, Brutal Reasoning. Animals, Rationality, and Humanity in Early Modern England, Ithaca (NY) 2006, and Markus Wild, Die anthropologische Differenz. Der Geist der Tiere in der frühen Neuzeit bei Montaigne, Descartes und Hume, Berlin/New York 2006.

47 See, for example, Peter Sahlins, The Beast Within: Animals in the First Xenotransfusion Experiments in France, ca. 1667–68, in: Representations 129/1 (2015), 25–55; id., 1668. The Year of the Animal in France, New York 2017; Hubert Steinke, Irritating Experiments. Haller's Concept and the European Controversy on Irritability and Sensibility, 1750–90, Amsterdam 2005; Donald Henderson, Smallpox. The Death of a Disease, New York 2009, 31–56.

48 Lucinda Cole, Imperfect Creatures. Vermin, Literature, and the Sciences of Life, 1600–1740, Ann Arbor 2016; Mary Fissell, Imagining Vermin in Early Modern England, in: History Workshop Journal 47 (1999), 1–29.

49 Mary Douglas, Purity and Danger. An Analysis of Concepts of Pollution and Taboo, London/New York 1984, 30–41.

50 Monika Urban. Von Ratten, Schmeißfliegen und Heuschrecken. Judenfeindliche Tiersymbolisierungen und die postfaschistischen Grenzen des Sagbaren, Konstanz 2014, 119–123; Jobst Paul, Das „Tier"-Konstrukt und die Geburt des Rassismus. Zur kulturellen Gegenwart eines vernichtenden Arguments, Münster 2004.

This dualistic conceptualization was dramatically re-enforced by the possibilities of visualization of non-human animals as vectors or hosts of epidemics and pandemics.[51] Scientific photography, especially micro photography, significantly influenced the identification of the agents of infection events. Diagrammatic images of animal disease carriers also followed this line, as did epidemic cartography.[52] Now the virus itself became the dangerous object, targeting both humans and non-humans at the same time and in relation to each other.[53] The presentation of empirical evidence as well as its popularization was to no small degree dependent on their graphic display. These "epidemic villains" as enemies of humankind were regularly depicted as anthropomorphic phantasms, endowed with not-very-subtle colonial and racist features.[54] But also animals as victims of viruses set the scene for moral expulsions. These ascriptions traded "upon a discourse of purity and pollution, whereby viruses transgress species divides."[55] As the history of preventing foot-and-mouth disease – an illness not normally deadly to animals – shows, fighting a virus usually now also meant killing the infected animals. But since this was not always the case, the question of what specifically makes infected animals a threat beyond their sickness remains a valid one.[56]

In order to contextualize contemporary discourses on animals and epidemics, it is also vital for historians to look at the perceptions of epizootic diseases, such as rinderpest, bovine tuberculosis, splenic fever, foot-and-mouth disease, and sheep pox.[57] We must ask how significant the environmental factor was for the event, as well as how infection levels between the species changed and triggered epidemics. It seems relevant to investigate the parallel development of epizootic diseases and epidemics and how it has been reported in medical and veterinary research and picked up by practitioners. An integrated perspective of both human and veterinary medicine that complements the spectre of contemporary narratives with the concepts of animal *agency* in the infection

---

51 Lynteris, Introduction (note 26), 15–18. See also Linda Kalof, Looking at Animals in Human History, London 2007.

52 Lynteris, Introduction (note 26), 15.

53 Rae-Ellen W. Kavey/Allison Kavey, Viral Pandemics. From Smallpox to COVID-19, London 2021.

54 Lynteris, Introduction (note 26), 16. See also Valeska Huber, Pandemics and the Politics of Difference: Rewriting the History of Internationalism through Nineteenth-Century Cholera, in: Journal of Global History 15 (2020), 394–407.

55 Gregg Mitman, The Unruliness of a Virus, in: Alagona et al., Reflections (note 3), 640–644, 641.

56 On the history of foot-and-mouth disease, see Abigail Woods, A Manufactured Plague. The History of Foot and Mouth Disease in Britain, 1839–2001, London 2004.

57 Dominik Hünniger. Umweltgeschichte kulturhistorisch. Tierseuchen in den Lebenswelten des 18. Jahrhunderts, in: Manfred Jakubowski-Tiessen/ Jana Sprenger (eds.), Natur und Gesellschaft. Perspektiven der interdisziplinären Umweltgeschichte, Göttingen 2014, 173–190; Timothy P. Newfield, Epizootics and the Consumption of Diseased Meat in the Middle Ages, in: Francesco Ammannati (ed.), Religion and Religious Institutions in the European Economy 1000–1800, Florence 2012, 619–640. See also Saurabh Mishra, Beastly Encounters of the Raj: Livelihoods, Livestock and Veterinary Health in India, 1790–1920, Manchester 2015.

events would follow human-animal studies in seeking its sources in the archives of both "culture" and "nature". It would also contribute to a more rigorous historicization of human-animal relations.[58]

One such attempt to combine the perspectives of human and animal diseases is provided by the One Health approach, introduced by public health officials in the early 2000s.[59] However, this approach has not been univocally welcomed. Human-animal studies scholars have, for example, criticized its blindness towards social, economic, and political processes that reproduce Western biomedical epistemologies. This blindness is seen to lie in the fact that, despite its insistence on entanglement, One Health operates with deep-seated conceptual differences and thereby assigns a privileged place to (some) humans. One Health, critics argue, strives to reduce diversity and to gloss over contingent and local interspecific relationships. Furthermore, One Health is based on a binary division between human and non-human, and between sick and healthy bodies, leaving little room for multispecies or relational perspectives.[60]

The question remains, then, whether this approach is suitable for the historical review of past zoonoses or for a critical assessment of political and social challenges, or whether it ultimately represents a health policy platform of the present. Another team, led by British veterinary historian Abigail Woods, assumes that medical history has paid too little attention to animals, although animals have been indispensable to the development of modern medicine, and that it has remained staunchly anthropocentric in its perspective. In this respect, their approach overlaps to a certain extent with that of One Health, which takes a multidirectional perspective in order to find solutions.[61] The animal history that Woods and her colleagues advocate also insists on a multidimensional perspective to gain a more complete picture of human history.

Choosing such an multidimensional approach can also be interpreted as a plea to understand One Health no longer as a diagram of overlapping zones, but rather as "entanglement" – as an interwoven structure, as assemblages that co-constitute one another. Veterinary ethicist Martin Huth has proposed the term "entangled health"

---

58 Philip Howell, The Triumph of Animal History?, in: Kean/Howell (eds.), The Routledge Companion to Animal-Human History (note 21), 521–541.

59 See Woods et al. (eds.), Animals and the Shaping of Modern Medicine (note 26).

60 Stephen Hinchliffe, More than One World, More than One Health: Re-Configuring Inter-Species Health, in: Clare Herrick/David Reubi (eds.), Global Health and Geographical Imaginaries, New York 2017, 159–175; Alicia Davis/Jo Sharp, Rethinking One Health. Emergent Human, Animal and Environmental Assemblages, in: Social Science & Medicine 258 (2020), 113093, https://doi.org/10.1016/j.socscimed.2020.113093 (4 June 2023); Nicolas Lainé/Serge Morand, Linking Humans, their Animals, and the Environment again: a Decolonized and More-Than-Human Approach to "One Health", in: Parasite 27 (2020), https://doi.org/10.1051/parasite/2020055 (4 June 2023); Melanie Rock/ Gwendolyn Blue, Healthy Publics as Multi-Species Matters: Solidarity with People's Pets in One Health Promotion, in: Humanities and Social Sciences Communications 7/1 (2020), 1–8.

61 Woods et al. (eds.), Animals and the Shaping of Modern Medicine (note 26).

for this, as he believes that health is more than just locating diseases, but also involves understanding ecologies of viruses, virus carriers, vulnerable bodies, and reagents. His approach is thus relational, taking into account the role of regimes of violence, infrastructures, scientific paradigms, knowledge production, and economic structures.[62] Temporalities and contingencies would also need to be considered, and it would be necessary to stop viewing pathogens as ahistorical entities detached from certain social, economic, environmental, and political relationships and historical situations. How humans and animals suffer from epidemics should be evaluated differently depending on the social, spatial, and ecological setting. Urban environments specifically played a major role in the outbreak, zoning, and containment of diseases.[63] Environmental historians have therefore also analyzed how climatic, topographic, or ecological changes in specific regions have impacted on animals, both human and non-human.[64]

Thus, in times of epidemic outbreaks, human-animal relationships are affected by (human made) politics, economies, and knowledge, as well as by the surrounding environment. As these features change, the ontological status of animals in this relationship changes with them, shifting from companion to investment, from experimental object to patient or productive unit in the pharmaceutical industry.

Finally, the understanding of disease, its causes and control, changes over time – as does the human-animal relationship and the context of their encounter, especially in times of epidemics. For this reason, a *longue durée* perspective is indispensable.

5. Case Studies and the *Longue Durée*: The Outline of this Volume

From a historical perspective, this volume examines time-specific perceptions of human-animal relations and the epidemiological explanatory approaches and practices that

62 Martin Huth, Entangled Health-Reconsidering Zoonosis and Epidemics in Veterinary Ethics, in: Svenja Springer/Herwig Grimm (eds.), Professionals in Food Chains, Wageningen 2018, 272–277.

63 On this topic, see, for example, Giovanni Colavizza, Epidemics in Venice. On the Small or Large Nature of the Pre-modern World, in: Bojan Bozic et al. (eds.), Computational History and Data-Driven Humanities. Second IFIP WG 12.7 International Workshop, CHDDH 2016, Dublin, Ireland, May 25, 2016, Revised Selected Papers 2, 2016, https://doi.org/10.1007/978-3-319-46224-0_4 (4 June 2023); Michael Zeheter, Epidemics, Empire, and Environments. Cholera in Madras and Quebec City, 1818–1910, Pittsburgh 2015; Sean Kheraj, The Great Epizootic of 1872–1873. Networks of Animal Disease in North American Urban Environments, in: Environmental History (2018). See also the contributions by Rawcliffe, Skotnes-Brown, and DaSilva in this volume.

64 See, for example, Adam R. Hodge, "In Want of Nourishment for to Keep them Alive": Climate Fluctuations, Bison Scarcity, and the Smallpox Epidemic of 1780–1782 on the northern Great Plains, in: Environmental History 17/2 (2012), 365–403; John Robert McNeill, Yellow Jack and Geopolitics: Environment, Epidemics, and the Struggles for Empire in the American Tropics, 1650–1825, in: OAH Magazine of History 18/3 (2004), 9–13.

resulted from them. It aims to shed light on the underlying practices, discourses, knowledge formations, and medial representations of animals and epidemics by discussing particular historical examples. These case studies follow the different perspectives laid out in this introduction which classify animals either as causes or transmitters of disease, helpers in overcoming epidemics, or as victims and carefully filter out the specific agency that comes with it.

The periodicity and recurrence of epidemiological incidents in human history – for example, of plague, smallpox, malaria, typhus, (bovine) tuberculosis, the (Spanish) flu, avian flu, SARS, MERS, Ebola, and Zika – furthermore opens up the possibility for a comparative historical perspective.[65] This perspective focuses on the *longue durée* of human-animal relations as potentially dangerous for pathogenic transmission. It also wants to show the possibilities for a historical reading that doesn't ignore the animal side of things. For this approach, it seems crucial to employ the methodical equipment of historical animal studies, but also to widen its scope to include other perspectives, such as those of history of science, medicine, and veterinary medicine, as well as environmental history and zooarchaeology.

Using epidemics and pandemics as a *magnifying glass* for reflecting on human-animal relations as culturally, socially, and economically specific, helps us to uncover processes of cultural and social change within these relationships. From our viewpoint, this research area must be based on a fruitful dialogue between the humanities and science. In order to study the complex relationship between animals and epidemics in a historical perspective, we advocate a theoretical and methodological pluralism and encourage historians to "leave their academic silos."[66]

Complementing this introduction to an animal historical perspective on the history of epidemics, Matthias Glaubrecht's opening chapter therefore also introduces a zoological perspective that helps to make sense of the scientific framing of animals. As humans in the Anthropocene exert a greater influence on the biosphere of the Earth, zoonoses are emerging and proliferating ever more rapidly, as the ongoing Covid pandemic painfully shows. While two-thirds of human diseases originate from livestock and domestic animals, zoonoses may also jump from various wild animals to humans. Glaubrecht discusses how and to what extent human encroachment into remote wildlife habitats and wildlife trade have a bearing on zoonotic spread.

We then turn to a series of historical case studies that unpack the multi-relational nature of an epidemic's momentum. As Carole Rawcliffe shows in her case study of urban epidemics in late medieval England, medical scholars and ordinary townspeople

65 Jörg Vögele/Stefanie Knöll/Thorsten Noack (eds.), Epidemien und Pandemien in historischer Perspektive/Epidemics and Pandemics in Historical Perspective, Wiesbaden 2016.

66 Frank Uekötter, In Order to Understand COVID-19, Historians Need to Leave Their Academic Silos, in: Peter Alagona et al., Reflections (note 3), 672–675.

alike blamed the exhalations – the aforementioned miasmas – of geese and other poultry for the spread of the plague and demanded the animals' removal from the urban sphere. Driven by health concerns, such interpretations spread rapidly through personal interactions and pressured local authorities to act. Cities have always been places where numerous people and animals met. As spaces of dense interaction, they were also particularly affected by plague waves. Long before discussions about the Wuhan wet market, public places where living and dead animals were sold were suspected to facilitate the spread of epidemics.

The concrete legislative measures taken by authorities against animals to combat (potential) epidemics are at the heart of William Riguelle's chapter on the plague in seventeenth-century Netherlands and the Principality of Liège. He considers how prophylactic regulations were always part of a wider governmental regime, depending on which species of animals were deemed to have caused the outbreaks.

Subsequently, Dominik Hünniger leads us to a time before the microscopic age to explain how specific diseases and pandemics were rarely regarded as individual entities, but rather as a continuum of health hazards. He focuses in particular on scholarly debates about the eighteenth-century cattle plague and details how "insects" and "worms" were both considered causes and/or effects of the "plague".

In her chapter on "Cattle Politics", Lucinda Cole deals with veterinarians' responses to cattle diseases with high mortality rates that plagued cattle owners in the eighteenth and nineteenth centuries in many European countries. Significantly disrupting what was already an international cattle trade, governments across Europe enacted harsh regulatory measures, including widespread slaughters, quarantines, and laws designed to regulate or limit the movement of "foreign" cattle.

Axel C. Hüntelmann's chapter focuses on mosquitos, looking at their ontological shift from an annoyance to a fatal threat around 1900, which prompted new institutional actions against them. This ontological shift was complicated, affecting the complex relationship between humans (scientists) and beastly insects and transforming parasites at the interface of laboratory and field research, as well as between colonies and the metropole, and sometimes even encompassing the whole empire.

The colonial dimension of disease control is also important in Stephanie Zehnle's chapter on the emergence and combatting of HIV, which she traces to an inter-primate encounter with deep roots in African histories of warfare and slavery. She advocates a cross-reading of genetics, archival source material, and indigenous voices, testifying to the complex and entangled history of different primate species in which the dividing line between human and animal was a matter of constant negotiation.

In the early twentieth century, in the wake of the bacteriological turn and new sanitation regimes, urban authorities worldwide regarded rats and other unwanted animal inhabitants of cities as "epidemic villains." Jules Skotnes-Brown's case study of the bubonic plague in Port Elizabeth/Gqeberha in South Africa in 1938 shows how the fight against animal "pests" became implicated in intra-human racial stereotyping. Alongside rats and fleas, Black Africans, too, came under general suspicion of spreading epidemics.

Matheus Alves Duarte Da Silva's chapter deals with measures to prevent the spread of the so-called sylvatic plague in Angola, Great Britain, and Brazil. It discusses the potential risks posed by wild rodents, their alleged infiltration across borders, and the emergence of new spaces of sanitary anxiety that were all part of a wider regime of control enforced by (imperial) governments. The war against the rats permanently marked them as disease reservoirs and, therefore, killable.

Delphine Berdah's chapter on the control of bovine tuberculosis explores a typical example of veterinary treatment between 1860 and 1960. In France and the UK from the mid-nineteenth century onwards, contagious animals were considered a threat to human health, either by spreading disease or by reducing the amount of available meat. Berdah analyses how veterinary expertise had emerged in order to face this danger. Socio-cultural imaginaries as well as professional and industrial issues are examined through a focus on bovine tuberculosis, a zoonosis which mainly affected children.

Brett Mizelle dives deep into the history of pigs and epizootic as well as zoonotic diseases. His chapter focuses the mass killings of pigs and other livestock in the name of disease prevention and eradication. Beyond such purely pragmatic considerations, recent instances of mass slaughter of pigs in Haiti and Egypt were motivated more by non-epidemiological reasons, such as neo-imperialist replacement ideas and the gentrification of impoverished neighbourhoods. Mizelle argues for a "multispecies justice" that aims both at combatting epidemics and improving the entangled lives of human and non-human animals.

Finally, Timothy Newfield's closing chapter provides a longitudinal study that sheds light on the periodic change and continuity central to this anthology. He takes us even further back into the past as he investigates animal plagues in western Eurasia from late antiquity to the Middle Ages (or rather, the other way around), thereby probing the limits of what we can glean about premodern animal plagues from written sources alone. This interdisciplinary *longue durée* perspective aims to tease out the relevance of recent and ongoing work in the paleo- and phylogenetic sciences, and hence to providing a framework for studying animal disease outbreaks in the distant past.

6. Conclusion

Through these epoch- and continent-spanning case and longitudinal studies, this volume shows historical animal studies' analytical potential to study epidemic experiences of the past. Against the previous marginalization of animals in historical syntheses, especially in the history of epidemics, it shows that non-human agents cannot be excluded from the historical analysis of plagues and epidemics. Animals played multiple – real or ascribed – roles in transmitting and spreading epidemics. This zoonotic paradigm highlights the significance of the study of human-animal relations in this field of research. However, rather unsurprisingly, history, as part of the humanities, until very recently tended to focus predominantly on humans as historical actors, even in the very physical field of plagues and their transmission. Clio turned a blind eye to human-animal cohabitation and its relevance for epidemiological aetiology, assessment, and management, in premodern as well as in modern times. Yet in historical hindsight, animals were much more than mere "epidemic villains." They were also a source of healing, as suppliers of vaccines and objects of pharmaceutical tests. Moreover, it is important to highlight the historical parallels between epidemics and epizootics in the discursive production of knowledge, as well as in the practical handling of these crises in form of biopolitical and bioeconomical agendas. Such an integrated human and veterinary medicinal perspective helps us to understand the historical contexts of epidemiological management and human-animal relations.

Now, as Covid-19 itself is increasingly historicised as the most recent chapter of the "pandemic century",[67] our own experience of contagion, social distancing, and lockdowns has sharpened our awareness of epidemics as interspecies entanglements on different fields, such as, for example, the debate over the zoonotic transmission of the coronavirus, the fatal consequences of human penetration into wildlife habitats, or the boom in and post-pandemic disposal of companion animals during the suspensions of social life. This volume's focus on the interdependence of animals and epidemics reflects our present experiences and redefines our approach to historical epidemiology and the history of medicine, as well as our own starting point, historical animal studies.

Photo credits

Fig. 1 "Détruisez les rats", colour lithograph by Obrad Nicolitch, Marseille, 1920. Wellcome Collection, 46901i, Public domain.

Fig. 2 Haggadah for Passover (the "Golden Haggadah"), c. 1320–30, fol. 12v. British Library, Public domain.

Fig. 3 Jan Smit, "Gods slaandehand over Nederland, door de pest-siekte onder het rund vee", etching, 1745 (detail). Wikimedia Commons, Public domain.

Fig. 4 Alfred Touchemolin, Vaccination, oil on canvas, c. 1895 (detail). © World History Archive, D98J0M.

Fig. 5 "Vaccination", coloured etching, published by John Ferdinand Smyth Stuart, c. 1802. Wikimedia Commons, Public domain.

67 Mark Honigsbaum, The Pandemic Century. One Hundred Years of Panic, Hysteria, and Hybris, London 2019.

Fig. 6 Cover of a brochure of the *Serum-Gesellschaft*, Berlin, c. 1900, Archive of the Paul Ehrlich Institute Langen, Dept. IX, no. 4, vol. 1. © Photo: Axel C. Hüntelmann.

Abstract:
This introductory chapter argues that animals have been important co-agents in historical epidemics, and that the history of epidemics provides a useful lens through which to examine changing human-animal relationships through the ages. Non-human animals have been identified and controlled over the centuries as potential agents of disease, but they were also seen as victims of epidemics or animal diseases worthy of protection, or even as saviours in the production of vaccines. The essay discusses different approaches to the topic, such as animal polity, biopolitics, and One Health, and argues for a multi-perspective, interdisciplinary view of the historical entanglements between humans and other animals in epidemic events.

Keywords:
epidemics | zoonoses | epizootics | human-animal relations | historical animal studies | epochs

Matthias Glaubrecht

Waves of Wild Viruses

How we Help Zoonotic Infectious Diseases to Spark Pandemics

1. The Theory of Black Swan Events, Or: The Dominant Role of the Unexpected

Zoologists, and in particular evolutionary biologists, might have an idiosyncratic perspective on the subject of viruses and the occurrence of zoonotic pandemics. For example, they can find some truth in an analogy involving the existence of white and black swans. Since ancient times it had been a fundamental certitude, at least for early European thinkers who had no chance to visit other parts of the world, that all swans are white. However, at the end of the seventeenth century, the first Dutch expeditions returned home with the news that, along the west coast of Australia, all the swans were black. Since then, in English, a "black swan" has referred to a rare event of an unpredictable nature, with a major and even extreme impact, similar to the one black swans once had on Western philosophers' thinking.

In 2007, the former Wall Street banker and trader, now philosopher and essayist Nassim Taleb published a bestseller called *The Black Swan Theory*, which he defined as an event that comes as a surprise and is later inappropriately rationalized with the benefit of hindsight.[1] One typical feature of such Black Swan events is that they are only said to have been predictable after the fact. However, generally, we all act as if there is no such things as a Black Swan event, since we constantly underestimate not only the rarity, but the chance and contingency behind such catastrophies. According to this theory, our world is ruled by the rare, the unpredictable, and the highly unlikely.

The Covid-19 pandemic was at first, when it gained momentum early in 2020, often held to be a Black Swan event, although it was not unpredictable or even surprising at all, as we know today. In fact, the occurrence of emerging infectious diseases (EIDs) among free-living wild animals had often been predicted. Viral ecologists and others had warned of these zoonoses, in particular those that are associated with spillover from wildlife populations living in proximity to humans, either via host or parasite translocations and/or involvement of domestic animals, as many wildlife species are reservoirs of pathogens that threaten domestic animals and humans.[2] Therefore, not

---

1 Nassim Taleb, The Black Swan. The Impact of the Highly Improbable, New York 2007.

2 See, e.g., Peter Daszak/Andrew A. Cunningham/Alex D. Hyatt, Emerging infectious diseases of wildlife –threats to biodiversity and human health, in: Science 287 (2000), 443–449; Nathan D. Wolfe/Claire Panosian Dunavan/Jared Diamond, Origins of major human infectious diseases, in: Nature 447 (2007),

only has the entire twentieth century been properly called a "pandemic century," but the emergence of infectious diseases and the number of pandemics has actually increased, in particular over the last couple of decades. Previously isolated zoonotic pathogens have now regularly infected and been transmitted between humans, and some have spread rapidly among populations and across borders. Between 1980 and 2017, outbreaks of more than two dozen such diseases were reported worldwide, thus indicating a growing risk of a once-in-a-century pandemic caused by a fast-moving virus. At the same time, the Covid-19 pandemic has revealed a collective failure to take pandemic prevention, preparedness, and response seriously.[3]

Although not a surprise to experts, the emergence of Covid-19 nevertheless had a major impact around the world. As we suffered through the waves of a mutating virus, we realized that they come at enormous cost, even apart from economic aspects. Contrary to the official and erroneous figures of about six million deaths, recent estimates suggest that at least three times as many lives were lost, raising the figure to about 18 million people who died in 2020 and 2021 from or with a coronavirus infection.[4] Another important lesson from the Covid pandemic is that, when we look back into the past and ask about the origin of these zoonoses, which are caused either by particular viruses or by bacteria, we realize that at its core, there is always a complex interaction between animal species and environmental and socio-economic factors.

In this essay, which also serves as a summary of a more extensive study,[5] I will briefly outline some of the basic features and commonalities of zoonoses, highlighting a couple of case studies to illustrate the history of infectious diseases, and then focusing on the human factor and, in particular, the ecology of pandemics, in order to see what insights we can gain and which lessons we can learn. The patterns this exercise reveals have the potential to help us to better understand also the origin of Covid-19, which was almost certainly not in a laboratory, contrary to highly contentious conjectures.[6]

279–283; Nathan Wolfe, The Viral Storm. The Dawn of a New Pandemic Age, New York 2011; David Quammen, Spillover. Animal infections and the Next Human Pandemic, New York 2012.

3 See Mark Honigsbaum, The Pandemic Century. One Hundred Years of Panic, Hysteria and Hubris, New York 2020; Christopher Elias/John N. Nkengasong/Firdausi Qadri, Emerging infectious diseases. Learning from the past and looking to the future, in: New England Journal of Medicine 384 (2021), 1181–1184; Neil M. Vora et al., Want to prevent pandemics? Stop spillovers, in: Nature 605 (2022), 419–422.

4 Haidong Wang et al., Estimating excess mortality due to the Covid-19 pandemic: a systematic analysis of Covid-19-related mortality, 2020–21, in: The Lancet 399 (2021), 1513–1536. See also Richard Van Noorden, Major study errs on Covid deaths, in: Nature 606 (2022), 242–244.

5 See for the more elaborate study in Matthias Glaubrecht, Die Rache des Pangolin. Wild gewordene Pandemien und der Schutz der Artenvielfalt, Berlin 2022.

6 Summarized in Alina Chan/Matt Ridley, The Search for the Origin of Covid-19, London 2021.

2. Looking at the Virosphere from an Evolutionary Biology Perspective

From an evolutionary biologist's perspective, the Covid-19 pandemic provided a case study, not only in terms of the wealth of data it provided on the biogeographical pattern of the spread of the virus, which originated in China already at the end of 2019, but also in terms of several phylogenetic aspects. Sophisticated comparisons of the various viral sequences even allowed pathogenic lineages to be traced backwards into the past in order to search for routes of transmission, and eventually the regional and organismal origin of SARS-CoV-2, which was evidently identified at a market in Wuhan as the epicenter of this pandemic.[7]

What also becomes clear is that coronaviruses are no exception among these pathogens, but rather resemble the tip of an iceberg. Viruses are tiny and invisible to the naked eye, but have a tremendous effect on us – a piece of bad news wrapped up in protein, according to an apt description by Peter and Jean Medawar.[8] Surprisingly, virologists don't even know the order of magnitude of viruses out there in the so-called virosphere, which might amount to at least about 1,500 relevant pathogen species, with an average of two new species of human viruses reported every year.[9] Fewer than about 250 of these viruses are known to cause zoonoses. For example, one database covering the period from 1940 to 2004 lists 335 emerging infectious diseases. These EIDs are dominated by zoonoses (60 percent of all EIDs) and the majority of these (over 70 percent) originate in wildlife, such as Ebola and SARS.[10]

From the accumulating evidence, we have learned that over the last two decades, EID events dominated by zoonoses not only have risen significantly, but demonstrated non-random global patterns, with the zoonotic risk being elevated in forested tropical regions experiencing land-use changes and where wildlife biodiversity (measured, e. g., as mammal species richness) is high.[11] On a global scale, it is mainly mammals, along with some birds, in human-dominated habitats that cause most of the diseases. It was found that the number of zoonotic viruses detected, especially in mammalian species, scales positively with global species abundance, suggesting that the risk of virus

7 Michael Worobey et al., The emergence of Sars-CoV-2 in Europe and North America, in: Science 370 (2020), 564–570; Jonathan E. Pekar et al., The molecular epidemiology of multiple zoonotic origins of Sars-CoV-2, in: Science 377 (2022), 960–966; Michael Worobey et al., The Huanan Seafood Wholesale Market in Wuhan was the early epicenter of the Covid-19 pandemic, in: Science 377 (2022), 951–959.

8 This characterisation stems from Peter and Jean Medawar, here cited from Kyle Harper, Plagues Upon the Earth. Disease and the Course of Human history, Princeton 2021, 26.

9 Mark E. J. Woolhouse et al., Temporal trends in the discovery of human viruses, in: Proceedings of the Royal Society B, 275 (2008), 2111–2115. See also Karin Mölling, Supermacht des Lebens. Reisen in die erstaunliche Welt der Viren, München 2015.

10 Kate E. Jones et al., Global trends in emerging infectious diseases, in: Nature 451 (2008), 990–993.

11 Toph Allen et al., Global hotspot and correlates of emerging zoonotic diseases, in: Nature Communications 8 (2017), 1124.

transmission is highest from animal species that have increased in abundance and even expanded their range by adapting to human-dominated landscapes. Next to primates, domesticated species, as well as bats and especially rodents, were identified as having more zoonotic viruses than other species. Pathogenic hosts that thrive and can make us ill are mostly small and abundant and have fast, short lives (such as rats and mice). When it comes to the domesticated animals that help to spread viruses, about a dozen species harbor over 50 percent of all currently known zoonotic viruses.[12]

Studies have also revealed that zoonoses originate not only significantly and overwhelmingly in tropical areas, but also in temperate zones; interestingly, EIDs are caused not by ecological "specialists," but more often by "generalists" that occur nearly everywhere.[13] For example, coronaviruses are generalists that find refuge in a wide array of wild and farmed animals. They therefore have not only the potential to spill over from an animal reservoir and vector to humans, but also to spill back from humans to animals, potentially creating additional waves of infectious viruses and increasing the risk of pandemics.[14] When we look at the drivers responsible for the emergence of these diseases globally, almost half of all EIDs are driven by what are euphemistically called "land-use changes", i. e., by agricultural intensification, by our use of forests and hunting and our treatment of wildlife.[15] Among threatened wildlife species, those with reduced populations owing to exploitation and loss of habitat shared more viruses with humans. This provides further evidence that exploitation, as well as anthropogenic activities that decrease wildlife habitat quality, have increased opportunities for animal-human interactions and facilitated zoonotic disease transmission to humans.

3. Man as Evolutionary Factor

Although we humans are, from a geo-historical perspective, only a „nine day wonder" in the course of evolution, mankind is currently leaving an enormous ecological footprint on the surface of the Earth, as it is immediately visible, to give just one example, at night by our traces of light on images taken from satellites. Over the past century so many components of the Earth system have changed that they no longer occur within the

---

12 Christine K. Johnson et al., Global shifts in mammalian population trends reveal key predictors of virus spillover risk, in: Proceedings of the Royal Society 287/B (2020), 20192736.

13 Rory Gibb et al., Zoonotic host diversity increases in human-dominated ecosystems, in: Nature 584 (2020), 398–405.

14 Iryna V. Goraichuk et al., Zoonotic and Reverse Zoonotic Transmissibility of SARS-CoV-2, in: Virus Research 302 (2021), 1–14; Smriti Mallapaty, The hunt for coronavirus carriers, in: Nature 591 (2021), 26–28; Cecilia A. Sánchez et al., A strategy to assess spillover risk of bat Sars-related coronaviruses in Southeast Asia, in: Nature Communication 13 (2022), 4380.

15 Felicia Keesing et al., Impacts of biodiversity on the emergence and transmission of infectious diseases, in: Nature 468 (2010), 647–652.

ranges evident during the Holocene, but warrant recognition as a new geological epoch – the Anthropocene, or the era of man, as currently discussed by geologists.[16]

However, we are influencing not only the geosphere of our planet, but we for a long time have also been changing very much the entire biosphere of Earth and its ecological processes. Hence, at least since the so-called "Great Acceleration" within the new era of the Anthropocene, i. e., since about 1950, humans have become a major and decisive evolutionary factor. One indication of our new role, therefore providing one signature of the Anthropocene, is the fact that, by 2020, man has produced an anthropogenic mass – made of bricks, concrete, metals, plastic, and all those things we have fabricated – equivalent to the entire biomass produced by plants, animals, and all living organisms on this planet.[17]

We also already dominate two-thirds of the land surface, using it for our cities and settlements, our industrial plants and traffic routes, but above all as agricultural land to grow food or energy crops, for ourselves as well as for livestock. In doing so, we are overtaxing the environment both on the land and in the water. A study that quantified the recent dynamics of global land-use change at an unprecedented spatial resolution found that the surface of the Earth in the past half-century has changed more dramatically than had long been assumed. In the decades from 1960 to 2019 alone, land-use change affected 43 million square kilometers, or almost a third (32 percent) of all land area, a figure four times greater than previously estimated, and which includes diverging processes and phases explained by effects of global trade on agricultural production.[18]

For too long, and with ever-increasing ferocity during the past decades of exponential human population growth, humankind has been waging a genuine war against nature, of which we ourselves are nevertheless also a part. The plundering of raw materials and the ruthless exploitation of biological resources are directly or indirectly destroying countless living creatures. This plundering of the true and unique biological treasure of Earth, the diversity of species, results in a loss of its components without which the ecosystems we rely on for our food, our water, and so much more will not function. By destroying their habitats all over the world, on both a small and a large scale, we are endangering the survival of many animal and plant species, for which we simply leave no room. Experts refer to this as "biological annihilation" or "defaunation", i. e.,

---

16 See on the Anthropocene e. g. Colin N. Waters/Simon D. Turner, Defining the onset of the Anthropocene, in: Science 378 (2022), 706–708.

17 On the anthropogenic mass see Emily Elhacham et al., Global human-made mass exceeds all living biomass, in: Nature 588/7838 (2020), 442–444. See on the signatures of the Anthropocene e. g. the WWF, Living Planet Report 2020, Gland 2020.

18 See Karina Winkler et al., Global land use change are four times greater than previously estimated, in: Nature Communications 12 (2021), 2501. See also on man's historical influence Erle C. Ellis et al., People have shaped most of terrestrial nature for at least 12,000 years, in: Proceedings of the National Academy of Sciences 118 (2021), e2023483118.

the extirpation or extinction of many species in the world, which is currently causing a global loss of biodiversity. At present, we are already in the midst of a massive decline of populations and species, with a significantly higher extinction rate than the long-term average. Driven essentially by habitat loss and degradation, direct exploitation through legal and illegal hunting and fishing, as well as pesticides and pollution, one million species out of a total of eight million could go extinct worldwide within decades, as the Intergovernmental Panel for Biodiversity and Ecosystem services (IPBES) has warned.[19]

This loss of species has become another distinctive feature or signature of the Anthropocene, resulting in a "sixth mass extinction," or, potentially, "the end of evolution," as I have called it. Although, of course, there is no end to evolution per se, we will nevertheless lose a major fraction of those organisms and ecosystems that came into existence during the lifetime of hominin lineages from which we as *Homo sapiens* only most recently derived.[20] However, collectively we are still mostly ignorant of the dimension and dynamics of the loss of biological diversity or the "extinction crisis." We are imperiling a considerable fraction of the contemporary biota and its diversity and, in addition, even endangering the future existence of our own species. In fact, alongside climate change, this dramatic decay of biodiversity, which also triggers the loss of ecosystem services, is another and by no means lesser threat to humanity and will remain one of the major challenges of the twenty-first century.

It is important to consider some of the consequences of this, as humans are not only responsible for changing the species composition of the planet, but the entire nature of ecosystems. While the occurrence and distribution of countless species is currently shrinking, and in some regions many are even disappearing forever, the population numbers of some other species, such as farm animals, which live in proximity to an exponentially growing human population, are increasing. Faced with the intensity of anthropogenic influence on the ecological system, from a zoological point of view, we must understand these processes are also linked to the emergence and proliferation of zoonoses, those infectious diseases that spread due to pathogens transferred between animals and humans.[21]

---

19 Intergovernmental Science-Policy Platform on Biodiversity and Ecosystem Services (IPBES), The global assessment report on biodiversity and ecosystem services, Bonn 2019, https://ipbes.net.

20 Summarized and with extensive references e. g. in Matthias Glaubrecht, Das Ende der Evolution. Der Mensch und die Vernichtung der Arten, München 2019. For a brief review see Matthias Glaubrecht, On the end of evolution. Humankind and the annihilation of species, in: Zoologica Scripta 52 (2023), 215–225. See also for a summary and overview e. g. Robert H. Cowie/Philippe Bouchet/Benoît Fontaine, The sixth mass extinction: fact, fiction or speculation, in: Biological Reviews 97 (2022), 640–663.

21 As argued extensively in Glaubrecht, Die Rache des Pangolin (note 5).

4. A Brief Look at the Long History of Zoonoses

Looking at the history of some of those human and wildlife EIDs, we find that zoonoses date back to the early human colonization of the globe and the subsequent dissemination of exotic pathogens.[22] For example, the shift from hunter-gatherer to agrarian societies favored the spread of infectious diseases, as expanded contact and trade between communities increased interactions between humans and animals, thus facilitating the transmission of zoonotic pathogens. Later in history, the emergence of cities and the extension of territories as well as the intensification of trade and travel, in concert with the effect of an increased human population on ecosystems, increased the emergence and spread of EIDs, leading to a higher risk of spillovers and outbreaks of epidemics and even pandemics, in which a zoonosis affects more than one continent, and today spreads globally.

One example that can illustrate the evolutionary timeframe of human EIDs is the bacterial pathogen *Mycobacterium tuberculosis* causing tuberculosis (TB), which originated and co-evolved with humans for most likely at least the last 70,000 years. It should be considered in concert with its immediate kin leprosy, which is caused by two related species with a zoonotic past, *Mycobacterium leprae* and *M. lepromatosis*. Tuberculosis is often considered a zoonosis that originated from wild bovids, although today there are also animal-adopted strains, like *Mycobacterium bovis*, which derived only secondarily from humans. In any case, TB already occurred in hunter-gatherer populations in Africa and left the continent with humans. Today, it is estimated to be the most deadly disease in human history, responsible for the death of more than one billion people during the last two millennia, and still infecting a quarter of the world's population today.[23]

Another pathogen that was recently found to have been present among our neolithic ancestors for the past 20,000 to 12,000 years is the hepatitis B virus, which remains a major health problem worldwide, causing close to one million deaths each year. A study based on the virus's genomes from close to 140 ancient Eurasians and Native Americans

22 See, for example, David P. Clark, Germs, genes & civilization. How epidemics shaped who we are today, New Jersey 2010. Nicholas A. Christakis, Apollo's arrow. The profound and enduring impact of coronavirus on the way we live, New York 2020. Kyle Harper, Plagues upon the Earth: Disease and the course of human history, Princeton 2021.

23 See for a brief review of the history of *Mycobacterium* and relevant literature in Glaubrecht, Die Rache des Pangolin (note 5), 243–260; and also Monica Green, The great dying: The epidemiological and medical implications of Old and New World encounters in the pre-and post-contact eras, in: Isis Critical Bibliography (online version Juni 2021). Robert Loddenkemper et al., History of tuberculosis, in: Giovanni Battista Migliori et al. (eds.), Tuberculosis (European Respiratory Society Monograph, vol. 82), Sheffield 2018, 8–27; Luca Freschi et al., Population structure, biogeography and transmissibility of *Mycobacterium tuberculosis*, in: Nature Communications 12 (2021), 6099.

highlights the dispersal routes and shifts in viral diversity that mirror well-known human migrations and demographic events, as well as some unexpected patterns.[24]

In contrast, many of the major infectious diseases, overwhelmingly of "Old World" origin, including some now confined to humans and absent from animals, are fairly new, having arisen only after the advent of agriculture (the so-called "neolithic revolution") and likely originating from either domestic animals or wild primates.[25] Although it was generally accepted that this might also apply to measles (which is nevertheless still listed as restricted to humans in many medical textbooks), the exact circumstances of the emergence of this disease remained controversial. A recent study, based on the sequencing of the genome of a 1912 measles virus and molecular-clock modeling, has now determined the divergence date of the measles virus and its closest relative, the rinderpest virus. According to this study, both pathogens diverged from a shared common cattle pathogen around 2,500 years ago, thus indicating that the measles potentially arose as early as the sixth century BCE, most likely coinciding with the rise of large cities.[26]

The study stuggests that the ancient Greek polis in Athens, with its considerable human population, or at least dense temporary aggregation of people during the Peloponnesian War (431–404 BCE), plus a critical mass of domestic cattle for the first time in history, provided a particularly fertile new environment for evolving zoonotic pathogens. This would offer another explanation for the occurrence of mysterious epidemics, such as the plague that devastated Athens during the second year (430 BCE) of the war, killing around one-quarter of its population, and returning twice more (in 429 BCE and in the winter of 427/426 BCE), also affecting, albeit less severely, much of the eastern Mediterranean. In a similar way, considerable swaths of the human population were affected when later, for example, Spanish conquistadors introduced measles, smallpox, and other diseases to the Americas, resulting in catastrophic depopulation, with an estimated 50 to 100 million deaths among indigenous inhabitants, and whose impacts were long and grossly underestimated.[27]

Using a similar approach – involving the use of museum tissue material, genome sequencing, and molecular-clock modeling – other EIDs have also been studied, such as the plague events in the fourteenth century (caused by the bacterium *Yersinia pestis*)[28]

---

24 Arthur Kocher et al., Ten millennia of hepatitis B virus evolution, in: Science 374 (2021), 182–188.

25 See e. g. Wolfe/Panosian Dunavan/Diamond, Origins of major human infectious diseases (note 2).

26 Ariane Düx/Sebastian Lequime/Livia Victoria Patrono/Bram Vrancken/Sébastien Calvignac-Spencer, Measles virus and rinderpest virus divergence dated to the sixth century BCE, in: Science 6497/368 (2020),1367–1379.

27 See for review Glaubrecht, Die Rache des Pangolin (note 5), and Monica Green, The Great Dying (note 23).

28 For a summary and review of the literature see Glaubrecht, Die Rache des Pangolin (note 5), 266–301; for a most recent study see e. g. He Yu/Alexandra Jamieson/David Orton, Palaeogenomic analysis of black rat (*Rattus rattus*) reveals multiple European introductions associated with human economic history, in: Nature Communications 13 (2022): 2399, and Aida A. Valtuena et al., Stone age *Yersinia pestis* genomes

and the Spanish Flu of 1918 (caused by the influenza virus H1N1).[29] These studies have provided many new insights, for example, as to the dating of the origin and the causation of these zoonotic pandemics, which were traced either to wild animals in close contact with humans (e. g., rodents such as marmots and rats) or to farm animals, especially swine. It was not only shown that the plague originated in marmots of the Tian Shan Mountains and around Lake Issyk-Kul in Central Asia (today's Kyrgyzstan), but additional evidence also suggests that it emerged about a century earlier than previously assumed.[30] Interestingly, molecular genetic analyses revealed that the 1918 pandemic influenza virus had originated shortly before in American wild birds, in particular geese, when a human H1 virus (which had emerged a decade before) acquired avian N1 neuraminidase and other protein genes via reassortment. The resulting pandemic virus then jumped directly to swine, to be displaced in humans only around 1922 by another reassortant virus, which was also of animal origin.[31]

In summary, EIDs have afflicted humans throughout history, and zoonoses have changed their course repeatedly. However, the probability of cross-species transmission of pathogens was raised dramatically by increased interactions with animals, first through hunting, then farming, later by the trade and travel of animals and foods, and most recently by wet markets and the exotic pet trade.

5. Lessons from Coronavirus Pandemics

Coronaviruses are in no way exceptions to the general pattern discernible in the most recent studies on the mechanisms of pandemic-causing zoonoses. However, it was long unclear that a major pandemic, the so-called Russian Flu that killed up to an estimated one million people between 1889 and 1892, was most likely caused by a bovine coronavirus that spilled over to humans. Evidently, the endemic human coronavirus

---

shed light on the early evolution, diversity, and ecology of plague, in: Proceedings of the National Academy of Sciences 119/17 (2022), e2116722119.

29 For a summary and review of the most recent literature see Glaubrecht, Die Rache des Pangolin (note 5), 334–361; for a most recent study see e. g. Livia V. Patrono et al., Archival influence virus genomes from Europe reveal genomic variability during the 1918 pandemic, in: Nature Communications 13 (2022), 2314. See also John M. Barry, The Great Influenza. The Story of the Deadliest Pandemic in History, New York 2004; John M. Barry, How the horrific 1918 flu spread across America, in: Smithsonian Magazine 17 (2017), https://www.smithsonianmag.com/history/journal-plague-year-180965222/ (12 June 2023); Laura Spinney, 1918. Pale Rider. The Spanish Flu of 1918 and How it Changed the World, London 2018.

30 Maria A. Spyrou et al., The source of the Black Death in fourteenth-century central Eurasia, in: Nature 606 (2022), 1–7. Nahyan Fancy/Monica H. Green, Plague and the fall of Baghdad (1258), in: Medical History 65/2 (2021), 157–177.

31 Michael Worobey/Guan-Zhu Han/Andrew Rambaut, Genesis and pathogenesis of the 1918 pandemic H1N1 influenza A virus, in: Proceedings of the National Academy of Sciences 111/22 (2014), 8107–8112.

(HCoV-OC43, i. e. being isolated originally from transplants kept in organ culture) is most closely related to the bovine coronavirus BCoV and, therefore, is thought to have emerged from ancestors in domestic animals such as cattle or swine during the Russian Flu. What then caused one of the most severe influenza-like epidemics, in fact the first coronavirus pandemic of modern times to originate in Central Asia, and second in effect only to the true influenza pandemic known as Spanish Flu, is today responsible for only a mild, cold-like disease. Both these zoonoses have in common that their severity potentially derived from the fact that an animal host was infected simultaneously with different viral lineages that exchanged and combined genes, resulting in a novel, highly pathogenic virus. A similar mechanism is not unlikely to have caused the most recent Asian coronaviruses to spill over. In any case, the novel virus hit a naïve human population in repeated waves, before people gradually developed a sufficient natural immune response.[32]

Over the two decades preceding Covid-19, from SARS in 2003/2004 and MERS in 2012, we have learned a lot about zoonotic transmissions from animals. We have seen not only that these coronaviruses are well equipped to adapt rapidly to changing ecological niches by the high mutational rate of their RNA genome, but also that they repeatedly crossed the animal-human species barrier. These viruses are all bat-borne, and it remains an unresolved question why these lethal human pathogens apparently coexist peacefully in the mammals that serve as their natural reservoir. Interestingly, shortly before the emergence of Covid-19, it was predicted that bat coronaviruses could be a likely source of future spillovers into both human and livestock populations.[33] Just a couple of weeks after that paper appeared, the second SARS-CoV disease confirmed this prediction. When we today review the available evidence, it becomes clear that the most closely related variants of SARS-Cov-2 found in humans are widely distributed in particular among *Rhinolophus* bats in southern China and adjacent regions in Southeast Asia. Viruses isolated from these animals not only occur in caves in the Yunnan province (with sequences known as RaTG13 and RmYN02), where they were first (though not exclusively) found. Contrary to this erroneous assumption in the early stage of the pandemic, these particular pathogens also occur in bats distributed from Myanmar and Thailand to Cambodia, Laos, and Vietnam. In fact, the bat coronaviruses most

---

32 Leen Vijgen et al., Complete genomic sequence of human coronavirus OC43: molecular clock analysis suggests a relatively recent zoonotic coronavirus transmission event, in: Journal of Virology 79/3 (2005), 1595–1604; Harald Brüssow, What we can learn from the dynamics of the 1889 'Russian flu' pandemic for the future trajectory of Covid-19, in: Microbial Biotechnology 14/6 (2021), 2244–2253; Patrick Berche, The enigma of the 1889 Russian flu pandemic: A coronavirus?, in: Presse Medicale 51/3 (2022), 104111; Victor M. Corman et al., Hosts and sources of endemic human coronaviruses, in: Advances in Virus Research 100 (2018), 164–179.

33 Lin-Fa Wang/Danielle E. Anderson, Viruses in bats and potential spillover to animals and humans, in: Current Opinion in Virology 34 (2019), 79–89.

closely related to human SARS-CoV-2 were found to occur in the north of Laos, with sequences labeled “Banal-52” (which refers to an anal sampling taken from bats).[34]

In contrast to the SARS-CoV-2 pandemic, for which an intermediate host remains unknown (the pangolin, e. g., *Manis javanica*, was erroneously proposed to be one), in the first SARS event, a potential intermediate host was able to be identified. *Paguma larvata*, the masked palm civet, whose meat was sold in markets in the Guangdong province in Southern China, was found to harbor a virus very similar to SARS-CoV. In addition to an employee and a guest at a restaurant where masked palm civets were sold, a considerable number of merchants in animal markets tested positive for antibodies.[35] As strongly as these indications hint at their role as intermediate hosts, it remained unclear whether these civets were indeed a natural reservoir for the virus or were only infected by other species. Although they are widely distributed in Southeast Asia, civets are nevertheless very unlikely intermediate hosts. Contrary to bats, which are roosting and living close together, viverrids are arboreal loners. The fact that they do not live socially renders them unlikely vectors for infectious diseases. It should also be noted that civets are not very closely related to true cats (of the family *Felidae*), but as a family of their own (*Viverridae*) represent a separate lineage within the carnivorous mammals.[36] The same is even truer of the *Manidae*, or pangolins, which represent another isolated branch. Pangolins are distributed in Asia and Africa, with four species on each of the two continents, and are subject to heavy trafficking. When SARS-CoV-2-related viruses were isolated in seized pangolins in southern China early into the pandemic, pangolins were erroneously assumed to have been intermediate hosts. However, sequences characteristic of coronaviruses isolated from them were not very similar to those from humans. Since, in addition, these viruses could later only rarely be verified to occur in Southeast Asian pangolins, these animals might have only accidentially been infected with the generalistic pathogens. Given their behavioral and ecological properties, pangolins

---

34 For a review and recent literature therein see Juan Li et al., The emergence, genomic diversity and global spread of Sars-CoV-2, in: Nature 600 (2021), 408–418; Sarah Temmam et al., Bat coronaviruses related to Sars-CoV-2 and infectious for human cells, in: Nature 604 (2022), 330–336; Deborah Delaune et al., A novel Sars-CoV-2 related coronavirus in bats from Cambodia, in: Nature Communications 12/1 (2021), 6563; Supapron Wacharapluesadee et al., Evidence for Sars-CoV-2 related coronaviruses circulating in bats and pangolins in Southeast Asia, in: Nature Communications 12 (2021), 972. For an essentially pre-Covid review see Alice Latinne et al., Origin and cross-species transmission of bat coronaviruses in China, in: Nature Communications 11 (2020), 4235.

35 Yi Guan et al., Isolation and characterization of viruses related to the Sars coronavirus from animals in southern China, in: Science 302 (2003), 276–278; Ming Wang et al., Sars-CoV infection in a restaurant from palm civet, Emerging Infectious Diseases 11/12 (2005), 1860–1865.

36 For a phylogeny of the mammalis showing these family affiliations see e. g. Robin M. Beck et al., A higher-level MRP supertree of placental mammals, in: BMC Evolutionary Biology 6/1 (2006), 93.

are no longer considered very likely to transmit coronaviruses as natural intermediate hosts.[37]

In summary, the coronaviruses that cause Covid-19, as well as SARS and MERS, originate from a natural reservoir in *Rhinolophus* bats, several species of which are widespread in Southeast Asia. In contrast, these bats do not occur naturally in the Hubei province around the city of Wuhan in central China, where SARS-Cov-2 was first detected. While evidently masked palm civets (*Paguma larvata*) were involved in transmitting coronaviruses to humans, causing the first SARS pandemic in southern China in 2003 and 2004, valid evidence is lacking for either these viverrids or other mammals, such as pangolins (*Manidae*), having acted as intermediate host in the second SARS-CoV pandemic.

6. Covid-19 and the Huanan Market in Wuhan

As pointed out in the introduction, we are not used to assuming the unlikely. However, the "unlikely event" is that by mutations and by recombination viruses tend to evolve, i. e., to mutate, spill over, and spread. Transmitted from a wild animal reservoir to humans and/or the few domesticated livestock species, coronaviruses (as well as, e. g., influenza viruses) tend not only to simply mutate, but to recombinate, i. e. to exchange and recombine parts of their genome as a natural process in their evolution.[38]

In addition to these and other inherent properties of these viruses, viral evolution is now aided by humans' manipulation of environmental conditions. Thus, it is no coincidence that we have seen, among other diseases, the two recent SARS pandemics occur in China. Next to deforestation and other massive land-use changes, urbanization and direct human interventions into the environment – such as the translocation of wildlife via trade and the live animal markets that represent the high-risk endpoints of that trade – contribute significantly to the outbreak of zoonoses.[39] We should not

---

37 Maciej F. Boni et al., Evolutionary origins of the Sars-CoV-2 sarbecovirus lineage responsible for the Covid-19 pandemic, in: Nature Microbiology 5/11 (2020), 1408–1417; Arinjay Banerjee et al., Unravelling the zoonotic origin and transmission of SARS-CoV-2, in: Trends in Ecology and Evolution 36/3 (2020), 180–183; Spyros Lytras et al., The animal origin of Sars-CoV-2, in: Science 373 (2021), 968–970; Edward C. Holmes et al., The origins of Sars-CoV-2: A critical review, in: Cell 184 (2021), 4380–4391; Sarah Temmam et al., Bat coronaviruses related to Sars-CoV-2 and infectious for human cells, in: Nature 604 (2022), 330–336.

38 Iryna V. Goraichuk et al., Zoonotic and Reverse Zoonotic Transmissibility of SARS-CoV-2 (note 14), 3.

39 Kate E. Jones et al., Global trends in emerging infectious diseases, in: Nature 451 (2008), 990–993; Kevin J. Olival et al., Host and viral traits predict zoonotic spillover from mammals, in: Nature 546 (2017), 646–650; Rory Gibb et al., Zoonotic host diversity increases in human-dominated ecosystems, in: Nature 584 (2020), 398–405; Christine Johnson et al., Global shifts in mammalian population trends reveal key predictors of virus spillover risk, in: Proceedings of the Royal Society B, 287 (2020), 20192736; Aaron

forget that Wuhan, with its around 11 million inhabitants, is located along the Yangtze River in central China, flanked to the east by Shanghai with about 25 million people, and to the west by the largest urban agglomeration worldwide, the city of Chongqing with more than 33 million inhabitants.

If we take a closer look at the human-animal interface, we find that not only are *Rhinolophus* bats absent in and around Wuhan, but that neither pangolins nor civets *Paguma larvata* – the two potential intermediate hosts – were evidently involved with animal trade in the city's animal markets. The human community transmission of the emerging disease at the end of December 2019 resulted in the closure of the adjacent Huanan wet market, whose stalls were cleared and cleaned, thus, erasing all potential traces. However, there exists an inventory of all the animals present at the market in the two years prior to the emergence, including both wild-caught and farmed non-domesticated species. Unfortunately, this list and report was published only later into the Covid-19 pandemic.[40] Reviewing all available evidence not only allows us to reconstruct the wild animal sales, but, even more, to localize the individual stalls involved, resulting in concert with other data in a heat map based on the ground plan of the Huanan market that pinpoints its southwestern corner as the most likely spillover source.

Based on the most comprehensive review and analyses of different datasets, which combine epidemiological data (including addresses of people and smartphone activities) with phylogenetic sequence data, it was possible to reconstruct what happened in Wuhan during the critical days in the final weeks of 2019. For example, based on the genetic diversity of the virus, we know that two distinct viral lineages resulted from at least two separate cross-species transmission events into humans, with the first occurring around mid-November 2019, and the second within weeks of the first. This not only defines a narrow window between when SARS-CoV-2 first jumped to humans and when the first cases of Covid-19 were reported, indicating that the emergence of the Covid pandemic resulted from multiple zoonotic events; but the analyses of all available data also reveal that these spillovers were geographically centered on the Huanan wholesale seafood market in Wuhan as the early epicenter of the pandemic. Although the exact circumstances (as well as potential intermediate hosts) remain obscure, it is evident that

---

T. Irving et al., Lessons from the host defences of bats, a unique viral reservoir, in: Nature 589 (2021), 363–370; Zoë L. Grange et al., Ranking the risk of animal-to-human spillover for newly discovered viruses, in: Proceedings of the National Academy of Sciences of the United States of America 118/15 (2021), e2002324118.

40 Xiao Xiao/Chris Newman/Zhao-Min Zhou, Animal sales from Wuhan wet markets immediately prior to the Covid-19 pandemic, in: Scientific Reports 11 (2021), 11898. See also the summary in Edward C. Holmes et al., The origins of SARS-CoV-2: A critical review, in: Cell 184 (2021), 4380–4391.

the emergence of SARS-CoV-2 occurred via and in close connection with the wildlife trade, both illegal and legal, in China.[41]

7. The Human Factor

Zoonoses in general are characterized by a complex global viral ecosystem – with some keystone species, such as bats and rodents, as well as some domesticated and domestic animals, in particular swine, poultry, and cattle, as the most suitable reservoirs that interact with other wild animals as intermediate hosts. These animals, which harbor agents causing human diseases, are favored by the conversion of natural habitats to our use. Thus, agricultural intensification, and in particular deforestation, are central among the socio-economic and ecological factors involved with EIDs. We have lost already half of the natural vegetation on the surface of the Earth, especially in the form of forests and woods, and this process is continuing in accordance with and paralleled by the increase of agricultural and urban areas.[42] Looking on a global scale at how we have changed the surface of the Earth over the last 10,000 years, we see that tropical and temperature woodlands have been particularly affected, and that their loss is correlated with an intensification of dense and mixed settlements in urban areas over the last century.[43] Especially over the past decades, that trend has increased exponentially in Asia, in regions from India to Southeast Asia and, in particular, China. This will not only continue over the next decades, but will also extend to Africa. Studies that have tried to estimate and evaluate the risk of spillover consistently find that it is related to highly biodiverse wildlife regions, with the risk most elevated in forested tropical areas undergoing intensive land-use changes.[44]

---

41 Michael Worobey et al., The Huanan Seafood Wholesale Market in Wuhan was the early epicenter of the Covid-19 pandemic, in: Science 377 (2022), 951–959; Jonathan E. Pekar et al., The molecular epidemiology of multiple zoonotic origins of Sars-CoV-2, in: Science 377 (2022), 960–966; Smriti Mallapaty, Covid-origins study links raccoon dogs to Wuhan market: what scientists think, in: Nature 615 (2023), 771–772.

42 Bryon A. Jones et al., Zoonosis emergence linked to agricultural intensification and environmental change, in: Proceedings of the National Academy of Science 110 (2013), 8399–8404; Felicia Keesing et al., Impacts of biodiversity on the emergence and transmission of infectious diseases, in: Nature 468 (2010), 647–652; Nicole L. Gottdenker et al., Anthropogenic land use change and infectious diseases: A review of the evidence, in: Ecohealth 11 (2014), 619–632; Toph Allen et al., Global hotspot and correlates of emerging zoonotic diseases, in: Nature Communications 8 (2017), 1124.

43 Erle C. Ellis et al., People have shaped most of terrestrial nature for at least 12,000 years, in: Proceedings of the National Academy of Sciences 118 (2021), e2023483118.

44 Zoë L. Grange et al., Ranking the risk of animal-to-human spillover for newly discovered viruses, in: Proceedings of the National Academy of Sciences 118/15 (2021), e2002324118. Cecilia A. Sánchez et al., A strategy to assess spillover risk of bat Sars-related coronaviruses in Southeast Asia, in: Nature Communication 13 (2022), 4380.

Consequently, since emerging diseases and the biodiversity crisis are directly linked, land-use and habitat change make pandemics more likely. Nevertheless, understanding these interdependencies also offers us a chance to predict future spillovers, and eventually even to prevent pandemics. The takeaway message is that the probability of zoonoses increases in human-dominated ecosystems, in managed and secondary environments, and in particular in urban areas, with their particular mix of wild and domesticated animals. We should not forget that it is the species that thrive in human habitats and that we directly use that make us ill.

In summary: There are many risk factors we can list with respect to human-animal transmission, but our use of land and animals is in fact the most risky endeavor that we have entered into in recent decades. Thus, along with the still rapidly increasing human population, it is the ecology of rural and urban areas, in particular how we deal with farmed animals, wildlife, and wildlife markets and traders, that will determine the emergence of zoonoses in the future.

8. Coda: Black Swan, Or: The Elefant in the Room – What We Need To Do

We have always lived in a viral world, but over the last couple of decades we have increased the opportunities for animal-human interaction, and thus facilitated zoonotic disease transmission. Since the early twentieth century, not only has the number of incidents and events increased, but also their costs in terms of lives and economy continue to be underestimated. It is therefore reasonable to presume that we will see many more of these emergent infectious diseases in the near future.

Since these outbreaks are actually not rare Black Swan events, as was assumed before, we need to focus much more of our attention on the economic consequences of zoonoses. From what we have learned about how pathogens emerge and travel from a local to a global scale, it becomes clear that we should not only invest in the development of medication and vaccination but that we should primarily focus on how to prevent diseases. First of all, we need to implement surveillance programs to rapidly detect the emergence of pathogens with a potential for zoonotic transmission at the animal-human interface. The costs of prevention have been recently estimated at about 20 billion USD, which is nevertheless only one-tenth of the annual economical losses caused by diseases such as Covid-19.[45]

Returning to the initial idea of pandemics being a Black Swan, it would in fact be more appropriate to think of them as an elephant in the room, since zoonoses have always been there. Accordingly, we should not focus so much on prediction but on prevention,

45 Aaron S. Bernstein et al., The costs and benefits of primary prevention of zoonotic pandemics, in Science Advances 8 (2022), eabl4183.

investing more into surveillance at the human interface. While it is impossible and impractical to surveil all wildlife species in nature for potential pandemic viruses, we need to better manage farmed animals and should separate ourselves from wildlife wherever possible. One way to do this is to strongly regulate and monitor wildlife hunting and trade. But, most importantly, we need to protect undisturbed natural areas, at least what is left of them, and we need to restore many more degraded habitats. In particular, we must stop deforestation, especially in the biodiverse regions of the tropics, and we must improve our agricultural practices to benefit both the environment and public health. If we do not do this, the costs will be enormous, as we have seen with Covid-19 and earlier pandemics.

The rich animal and plant life is the greatest and truest wealth we have on this planet. However, these biological treasures are under threat, on both a global and a historical scale. Biodiversity loss threatens to become a global crisis of life, a drama of planetary dimensions, and it is, next to anthropogenic climate change, another and by no means lesser threat to humanity.[46] Emerging infectious diseases, and in particular zoonoses, are as intimately tied to our history as they are correlated with the biodiversity crisis. We must, therefore, not underestimate the effects of this staggering loss of species and ecosystem richness, for it is of enormous ecological topicality and has considerable social impact.[47]

We can still take countermeasures, but we must quickly change how we think about nature and its richness, as well as about our way of living; and, in particular, we must transform our economy and thus human ecology.

Abstract:
Although humans are, from a geological perspective, only a “nine day wonder” in the course of evolution, we have long influenced not only the geosphere, but also the biosphere of Earth. At least since the so-called “Great Acceleration” within the new era of the Anthropocene, humankind has become the decisive evolutionary factor for the survival of species. “Biological annihilation” and “defaunation” are causing a global decline in biodiversity, with the occurrence and distribution of countless species shrinking, and many even disappearing forever. In contrast, the populations of farm animals and a few other species who live in proximity to an exponentially growing human population are increasing. From a zoological point of view, both processes are linked to the emergence and proliferation of approximately 250 known and commonly occurring zoonoses, diseases that spread from animals to humans. About two-thirds of human diseases originate from farm animals (especially pigs, cattle, and chicken)

46 Glaubrecht, Das Ende der Evolution (note 20).
47 Glaubrecht, Die Rache des Pangolin (note 5).

with which humans have lived closely for millennia. In addition to ancient infectious diseases (such as tuberculosis, leprosy, and hepatitis B), our widespread childhood diseases (such as measles and rubella) were originally spread by domesticated animals. Together with other diseases, e. g., plague and smallpox, transmitted by animals closely associated with humans, zoonoses have periodically determined the history and fate of our increasingly densely settled species. Next to livestock and domestic animals, a second infection route of epidemic zoonoses leads from various wild animals to humans. Subsequently, mutations cause the pathogen to spread from human to human, as in the case of HIV or Ebola. Human encroachment into remote wildlife habitats plays a role, as do wildlife trade and markets. Taking a historical perspective on zoonoses, it becomes clear that viruses are not man-made (as it was conjectured for SARS-CoV-2), but more importantly that humans often play their part in pandemics, as can be seen in the origin and spread of coronaviruses.

Keywords:
Black Swan theory | zoonoses | emerging infectious diseases (EID) | pandemics | domesticated animals | wildlife trade and markets

Case Studies

Carole Rawcliffe

"The Abominable Offence and Poisoning of The Air"

Animals, Miasmas, and Urban Epidemics in Late Medieval Britain

In July 1444, a group of anxious citizens petitioned the mayor of London about the threat posed by poultry sellers in the central area near the Stocks Market and on other major thoroughfares (fig. 1). Begging him to have "tender consideration of the great and damaging and grievous hurt" suffered by residents and visitors alike, they drew attention to the health hazard posed by so many

> swans, geese, young herons and other poultry, whose dung and presence generates such a great stench and evil atmosphere that it causes *great and perilous infections* among the populace and has long done so. This has prompted innumerable complaints by lords and ladies, as well as neighbours and many other people. We ask that the poultry sellers should acquire premises in less central places near London Wall and elsewhere in the city to keep their birds [...] and that the dung should be removed from thence and immediately out of the streets twice a week at times when few people are passing by.[1]

This appeal is of interest for several reasons, not least being the direct connection made between polluted air, livestock, and the spread of disease. Like Venice, fifteenth-century London experienced outbreaks of plague on average at least every three and a half years; and although some of them had only limited local impact the fear of widespread mortality remained constant. Indeed, just two months later, in September 1444, the king postponed a visit to Bury St Edmunds (Suffolk) because pestilence had recently been reported in East Anglia.[2] The reference to "lords and ladies" reflects an understandable concern, apparent in many civic records, that the reputation of England's capital city might be damaged by foul smells and filthy streets, and that trade would decline as courtiers and other high-status visitors stayed away. Complaints about insanitary nuisances were not, however, voiced solely by the elite. The exasperation

---

1 Reginald R. Sharpe (ed.), Calendar of Letter-Books of the City of London: K, London 1911, 289. Young herons and swans made prestigious gifts, as in 1483, when the city of York presented six of each to Richard III; cf. Angelo Raine (ed.), York Civic Records I (Yorkshire Archaeological Society Record Series, 98), Wakefield 1938, 76. They were sold live in markets to ensure freshness for the consumer. See, for example, James D. Marwick (ed.), Extracts from the Records of the Burgh of Edinburgh A.D. 1403–1528, Edinburgh 1869, 67.

2 Carole Rawcliffe, Urban Bodies. Communal Health in Late Medieval English Towns and Cities, Woodbridge 2013, 68, 307.

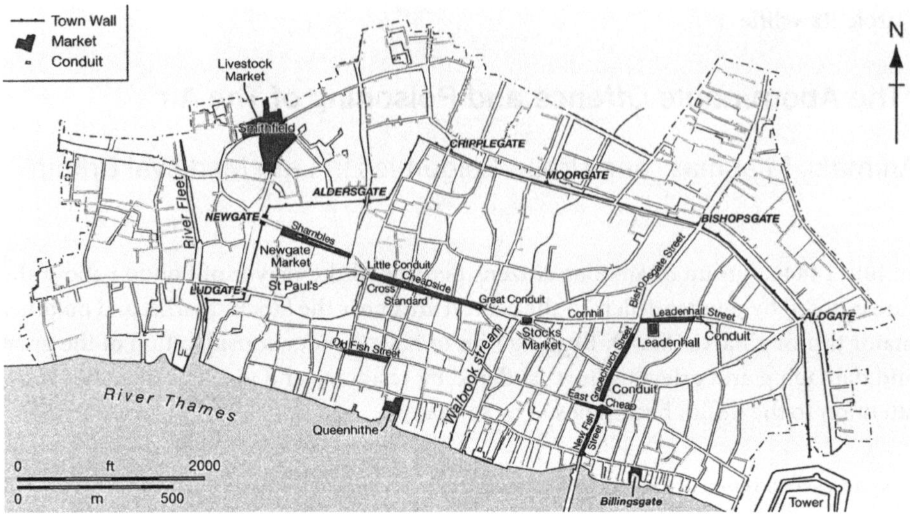

Fig. 1 Map of late medieval London, with the Stocks Market in the centre and the Smithfield cattle market of in the north-west.

felt by neighbouring householders in the face of official inertia, as previous petitions fell on deaf ears, confirms that ordinary people were as nervous about their health as aristocrats.

We should also note the proposed solution, which involved the type of zoning that already saw the relegation of such unpleasant trades as tanning and butchery to the urban periphery.[3] Significantly, the noxious waste generated by poultry keepers in their new quarters was to be removed regularly at twice-weekly intervals when the streets were empty in order to contain the risk of airborne infection.[4] That the inhabitants of these less salubrious parts of London might object just as strongly - but often less effectively - to environmental pollution is apparent from a list of presentments made in 1422 to the city's various local courts. Among the many miscreants accused of antisocial behaviour was a poulterer who had reputedly thrown "goose dung, heron dung and horse dung" into the streets of Farringdon ward.[5] The same source reveals that mounting

3 Rawcliffe, Urban Bodies (note 2), 148–151, 166–167, 206–210; ead., Great Stenches, Horrible Sights and Deadly Abominations. Butchery and the Battle against Plague in Medieval English Towns, in: Lukas Engelmann/John Henderson/Christos Lynteris (eds.), Plague and the City, London 2018, 18–38.

4 The removal of dung and other noxious waste at night or early in the morning so that fewer people would be harmed by the smell was common. See, for instance, Historical Manuscripts Commission, Twelfth Report, Appendix IX, London 1891, 440.

5 Arthur H. Thomas (ed.), Calendar of Plea and Memoranda Rolls of the City of London, 1413–1437, Cambridge 1943, 153. London ward moots had to report if anyone kept "swine, cattle, oxen, cows or calves,

heaps of manure near the Smithfield cattle market on the western margin of the city posed an even greater problem. Observing with some asperity that they had presented this "right grievous nuisance" for the previous sixteen years, local jurors attempted to shame the authorities into action by invoking "the reverence of God", "the safety of the king's subjects" and "the good name of the City", thereby hitting three birds with one stone.[6]

Anxiety about the role of urban animals as vectors of disease spread far beyond the capital. In 1485 jurors in the port of Great Yarmouth (Norfolk) bound over one Thomas Rant for keeping his pigs in such squalid conditions that anyone passing by risked infection because of the appalling stench ("*de fetore inde capiunt infeccionem*").[7] Given that sweating sickness, as well as plague, was then sweeping through the country, their alarm seems entirely justified.[8] But earlier complaints, such as those voiced by the residents of Hythe (Kent) in 1422 about a local pigsty, "which smells very badly and is abominable to all men coming to market as well as to all dwelling in the town" imply, even if they do not overtly state, the same fear of miasmatic air.[9] A jury elected to examine misdemeanours of this kind fifteen years later in Wakefield (Yorkshire) refused point blank to meet in the usual place because of the threat posed by the "smell and muck" of the pigs kept nearby.[10]

How did these ideas, initially confined to the pages of specialist medical literature, become so commonplace? This paper begins by exploring their origins in the work of Greco-Arab physicians and their dissemination at a popular level through the medium of vernacular plague tracts, government directives, and urban byelaws. Having established that demands for the control of animals and their waste products for reasons of public health had long predated the arrival of bubonic plague in 1348, we examine some of the directives that were - not coincidentally - issued during subsequent epidemics. Official initiatives had traditionally focused upon the state of the streets, but the pollution of urban waterways soon became an equally pressing issue. Measures adopted in King's Lynn (Norfolk) following improvements to the town's water supply during the 1420s

---

or ducks within the walls to the annoyance of their neighbours"; cf. Caroline M. Barron/Laura Wright (eds.), The London Jubilee Book, 1376–1387 (London Record Society, 55), Woodbridge 2020, 67, 107. Residents of Portsoken ward, on the eastern edge of the city, clearly objected to the rearing of poultry; in 1471/2 and 1472/3, for example, they indicted Wat White for the nuisance caused by his geese and ducks. See Christine L. Winter, The Portsoken Presentments. An Analysis of a London Ward in the 15th Century, in: Transactions of the London and Middlesex Archaeological Society 56 (2005), 97–161, on 121, 123.

6 Raymond W. Chambers/Marjorie Daunt (eds.), A Book of London English, Oxford 1931, 122–123.

7 Norfolk Record Office, Norwich (hereafter: NRO), Y/C4/190, rot.17r. Four other individuals were then presented for keeping "noxious" boars, pigs, and sows (rot.16v).

8 Rawcliffe, Urban Bodies (note 2), 370.

9 Historical Manuscripts Commission, Fourth Report, London 1874, 432.

10 Brian J. Barber (ed.), The Court Rolls of the Manor of Wakefield from 19 October 1436 to 6 September 1437 (Wakefield Court Rolls Series, 17), Leeds 2014, 63.

furnish an excellent example of the challenges that could arise, and the compromises that had to be negotiated, in a town where livestock keeping was common. A final section investigates the extent to which precept could be converted into actual practice in a society that not only relied on consensus and communal policing for the enforcement of health measures but also lived cheek by jowl with a large population of domesticated and semi-domesticated animals.

It is important to stress at the outset the wide variety of livestock upon which the inhabitants of late medieval towns depended for sustenance, labour, companionship, and transport. We have already encountered poultry. Sheep and cattle were not only brought into urban markets but regularly driven through the streets on their way to or from extramural pastures and might well be left to graze on open land within the walls. Winchester's butchers fattened their beasts in the city's ditches and on other areas close to the defences, which were badly damaged when sheep scrambled over them.[11] Even if they did not maintain a suburban smallholding, many householders found space for a pig or two, often allowing them to roam free in search of food, despite repeated instructions to the contrary.[12] Horses were ubiquitous, fouling watercourses, endangering children and "annoying the king's streets".[13] Goats appear sporadically in the surviving records, but there was no shortage of dogs.[14] Alongside the feral packs that roamed the streets, were the stocky, notoriously aggressive beasts kept by butchers for herding cattle, bullbaiting and bearbaiting, guard dogs (essential at a time before formal policing), elite hunting dogs owned by wealthy residents, and domestic pets that were rarely restrained.[15] Assemblages of skeletal remains discovered by archaeologists

11 Derek Keene, Survey of Medieval Winchester, 2 vols., Oxford 1985, vol. 2, 153, 256. The "ancient usages and customs" of Winchelsea ruled that sheep should not "run at large" in the streets; cf. British Library, London (hereafter: BL), Cotton MS Julius B IV, f.26r.

12 Dolly Jørgensen, Running Amuck? Swine Management in Late Medieval England, in: Agricultural History, 87/4 (2013), 429–451, provides a comprehensive account of urban pig keeping, which highlights the amount of waste involved. She does not, however, consider the relationship between this problem and fears of epidemic disease. Thus, for example, when noting that no fewer than 20 of the 34 presentments made by Nottingham jurors in October 1407 concerned the deposit of dung in highways (434–435), she fails to mention that England was then suffering from a devastating plague (for which see Rawcliffe, Urban Bodies (note 2), 67, 356, 364).

13 Alan Rogers (ed.), William Browne's Town. The Stamford Hall Book Volume I: 1465–1492, Stamford 2005, 70.

14 King's Lynn Borough Archives, King's Lynn (hereafter: KLBA), KL/C 17/19, m.6 (1426), and Winter, The Portsoken Presentments (note 5), 144 (1507/8), refer to goat keeping, as do several late fourteenth-century Winchester court rolls; cf. Keene, Survey of Medieval Winchester (note 11), vol. 1, 153. One negligent owner, repeatedly presented on this score, even left the body of a dead goat to rot in the street; cf. Derek Keene, The Medieval Urban Environment in Documentary Records, in: Archives 16 (1983), 137–144, on 141.

15 Carole Rawcliffe, Town Tykes and Butchers' Hounds. Urban Dogs at Work in the later Middle Ages, in: Medieval Prosopography 33 (2018), 45–62.

suggest that both dogs and cats were reared, or trapped, in significant numbers for their skins, the disposal of their bodies in wells and waterways constituting yet another routine hazard for town dwellers.[16]

These creatures prompted a whole roster of byelaws and litigation as they rooted, bit, mauled, chewed, trampled, urinated, and defecated their way through the thoroughfares, workshops, and dwellings of late medieval cities. Objections to their unfettered presence focused from an early date upon the damage that they caused, sometimes resulting in fatalities.[17] Their waste, left to accumulate in public places, created dangerous obstacles and disgusting smells.[18] There was, too, a growing feeling that urban life was – or should be – defined by the higher standards of hygiene and decorum that set it apart from the dirty, malodourous world of the countryside.[19] When banning pigs from the streets in 1481, the rulers of Frankfurt stressed its position as an Imperial city, whose status and reputation demanded that public places should remain clean.[20] Nearer home, from the late fourteenth century the street cleaners of London swore on oath to keep all thoroughfares free of "dung and all manner of filth for the good name of the City".[21]

Similar sentiments may be found even in small English towns such as Basingstoke (Hampshire), where in the early 1500s the inconvenience, "great soil" and congestion caused by "men of the country" and their unruly livestock on market days prompted rising levels of indignation.[22] We should also bear in mind the longstanding association made between wandering pigs and prostitutes, who spread their own moral miasma throughout society, as well as the increasingly harsh reaction against work-shy vagrants and "sturdy beggars" occasioned by successive outbreaks of plague.[23] To a notable extent,

16 James Drummond-Murray and Jane Liddle, Medieval Industry in the Walbrook Valley, in: London Archaeologist, Spring 2003, 87–94, on 92–93; Catherine Smith, Dogs, Cats and Horses in the Scottish Medieval Town, in: Proceedings of the Society of Antiquaries of Scotland 128 (1998), 859–885, on 873, 877; below notes 39 and 78.

17 Rawcliffe, Urban Bodies (note 2), 153–163.

18 Dolly Jørgensen, The Medieval Sense of Smell, Stench and Sanitation, in: Ulrike Krampl/Robert Beck/Emmanuelle Retaillaud-Bajac (eds.), Les cinq sens de la ville du Moyen Âge à nos jours, Tours 2013, 307–312.

19 Claire Weeda, Cleanliness, Civility, and the City in Medieval Ideals and Scripts, in: Carole Rawcliffe/Claire Weeda (eds.), Policing the Urban Environment in Premodern Europe, Amsterdam 2019, 39–68.

20 Annemarie Kinzelbach, Policing the Environment in Premodern Imperial Cities and Towns, in: Rawcliffe/Weeda (eds.), Policing the Urban Environment (note 19), 242.

21 Barron/Wright (eds.), London Jubilee Book (note 5), 55, 91; Reginald R. Sharpe (ed.), Calendar of Letter-Books of the City of London, D, London 1902, 192. See also, Ernest L. Sabine, Street Cleaning in Mediaeval London, in: Speculum 12 (1937), 19–43.

22 Francis Joseph Baigent/James Elwin Millard, A History of the Town and Manor of Basingstoke in the County of Southampton, Basingstoke 1889, 314. In sixteenth-century Manchester, then a small township, manure heaps in the highway were deemed "unseemly"; cf. John Parsons Earwaker (ed.), The Court Leet Records of the Manor of Manchester I, Manchester 1884, 18.

23 Rawcliffe, Urban Bodies (note 2), 104–115.

stray or intransigent animals assumed the undesirable characteristics attributed to their human counterparts. The mayor and aldermen of Norwich, then England's second city, clearly took all these issues to heart, protesting that "many swine and ducks commonly by the willful sufferance of their owners do wander about the streets ... to the great nuisance of the inhabitants [...] and *great rebuke and slander* of its rulers".[24] Underlying all these objections was an entrenched and pervasive belief that noxious dung, filthy straw, and the rotting bodies of animals dumped in waterways and public places were potentially lethal as well as profoundly unpleasant. Orders for the slaughter of pigs found roaming in the streets of Edinburgh may have been enacted "for the *common profit and honesty* of this town", but they were also part of a medically informed strategy directed against "the contagious plague of pestilence".[25]

1. Medical Ideas and Their Application

A Latin version of the pseudo-Hippocratic text *Airs, Waters, Places* had been in circulation from the twelfth century, underscoring the importance of fresh, temperate air for communal health. Its influence is apparent in the panegyrics that proliferated during the later Middle Ages, praising the cleanliness and invigorating environments of various European cities, while passing silently over less salubrious aspects of urban life.[26] More significant in the present context, however, was the work of the celebrated Greek physician Galen of Pergamon (*d.* 216), which underpinned most medieval ideas about human physiology. Since the effectiveness of all physical and mental processes initially depended upon what one ate, health was, to a notable extent, determined by diet, "the first instrument of medicine".[27] Having been cooked in the oven of the stomach, partially digested food was conveyed to the liver, where it was converted into humoral matter or natural spirit. It then travelled along the veins to the organs and extremities, being absorbed as essential nourishment. During this final stage of the digestive process, the natural spirit might easily be affected by the quality of the air drawn into the body

---

24 NRO, NCR, 16D/2, Assembly Book, 1510–1550, f.202r. The solution was to impound all stray animals until their owners paid an appropriate fine (f.169v). Pounds for the detention of vagrant livestock were already to be found in many English towns. Cf. Nathaniel Bacon, Annalls of Ipswiche, ed. William H. Richardson, Ipswich 1913, 147; Phyllis Mary Briers (ed.), Henley Borough Records. Assembly Books i-iv, 1395–1543 (Oxfordshire Record Society, 41), Banbury 1960, 34; Cheryl Butler, ed., The Book of Fines. The Annual Accounts of the Mayors of Southampton, Volume I, 1488–1540 (Southampton Records Series, 41) Southampton 2008, 116.

25 Marwick (ed.), Extracts from the Records of Edinburgh (note 1), 110, 140.

26 Weeda, Cleanliness, Civility and the City (note 19), 49–55.

27 For what follows, see Carole Rawcliffe, The Concept of Health in Late Medieval Society, in: Simonetta Cavaciocchi (ed.), Le interazioni fra economia e ambiente biologico nell'Europa preindusriale. Secc. XIII–XVIII, Florence 2010, 317–334.

through the open pores. For this reason, anything likely to raise one's temperature and encourage perspiration was to be avoided during epidemics.[28]

Although the concept of circulation as we know it today was not fully understood until the seventeenth century, it was assumed that some blood passed directly to the heart, whose function was to generate heat, the source of life itself. Flowing through the septum, from right to left, it mingled with cooling air from the lungs and entered the arterial system as a frothy substance known as vital spirit or *pneuma* because it transported life-giving warmth throughout the body.[29] The nature of the external environment played a crucial role at this stage, since corrupt air, such as that generated by dung heaps and contaminated water, could rapidly poison the entire system, while fresh breezes and fragrant aromas would strengthen it. Many authorities regarded odours as corporeal entities or "smoky vapours", somewhere between water and air, which transported "the print and likeness" of the thing from whence they came directly into the bodies of those who inhaled or absorbed them.[30]

When combined with air inhaled through the nostrils, the vital spirit that reached the brain underwent another transformation to become the highly refined and volatile animal spirit that energised both body and mind. It influenced behaviour according to information received from the senses, reacting with great acuity to sights and smells, which had a powerful impact upon mental as well as physical health. Whereas aromatic plants could be prescribed to rectify the humoral balance and soothe or stimulate the spirits, repellent odours had a contaminating *and* destabilising effect. Indeed, once they penetrated the inner recesses of the brain, their "darkness and stench" threatened the processes of thought and movement, and thus seemed particularly dangerous.[31] Repugnant sights, such as festering carrion, would likewise be absorbed into the body through the eyes, along with the very "form" or "similitude" of the object in question, eventually spreading corruption throughout the entire venous and arterial systems.[32] During a poultry epidemic in 1344, one Scottish chronicler reported that "men utterly shrank from eating, *or even looking upon*, a cock or hen, as though unclean and smitten by leprosy; and thus [...] nearly the whole of that species was destroyed".[33]

---

28 Johannes Jacobi, A Litill Boke Necessarye and Behouefull agenst the Pestilence, London 1485, f.3r.

29 Heather Webb, The Medieval Heart, New Haven (Ct) 2010, 26–31, 96–107.

30 Richard Palmer, In Bad Odour. Smell and its Significance in Medicine from Antiquity to the Seventeenth Century, in: William F. Bynum/Roy Porter (eds.), Medicine and the Five Senses, Cambridge 1993, 61–68; Rawcliffe, Urban Bodies (note 2), 120–121.

31 Bartholomaeus Anglicus, On the Properties of Things. John Trevisa's Translation of Bartholomaeus Anglicus' De proprietatis rerum, ed. Michael C. Seymour, 3 vols., Oxford 1975–1988, vol. 1, 561–562.

32 Dallas G. Denery, Seeing and Being Seen in the Late Medieval World. Optics, Theology and Religious Life, Cambridge 2005, 82–89.

33 William F. Skene (ed.), John of Fordun's Chronicle of the Scottish Nation, Edinburgh 1872, 358.

A clear exposition of these theories, initially outlined in several different Galenic texts, might be found in the *Canon* of Avicenna (Ibn-Sina, d. 1037). This influential work, which systematised and embellished Galen's teachings, formed the bedrock of the north European medical syllabus from the thirteenth century onward. A celebrated passage in book four describes the toxic effect of miasmatic exhalations upon the human body:

> Vapours and fumes rise [into the air] and spread in it and putrefy it with their debilitating warmth. And when air of this kind reaches the heart, it corrupts the complexion of the spirit that dwells within it; and, surrounding the heart, it then putrefies it with humidity. And there arises an unnatural heat; and it spreads throughout the body, because of which pestilential fever will occur, and will spread to a multitude of men who likewise have vulnerable dispositions.[34]

Starting with a report submitted in October 1348 by the Faculty of Medicine of the University of Paris, plague tracts invariably drew on, and developed, this passage.[35] The report, which had been commissioned by the king of France to explain the causes of the lethal epidemic then sweeping across Europe, stressed that "bad air is more noxious than food or drink in that it can penetrate more quickly to the heart and lungs to do its damage" and identified "bad, rotten and poisonous vapours" as the immediate source of infection.[36] The vernacular treatises that followed left no room for uncertainty in their uncompromising assertion that "pestilence is no other thing than a venomous infection of the air".[37]

As Guy Geltner reminds us, sensitivity to these environmental issues at all levels of society had long predated the "false watershed" of the Black Death.[38] It is clearly apparent, for example, in a Norwich court roll for 1288/9, which records the payment of fines by two antisocial residents. One had thrown the bodies of dead cats into a watercourse

---

34 Avicenna, Liber canonis medicinae, Lyon 1522, liber IV, f.329r.

35 Jon Arrizabalaga, Facing the Black Death. Perceptions and Reactions of University Medical Practitioners, in: Luis García-Ballester/Roger French/Jon Arrizabalaga/Andrew Cunningham (eds.), Practical Medicine from Salerno to the Black Death, Cambridge 1994, 237–288, notably 246–255; Jacobi, A Litill Boke (note 28), f.2r.

36 Rosemary Horrox (ed.), The Black Death, Manchester 1994, 160–161. Members of the Faculty identified ultimate (divine) and intermediate (planetary) causes as well.

37 George R. Keiser, Two Medieval Plague Treatises and their Afterlife in Early Medieval England, in: Journal of the History of Medicine 58 (2003), 292–324, on 312.

38 Guy Geltner, Roads to Health. Infrastructure and Urban Wellbeing in Later Medieval Italy, Philadelphia (Pa) 2019, 27–31. The assumption that campaigns "to promote health by distancing human bodies from harmful biological entities" date from the rise of "urban modernity" in the later nineteenth century persists, even today, despite the wealth of evidence presented by Geltner and other medievalists. Chris Pearson, Dogopolis. How Dogs and Humans Made Modern New York, London, and Paris, Chicago (Il) 2021, 14, offers a classic case of "presentism".

"so that the air is poisoned (*iter quod aer corrumpitur*)", while the other was found to have left a stinking dung heap in the highway "whereby the air is abominably poisoned (*per quod aer pessime corrumpitur*)".[39] Evidence of this kind confirms that attempts to eliminate the dangerous miasmas caused by animals and their waste products were being made by urban communities well before the first outbreak of bubonic plague.[40] Not surprisingly, the crown addressed the worst cases of official neglect with considerable force, spelling out the risks involved. A strongly worded letter sent in 1298 by Edward I to the bailiffs of St Mary's abbey, York, is typically blunt:

> The air is so corrupted and infected by the pigsties situate[d] in the king's highways and in the lanes of that town and by the swine feeding and frequently wandering about in the streets and lanes and by dung and dunghills and many other foul things (*feditates*) placed in the streets and lanes, that great repugnance (*horror abhominabilis*) overtakes the king's ministers staying in that town and also others there dwelling and passing through, the advantage of more wholesome air is impeded, the state of men is grievously injured, and other unbearable inconveniences and many other injuries are known to proceed from such corruption ... to the peril of their lives and to the manifest shame and reproach of the bailiffs and other the inhabitants.[41]

Despite Edward's order that any pigsties abutting major thoroughfares should be demolished, wandering pigs restrained "on pain of grievous forfeiture", and the streets kept clean, York lost none of its unsavoury reputation. As parliament prepared to meet there in 1332, his grandson, "detesting the abominable smell abounding in the said city more than in any city in the realm from dung and manure and other filth and dirt", demanded immediate measures to safeguard the health of inhabitants and visitors alike.[42]

The arrival of plague lent an even greater sense of urgency to these directives, which became correspondingly more explicit about the medical rationale involved. On learning "that dung-heaps, swine, hog-sties and other nuisances in the streets, lanes and suburbs of Dublin infect the air and produce mortality, fevers and pestilence throughout the city", Henry VII wrote sharply in November 1489 to the mayor and bailiffs. Warning that

39 William Hudson (ed.), Leet Jurisdiction in the City of Norwich during the XIIIth and XIVth Centuries (Selden Society, 5), London 1892, 23, 29.

40 For the role of these local courts, see Carole Rawcliffe, The View from the Streets. The Records of Hundred and Leet Courts as a Source for Sanitary Policing in Late Medieval English Towns, in: eadem/Weeda (eds.), Policing the Urban Environment (note 19), 69–95.

41 Calendar of Close Rolls, 1296–1302, London 1906, 218. Measures against vagrant pigs were introduced three years later as part of a comprehensive package of civic improvements; cf. Michael Prestwich (ed.), York Civic Ordinances, 1301 (Borthwick Papers, 49), York 1976, 16. They had already been banned from the streets of London by 1276; cf. Richard R. Sharpe (ed.), Calendar of Letter-Books of the City of London, A, London 1899, 216–217, 220.

42 Calendar of Close Rolls, 1330–1333, London 1898, 610.

"the fear of pestilence prevents the coming thither of lords, ecclesiastics and lawyers", with inevitable "impediments to business", he commanded them "to cause forthwith the removal of all swine and to have the streets and lanes freed from ordure, so as to prevent loss of life from pestilential exhalations".[43] His concerns may have been primarily – and characteristically – about the loss of revenue, but that, in turn, was an inevitable consequence of poor hygiene and endemic disease. Regulations already in place for the restraint of wandering pigs and their removal from "void" urban spaces had clearly proved ineffective; and in 1491 the keeping of both cattle and swine within the walls was completely forbidden by the civic authorities.[44] Not coincidentally, the extramural hospital of St Stephen was then ordered to admit free of charge any resident of Dublin suffering from leprosy, which was regarded as another dangerous source of miasmatic air.[45]

Since mandates of this kind were proclaimed through the streets and in public places, ordinary people would have been constantly reminded that livestock posed a particular threat during epidemics. In response to a serious outbreak of pestilence in 1512/13, King James IV of Scotland ordered the proclamation at the market cross in Edinburgh of a series of measures that had already been rolled out by the provost during previous epidemics. As well as the stringent application of quarantine (now on pain of death), he demanded the immediate slaughter of "all vile and suspect beasts, [such] as dogs, swine and cats" running at large, the cleansing of streets, lanes, closes, and gutters within the next four days and a total ban on the positioning of manure heaps anywhere near the city gates. Offenders faced a substantial fine of 66*s* 8*d* for any infringements, which would surely have converted those who remained sceptical of the science involved.[46] It is worth noting at this point that the "great dog massacres" described so eloquently by Mark Jenner as a means of combatting plague were a later sixteenth century development, although dogs were occasionally singled out as carriers of disease in medieval England.[47]

---

43 John T. Gilbert (ed.), Calendar of the Ancient Records of Dublin, I, Dublin 1889, 139–140.

44 Ibid., 221, 229, 298, 306, 333, 375; Ian Cantwell, Anthropozoological Relationships in Late Medieval Dublin, in: Dublin Historical Record 54:1 (2001), 73–80. Previous byelaws for the slaughter of wandering pigs seem to have been more concerned with damage to property than the risk to health.

45 Gilbert (ed.), Calendar of the Ancient Records of Dublin (note 43), 372.

46 Marwick (ed.), Extracts from the Records of Edinburgh (note 1), 140–141.

47 Mark Jenner, The Great Dog Massacre, in: William G. Naphy/Penny Roberts (eds.), Fear in Early Modern Society, Manchester 1997, 44–61. As Jenner observes, plague offered a useful pretext for eliminating disorderly animals that caused a public nuisance. In medieval German cities, magistrates established the office of 'dog-slayers' ("Hundeschläger") for sanitary reasons, e. g. for fear of rabies. Cf. Eberhard Isenmann, Die deutsche Stadt im Mittelalter 1150–1550. Stadtgestalt, Recht, Verfassung, Stadtregiment, Kirche, Gesellschaft, Wirtschaft, Cologne/Weimar/Vienna 2014, 68; Georg Wachta, Tiere und Tierhaltung in der Stadt sowie im Wohnbereich des spätmittelalterlichen Menschen und ihre Darstellung in der bildenden Kunst, in: Das Leben in der Stadt des späten Mittelalters. Internationaler Kongress Krems an der Donau 20. Bis 23. September 1976, Wien 1977, 229–260, 240.

When plague was raging in 1433/4, for instance, the mayor of Exeter pointed to the "great damages" caused "in the infectious times of sickness by keeping of dogs within this city". He ordered a cull of strays and banned the ownership of hounds that "in the day time run from house to house where the sickness is", thereby spreading the miasmas of pestilence.[48]

The rulers of York also hoped to purify the air when resuming their long campaign against pig keeping in 1498. Their target was the noxious stench of urban pigsties, for even the most docile and sedentary of animals was liable to contaminate its surroundings if left in squalid conditions. By demanding that no butcher or any other resident should keep "swine in swine-sties or in any other house or place within the city or suburbs ... *for the foul corruption that comes of them*", magistrates yet again highlighted the risks involved.[49] Backed up by the threat of incremental fines beginning at 40*d* and doubling for each successive offence, the ruling was made in response to an outbreak of plague then spreading across the north east, and invariably lost some of its force with the passage of time.[50] Nevertheless, as the above-mentioned protests about noxious pigsties in Yarmouth and Wakefield clearly demonstrate, ordinary householders as well as magistrates expected owners to rear their animals in clean conditions and avoid poisoning the environment. Having been reprimanded by Edward III in the aftermath of the Black Death about the filthy and dangerous state of their streets,[51] the rulers of Norwich introduced their first ban on vagrant boars, sows, and piglets in 1354. Although any animal found at large could be killed on sight, an amnesty obtained on Saturdays between noon and dusk, when pigsties had to be mucked out, leaving their occupants free to roam.[52] Some owners got round the problem of waste disposal by keeping their livestock near streams, canals, or rivers, so that the dung and straw could be thrown directly into running water, but such reckless behaviour further increased the risk of epidemic disease.

---

48 John Vowell, *alias* Hooker, Description of the Citie of Excester, III (Devon and Cornwall Record Society, original series, 14), Exeter 1919, 898.

49 Joyce W. Percy (ed.), York Memorandum Book B/Y (Surtees Society, 186), Gateshead 1973, 217–218. The keeping of intramural pigsties had already been banned in 1481; cf. Raine (ed.), York Civic Records I (note 1), 38.

50 For the 1498 plague, see Rawcliffe, Urban Bodies (note 2), 107, 371.

51 Calendar of Patent Rolls, 1350–1354, London 1907, 283–284.

52 William Hudson/John Cottingham Tingey (eds.), Records of the City of Norwich, 2 vols., Norwich 1906–1910, vol. 2, 205–207. Similar measures, allowing for the cleansing of sties on Saturdays, had been in force in King's Lynn from at least 1331; cf. Holcombe Ingleby (ed.), The Red Register of King's Lynn, 2 vols., King's Lynn 1919–1922, vol. 2, 203.

2. Water Pollution and Disease

Concern about the effects of animal waste went far beyond the accumulation of dung or dirt in city streets. Blocked, overflowing drains and stagnant, infected water ranked as a major source of plague because of the stench and the risk to anyone who drank from such contaminated sources, or used them for cooking. Echoing authors from Hippocrates onward, successive plague tracts warned against "the corruption of stinking ditches and waters found many times in corrupt places".[53] In his treatise of 1485 on the sweating sickness, the Norman physician Thomas Forestier singled out "stinking carrion cast in the water near to the cities or towns" as a particular hazard, but stressed how easily "other foul things" could lead to widespread sickness and death.[54] From the time of the second major plague pandemic of 1361/2, the pollution of the Thames and other English rivers by butchers was subject to stringent regulation by the crown and parliament.[55] But ordinary householders were also culpable; the reckless disposal of their dead or dying animals, including horses and sheep, prompted handwringing by neighbours and magistrates alike. An attempt to clean up the borough of Leicester during the "great pestilence" of 1467 dealt, predictably, with illicit dung heaps and the ubiquitous problem of wandering cattle, pigs, and poultry. An additional ordinance under the rubric "corruption in the streets" ruled that

> no man nor woman suffer any corruption to lie before his door or cast any out of his door by night or by day, that is to say horse, swine, dog or cat [...] within the four gates, or within the four streets of the suburbs, but dispose of it away in the field [far] from the course of the people on pain of imprisonment.[56]

Rather than transport their dead livestock to inconvenient places, some people simply threw them in the nearest stretch of water. The warning in the Towneley play of the raising of Lazarus that all men were mortal and would one day "stink as a dog in a dyke" drew upon a commonplace of urban life.[57] Residents of York were forbidden in 1517

53 Joseph P. Pickett, A Translation of the "Canutus" Plague Treatise, in: Lister M. Matheson (ed.), Popular and Practical Science of Medieval England, East Lansing (Mi) 1994, 271–272, 274; Arrizabalaga, Facing the Black Death (note 35), 255.

54 BL, Additional MS 27582, f.71v.

55 Rawcliffe, Butchery and the Battle against Plague (note 3), 20–22.

56 Mary Bateson (ed.), Records of the Borough of Leicester II, London 1901, 290. For the 1467 plague, see Rawcliffe, Urban Bodies (note 2), 369. A London shopkeeper was then ordered to close his premisses and threatened with the loss of citizenship because he refused to remove a dead dog lying outside; cf. Clare A. Martin, Transport for London 1250–1550 (unpublished PhD thesis), Royal Holloway University of London 2008, 167.

57 Martin Stevens/Arthur Clare Cawley (eds.), The Towneley Plays, I (Early English Text Society, supplementary series, 13), London 1994, 429, line 156.

from dumping the contents of privies and the bodies of dogs along the common quay on the River Ouse, while anyone who blocked one of Winchester's many open streams with a dead animal faced a penalty of 12*d* for each offence.[58]

Nor was it only in death that livestock contaminated urban streams, rivers, aqueducts, and gutters. In 1364, for example, Winchester magistrates ordered Alice atte Churche and Richard Beyghe to dismantle an insanitary poultry yard "of geese and other fowl" which annoyed the neighbours and disrupted the adjacent market, presumably because of the stench. Alice faced an additional fine of 3*s* 4*d* should she fail to repair a drain, from which "dung and other filth (*finum et alia putrida*)", was pouring from the yard into the market to the further harm of residents and visiting merchants.[59] Winchester boasted an abundant natural water supply, and it is easy to see how quickly the streams that fed homes and workshops would have been contaminated by effluence. This case and the anxiety that it caused were far from unusual, as urban communities sought to protect themselves from the perils of miasmatic air and infected water. The complaints, noted above, by residents of Basingstoke went beyond snide remarks about uncouth yokels to focus upon the piles of manure left uncollected in their market by negligent bailiffs, and, significantly, the need for gratings to be placed over adjacent gutters to prevent the water in them from becoming filthy, noisome, and "hurtful to the people".[60]

The potentially fatal interconnection between animals, dung, and the pollution of streets and water supplies emerges clearly from the regulations promulgated - and regularly reiterated - by the rulers of late medieval English towns. A draconian set of byelaws introduced by the reforming mayor of Coventry in 1421 (a plague year) sought to eliminate wandering pigs, dogs, and ducks, as well as the keeping of swine in stalls near the highway, while banning the disposal of dung from stables and "other filth" in the river Sherbourne under pain of fines as high as 20*s*. Failure to use the designated dumps for manure and noxious waste that had been established beyond the gates could alone incur a penalty of 2*s*, which was more than a labourer's weekly wage. At the same time, compulsory measures were introduced for cleansing the river and town ditches of the accumulated filth which caused flooding and contamination.[61] By 1443 the amercement for owning a pig that caused any kind of nuisance stood at 6*s* 8*d*.[62] Such heavy fines served to underscore the severity of the offence and would in

58 Angelo Raine (ed.), York Civic Records III (Yorkshire Archaeological Society Record Series, 106), Wakefield 1942, 59; William H.B. Bird (ed.), The Black Book of Winchester, Winchester 1925, 121.

59 John S. Furley (ed.), Town Life in the XIV Century as Seen in the Court Rolls of Winchester, Winchester 1946, 132–133.

60 Baigent/Millard, History of Basingstoke (note 22), 316, 321.

61 Mary Dormer Harris (ed.), The Coventry Leet Book I (Early English Text Society, original series, 134), London 1907, 27, 29–31. Privies over water courses were also to be removed, under pain of a 40*s* fine. Some of these orders were reissued eight years later (119).

62 Dormer Harris (ed.), Coventry Leet Book I (note 61), 217.

practice have been subject to negotiation. Although their scale of fines was somewhat lower, Worcester's magistrates adopted a similar approach to sanitary policing. An ordinance of 1467 banned vagrant pigs, together with the disposal of dung on the quays and approaches to the river Severn, threatening miscreants with a far from negligible penalty of 3*s* 4*d* whenever they did so.[63]

Designed to avoid these very problems, and thus to protect against the spread of pestilence, the conduits, canals, lead or wooden pipes, and other hydraulic devices that proliferated in English towns from the thirteenth century onward still had to contend with the unwelcome presence of animals.[64] A major investment by the residents of King's Lynn in improvements to their water supply during the 1420s prompted the introduction of comprehensive measures to keep the town clean and avoid any blockages or pollution of the new system (fig. 2).[65] An analysis of complaints made to the town's leet courts in 1403 casts an interesting light on the impact that animals already had on Lynn's congested streets and waterways: thirteen individuals were presented for rearing pigs (some of which constituted a "grave nuisance"), seven for keeping an unspecified "beast" and four for owning at least one cow. These numbers pale into insignificance when compared with the seventy-two cases of negligent horse ownership reported by jurors, especially since presentments involving any kind of livestock were almost invariably accompanied by further allegations regarding the pollution of watercourses and public thoroughfares with dung and other noxious matter. If we also consider the two farriers who phlebotomised horses in the open street and the owner of a "common stable" who threw so much refuse into one of the fleets that "it impeded the flow of water to the grave nuisance of the entire community", the scale of the challenge becomes apparent.[66] These cases were, moreover, the tip of an iceberg, since it is clear that many more people kept animals than were customarily charged and fined for doing so.

It was in this wider context that, in October 1425, orders were issued for the seizure of any pigs, sows, or horses found wandering at large, and the imprisonment of their owners should they resist.[67] That precept did not always equate with practice or constitute a meaningful deterrent is apparent from presentments made by local juries in the following year, when ten people were accused of letting their swine run free but fined only modest amounts. Even the notorious Robert Thakker, whose many delinquent animals had left an incriminating trail of dung and filth around the streets and water gate, escaped with no more than a 20*d* penalty.[68] It does, however, seem that the authorities were

63 Toulmin Smith/Lucy Toulmin Smith (eds.), English Gilds (Early English Text Society, original series. 40), London 1870, 398.

64 Roberta J. Magnusson, Water Technology in the Middle Ages, Baltimore (Md) 2002.

65 Rawcliffe, Urban Bodies (note 2), 182–183.

66 KLBA, KL/C 17/14.

67 KLBA, KL/C 7/2, Hall Book, 1422–1429, p.104.

68 KLBA, KL/C 17/19, m.1r.

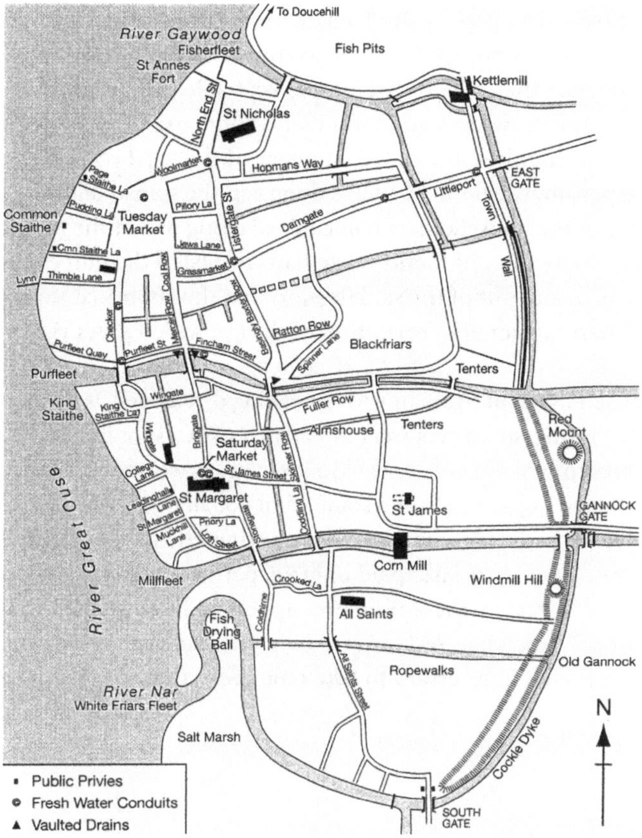

Fig. 2 Late medieval King's Lynn.

already planning a more pragmatic measure introduced in 1427, whereby householders who kept livestock in the town would have to pay higher contributions on a *per capita* basis toward the cost of street cleaning.[69] As well as reporting the names of these people, the jurors provided a careful record of the *number* of animals that each of them owned. In only a few cases, such as that of Thomas Bateman, who blocked a lane with the filth from his pigsty "to the grave nuisance of the people", are precise figures lacking.[70] The totals are striking and suggest that the jurors must have been extremely diligent

69 KLBA, KL/C 7/2, Hall Book, 1422–1429, p.134. The budget was then £13 6*s* 8*d* a year.

70 KLBA, KL/C 17/19. The thoroughness of the survey is apparent from a comparison with the leet roll for 1416, when jurors presented only nine people (including one of the constables) for owing pigs, six for keeping an unspecified "beast", eleven for having at least one cow, and sixteen horse owners. Sixteen cases involving the illicit disposal of cow and horse dung by other individuals confirm that far more residents owned livestock than those reported by their neighbours; cf. KLBA, KL/C 17/16.

in compiling their census: thirty-two people reared a bare minimum of ninety-seven pigs and four unidentified "beasts" between them; thirty-three residents accounted for thirty-eight cows; and no fewer than ninety-five people kept at least 133 horses. A couple of individuals had a few goats, while two others owned nine oxen.[71] Although rarely made explicit in the terse, highly abbreviated language of the legal record, the connection between the irresponsible disposal of all this dung and the spread of disease was clearly understood. Some of the householders named lived along one of the town's more vulnerable waterways, where piles of foetid waste had "impeded the entry and exit of tidal water which flows in and out of the said fleet, so that the abominable and stinking matter deposited [there] generates corruption of the air, which gives rise to many great infirmities".[72]

Yet again, vagrant pigs carried much of the blame for spreading dirt as well as damaging infrastructure and in 1428 negligent owners were threatened with a spot fine of 12*d* or imprisonment for every breach of the regulations.[73] In practice, as we have seen, not everyone who broke the law had to pay so much and some – but not all – got away lightly. William Fillipot, whose fifteen wandering ducks and four peripatetic pigs presented a "grave nuisance to the people" two years later paid only 9*d*, perhaps as a concession to his financial circumstances.[74] Even so, these measures appear to have worked well enough, and it was not until 1517, when new orders for the cleansing of waterways were promulgated, that the authorities felt it necessary to take renewed action.[75]

3. Conclusion

Given the continuing dependence of urban populations on animals, a permanent ban on the keeping of livestock was unrealistic and doomed to failure in the long term. Despite the stringent ruling of 1498, noted above, pigs eventually returned to Tudor York, just as they had done two centuries before. Several people were fined modest sums by the chamberlains for keeping them "contrary to the form of the ordinance of this city" during the 1520s; the authorities probably regarded these payments as a kind of tax, which they were happy to collect unless outbreaks of pestilence or other

71 The oxen would have been used for transport. In Winchester, where oxen were stabled alongside horses, many owners were presented for dumping "*finem equorum et taurorum*" in streets and watercourses. Cf. Keene, Survey of Winchester (note 11), vol. 1, 154.

72 KLBA, KL/C 17/19, m.6v.

73 KLBA, KL/C 7/2, Hall Book, 1422–1429, p.178.

74 KLBA, KL/C 17/21. Five people were then presented for owning ducks, which had not previously been recorded.

75 KLBA, KL/C 7/5, Hall Book, 1497–1544, f.180r. Articles of the leet drawn up in c. 1460 reminded jurors to report anyone whose pigs wandered the streets; cf. NRO, NCR, 5C/10.

extraordinary events, such as royal visits, demanded more extreme measures.[76] A few days before Henry VIII's arrival in September 1541, York residents were ordered to "remove all their cattle and swine out of this city [...] and so to keep them out [...] until such time that the King's Majesty and the Queen's Grace and their most honorable retinue have departed". Anyone who attempted the risky exercise of hiding a cow in their own home faced a substantial fine of 6*s* 8*d*.[77] Draconian penalties of the kind described above in Coventry certainly lost much of their force over time, and may, indeed, have proved counterproductive once life returned to normal in the aftermath of epidemics. The townspeople had lapsed into their old ways by 1480, when the prior of Coventry complained that, contrary to earlier regulations, they were blocking his floodgates and obstructing his watermill "daily with their dung, filth and sweepings thrown in the common river". Even worse, the health of his community had suffered because of the foul air generated by so much noisome refuse.[78] Perhaps those responsible were simply moving the problem further down river, in order to prevent their own stretch from becoming polluted with waste.

At best, magistrates, sought to keep principal thoroughfares, watercourses, and markets as clean and attractive as possible by relegating livestock, along with other environmental nuisances, to outlying areas. In many places, the modest fines routinely collected by local courts constituted a type of informal licensing system, whereby the owners of prohibited or vagrant animals contributed to communal coffers and helped to finance public works, such as refuse collection and piped water. In towns such as King's Lynn, they might even be required to pay more up front for these services because of the burden they placed upon them. Egregious and persistent nuisances, like Thomas Rant's miasmatic pigs, were, however, another matter, since they overstepped acceptable norms and posed an immediate threat to health. In this regard, it is worth noting that Rant was presented to the court by his neighbours, who were clearly unprepared to tolerate behaviour that not only seemed extremely dangerous and offensive, but also undermined the ties of mutual support and Christian brotherhood that bound communities together in the face of external threats like plague. All urban animals may

---

76 York Civic Archives, York, CB 2, ff.13r–14r, 18r, 51r, 52r, 137v.

77 Angelo Raine (ed.), York Civic Records IV (York Archaeological Society, 108) Wakefield 1945, 64, 65. In 1513 a large dunghill near the water gate at Southampton was removed in anticipation of Henry's arrival. See Butler, (ed.), Book of Fines (note 24), 82. Towns always presented their best face to visiting royalty. When the queen of Scotland visited Aberdeen in 1501 and 1511, for example, all pigs, pigsties and middens were removed from the streets. Cf. John Stuart (ed.), Extracts from the Council Register of the Burgh of Aberdeen, Aberdeen 1844, 70, 81. Even so, King Henry's fear of plague, which had killed his mother, was notorious.

78 Mary Dormer Harris (ed.), The Coventry Leet Book II (Early English Text Society, original series, 135), London 1908, 445. Archaeological evidence confirms that dead dogs and cats were also being dumped in the town's ditches, in defiance of current byelaws; cf. Paul Mason/Danny McAree/Iain Soden, Coventry's Medieval Suburbs, Oxford 2017, 107.

have posed a potential risk as vectors of disease, but some, including feckless humans, seemed far more dangerous than others.

Photo credits

Fig. 1 Map of late medieval London, drawn by Catherine D'Alton. (First published in Carole Rawcliffe, Urban Bodies. Communal Health in Late Medieval English Towns and Cities, Woodbridge 2013.)

Fig. 2 Map of late medieval King's Lynn, drawn by Catherine d'Alton. (First published in Rawcliffe, Urban Bodies.)

Abstract:
In 1444, a plague year in southern England, a group of Londoners complained about the filth generated by poultry sellers in the city centre, protesting that the presence of large numbers of swans, geese and other birds produced a terrible stench, which in turn spread "great and perilous infections". Concern that urban livestock, both alive and dead, would give rise to miasmatic air and thus cause epidemic diseases was widespread throughout late medieval England, reflecting a general awareness of current medical ideas about environmental health and the recommendations made by the authors of plague treatises. Official initiatives for the control of animals and their waste had traditionally focused upon the state of the streets, but (again in keeping with medical advice) came increasingly to address the pollution of urban waterways as well, thereby adopting a holistic approach to the problem of "venomous infection". Yet precept, however forcefully expressed, did not always accord with practice. Measures adopted in King's Lynn following a major investment in the town's water supply during the 1420s furnish an excellent example of the challenges that could arise, and the compromises that had to be negotiated, in a town where livestock keeping was common. The enforcement of sanitary measures in a society that depended heavily upon communal policing inevitably meant that a degree of consensus had to be reached, and animal keeping was often tolerated within accepted limits.

Keywords:
infection | miasma | plague | public health | waste disposal

William Riguelle

Purifying the Streets

Legislation Against Animals During Epidemics in the Towns of Southern Netherlands and the Principality of Liège, 1600–1670

In 1668, Maximilian Henry of Bavaria, Prince-Bishop of Liège, imposed several preventive measures to protect the city of Huy from the plague. Among other things, he banned all residents from keeping "dogs, cats, doves, pigeons, rabbits, goats, pigs and sheep, or other kinds of beasts [...]".[1] In the seventeenth century – as in the centuries before[2] – the authorities in the Netherlands and the Principality of Liège placed restrictions on the movement of certain animals in the streets when faced with the threat of epidemic. In Ostend, Bruges, Turnhout, Brussels, Huy, Liège, and Namur, the requirement to remove pigs, poultry, and dogs from the streets or to keep them enclosed was one of – and sometimes the first[3] – measures that administrators imposed to prevent "contagious disease".[4] Decaying animal carcasses were equally dreaded. Cats, chickens, or, much more rarely, dead rats were considered just as likely to cause a "great infection" and were to be thrown immediately into the river or taken out of the city.[5]

---

1 "Chiens, chats, colombes, pigeons, lapins, chèvres, porcs et moutons ni autre sorte de bestes [...]". Ordonnance prescrivant les mesures à prendre pour se préserver de la maladie contagieuse régnant à Huy, 18 October 1668, in: Mathieu-Lambert Polain (ed.), Recueil des ordonnances de la principauté de Liège (hereafter: ROPL), 2nd series, vol. 3, Brussels 1872, 337–338, article 4.

2 See Christian De Backer, Maatregelen tegen de pest te diest in de vijftiende en zestiende eeuw, in: De pest in de Nederlanden. Medisch historische beschouwingen 650 jaar na de zwarte dood, Brussels 1999, 183–209; Christelle Dethy, La lutte contre la peste à Mons sous Charles Quint, unpublished Degree Dissertation, Université Catholique de Louvain, academic year 1999–2000.

3 Bibliothèque de l'Université de Liège (hereafter: BUL), Liège, manuscripts, no. 238C.

4 Jacques Membré, La peste à Valenciennes. L'épidémie de 1668. Les bancs politiques, les remèdes préconisés, les comptes des pestiférés, in: Épidémies et endémies à Ath et en Hainaut du Moyen Âge au XIXe siècle, Chièvres 1998, 77–87, 78–79; Jacques Charlier, La peste à Bruxelles et ses conséquences démographiques, Brussels 1969, 58; Louis Huyghebaert, Saint Hubert. Patron des chasseurs, (s. l.) 1928, 144. It is important to remember that in the seventeen century, other infectious diseases were rampant in addition to the plague. These are not easy to identify given the generic use of the terms "contagion" and "peste" in these sources to refer to all epidemics. Nevertheless, contemporaries distinguished between them and treated them differently. See Françoise Jacquet-Ladrier, L'hôpital Saint-Roch et la lutte contre la peste à Namur, aux XVIIe et XVIIIe siècles, in: Annales de la Société belge d'histoire des hôpitaux, vol. XVIII, (1980), 59–70, 63.

5 Namur State Archives (hereafter: AEN), Ville de Namur, 48bis, 8 December 1634, fol. 26r; Charlier, La peste à Bruxelles (note 4), 58; "Mesures pour prévenir la propagation de la peste", 1 September 1603, in: Victor Brants (ed.), Recueil des ordonnances des Pays-Bas. Règne d'Albert et Isabelle. 1597–1621, vol. 1,

Thus, animals were an integral part of legislation during times of epidemic.[6] The rules regarding them shed light on how humans considered animals and the "status this consideration bestowed on them".[7] In this context, the control of animals cannot be separated from issues of public hygiene, nor from another figure roaming towns and cities: the vagrant. It is therefore important to include animals and their fate in analyses of other aspects of urban life in the seventeenth century.

The analysis focuses on the territory of present-day Belgium, which brought together two quite distinct socio-political realities in the seventeenth century: in the West, we find the Netherlands, administered by a sovereign issuing from the Spanish House of Habsburg. The capital was Brussels. In the East, we find the principality of Liège, an autonomous region directed by a prince-bishop, albeit a vassal of the Germanic Holy Roman Empire since the tenth century. If the legislation regarding animals was similar within these two territories, it is nevertheless necessary to distinguish the different levels of power. The central authorities of these two territories – a prince-bishop in Liège and a sovereign in the Netherlands – had competencies in a wide range of areas, including general administration and domestic policy. Their decisions took the form of edicts or ordinances – the vocabulary is unstable – formal documents imposing a legal provision. In Liège, the prince-bishop had a body responsible for drafting the acts: the Private Council, which exercised sovereign authority and was therefore involved in all acts of government. In the Spanish Netherlands, the heads of state, rarely present in the territory, were represented by a governor general assisted by the three collateral councils set up by Charles V in 1531, which remained until the end of the *ancien régime*: the Council of Finance, the Council of State, and the Private Council. The latter was a consultative body that transformed the will of the prince and the governor general into regulations. Its powers evolved during the early modern period and extended to police

---

Bruxelles 1909, 220–224. Rats rarely appear in legislative sources. For example, there is no mention of them in Liège.

6 However, historiography pays relatively little attention to the animal's fate in the context of epidemics. Jean Vitaux's recent *Histoire de la peste* lists eight historical preventive measures against the spread of the plague. Although the cleaning of streets is mentioned, none of the measures refers explicitly to animals. See Jean Vitaux, Histoire de la peste, Paris 2010, 145–146. In Belgium, several researchers have looked at the epidemics of the Middle Ages and modern times, mainly as part of local studies. Even though animals are often listed among the preventive measures adopted, no in-depth analysis has been made on this topic. See Françoise Jacquet-Ladrier, Les épidémies de Peste aux XVIe–XVIIe siècles. L'exemple de Namur, in: Cahiers de Sambre et Meuse 4 (2007), 122–141; Pierre Bauwens, Les deux dernières graves épidémies de peste à Huy (1634–1636 et 1668–1669), in: Annales du Cercle hutois des sciences et des beaux-arts (hereafter: ACHSBA) 48 (1994), 41–64. However, one exception in this historiographical landscape should be mentioned: Stéphane Audoin-Rouzeau, Les chemins de la peste. Le rat, la puce et l'homme, Rennes 2003.

7 Corinne Beck/Éric Fabre, L'animal, l'histoire et l'histoire naturelle. Un mariage à trois est-il possible?, in: Études rurales 189 (2012), 107–120, 107.

matters. At the local level, cities were administered by local councillors. In Liège, this was the City Council, composed of a noble and bourgeois oligarchy and presided over by the burgomasters. However, their intervention was limited with regard to the plague. In the Netherlands, most of the normative activity was in the hands of a magistrate, the local name for the *échevinage*. His powers and scope of action covered everything that concerned the administration and policing of the city, including public hygiene and therefore the divagation of animals.

Relying mainly on these authorities' legislative sources and on medical treatises, this chapter analyses how central and local authorities in the Southern Netherlands and the Principality of Liège legislated urban animals in times of plague.[8] More specifically, it focuses on orders issued in the seventeenth century, when the disease recurred irregularly until 1670.[9] From this corpus of documents, I examine the authorities' speeches, silence, methods of repression, and above all, their motives. Why did the authorities target animals? It also seems legitimate to think that, in view of the numerous utilitarian functions fulfilled by some animals, the authorities decided to target only some of them. A hierarchy of animal species according to their degree of "public nuisance" must therefore be established. In this case: what species were considered to be pests? How did the authorities organize their fight against these harmful species?

1. Miasmas, But No Fleas

The plague was "the archetype of the devastating scourge".[10] It quickly killed masses of people and was an object of great fear in the collective imagination. In his famous *Traité de la police*, Nicolas Delamare stated that, "of all the diseases that come to men, there is none more dangerous than this; it has often distressed and ravaged the entire Provinces in just a few months, leaving them deserted".[11] If the plague symbolized death and seriously destabilized human societies, it was because contemporaries had little concrete knowledge of its origins. Not until 1894 did Alexandre Yersin identify the *Yersinia pestis* as the bacterium responsible for the plague. In the same period (1898),

---

8 These two territories more or less cover today's Belgium.

9 After 1670, the disease never returned to the territory of modern Belgium. Claude Bruneel, La mortalité dans les campagnes. Le duché de Brabant aux XVIIe et XVIIIe siècles, Louvain 1977, 514; Maurice-Aurélien Arnould, Mortalité et épidémies sous l'ancien régime dans le Hainaut et quelques régions limitrophes, in: Paul Harsin/Étienne Hélin (ed.), Problème de mortalité. Méthodes, sources et bibliographie en démographie historique, Liège 1965, 465–481, 477.

10 Annick Le Guérer, Le déclin de l'olfactif, mythe ou réalité?, in: Anthropologie et Sociétés 14 (1990), 25–45, 34.

11 "De toutes les maladies qui arrivent aux hommes, il n'y en a point de plus dangereuse que celle-ci ; elle a souvent désolé et ravagé en peu de mois les Provinces entières, et les a rendues désertes". Nicolas Delamare, Traité de la police, vol. 1, Paris 1722, 648.

Paul-Louis Simond discovered that it was transmitted by fleas, whose role had been completely unknown to earlier hygienists.[12] Therefore, in Western Europe, the flea and the rat did not feature among the explanatory factors behind the scourge in the seventeenth century. The causes of the disease were sought elsewhere. In particular, it was believed to arise from tainted air, which in turn resulted from "planetary conjunctions or emanations from the soil".[13] Many members of the medical profession agreed on the harmful role of bad air. These include the Ghent physician Herman Van der Heyden, Dr Lazare Macquis, and Louis Overdatz, who published a treatise on the plague in Brussels in 1668 in which he stated that the disease originated from stale air.[14]

This theory had been formulated by scholars and physicians and was shared by the authorities in the Netherlands and the Principality of Liège, who relied on their advice[15] and feared the miasmas, the putrid vapours that polluted the air.[16]

Consequently, the authorities adopted a series of preventive public measures to eliminate anything that might contribute to a stale, infected atmosphere: fumigation; isolating those who had caught the plague; cleaning the streets; and banning residents from feeding pigs, rabbits, pigeons, or dogs in the city. Fear of the plague and the bad smells conveyed by dogs and cats led to many references to "filthy" or "stinking" animals which should be prevented from moving and breeding within towns. Fear of bad air also extended to any figure of aimless movement suspected of conveying it: infected objects, vagrants, the poor, or stray animals. Thus, the idea gained ground that the disease was brought into the city by infected objects, vagrants, the poor, or stray animals. Animals were presumed to be one of the epidemic's primary vectors, because, according to the Liège burgomaster, Mathias de Grati, they carried rotten vapours in their bowels and in

12 Robert Delort, La peste soit du rat!, in: L'Histoire 74 (1985), 50–55, 50.

13 Jean-Noël Biraben, Peste, in: François Bluche (ed.), Dictionnaire du Grand Siècle, Paris 1990, 1188–1189, 1188; Charles-Auguste Vandermonde, Dictionnaire portatif de santé, vol. 2, Paris 1783, 370. The appearance of the epidemic was also seen as the manifestation of divine anger unleashed because of the sins of humans. See Jean Delumeau, La peur en Occident (XIVe–XVIIIe siècles). Une cité assiégée, Paris 1978, 171; Jean de la Fontaine, Les animaux malades de la peste, 2nd collection, book 7, fable 1, 1678. See also the chapter by Carol Rawcliffe in this volume.

14 Herman Van der Heyden, Discours et advis sur les flus de ventre douloureux, soit qu'il y at du sang ou point, Gand, Servais Manilius, 1645, 38; Léon Bertrand, Contribution à l'étude de la peste dans les Flandres du XIVe au XVIIIe siècle, Évreux 1922, 42–53, 45; Louis Overdatz, Kort verhael vande peste met hare geneesmiddelen dienstigh voor alle arme verlaten menschen, Bruxelles 1668.

15 On this subject, see Charlier, La peste à Bruxelles (note 4), 23, 61.

16 On the miasma theory, see Alain Corbin, Le miasme et la jonquille. L'odorat et l'imaginaire social XVIIIe–XIXe siècles, Paris 1982.

their hair or feathers that were likely to rise into the air and pollute it.[17] Like clothing, fur, or bedsheets, animals were supposed to "hold" the plague and carry it into the city.[18]

Thus, a contagionist doctrine was added to the theories of the so-called aerists, who feared infection of the air. From the sixteenth century onwards, law-making was inspired by both of these conceptions[19] – as were medical recommendations for epidemics. In Liège, the physician Jean-François Bresmal stated that, in times of plague, it was advisable to kill "dogs, cats, pigeons and other domestic animals that might carry air".[20] At the end of the sixteenth century, the Antwerp physician Van Hakendover recommended that animals should not be kept if they gave off a bad smell.[21] The physicians also mentioned decaying carcasses and emphasized that foul air would be particularly found in places where human and animal corpses were abandoned.[22]

Although public health was cited as the main justification for excluding animals, it is not unreasonable to suggest that the authorities were also motivated by the belief that the animals were diseased, too. While some authors held that dogs and cats acted as plague vectors without themselves being infected,[23] others believed animals were vulnerable to being touched by the "contagious and contaminated" air and therefore by the disease. Antoine de Furetière's *Dictionnaire universel* states, for example, that the plague is "the mortal enemy to the life of men, animals and even plants and trees".[24] Jean Van der Cruyse, a parish priest from a small town north of Antwerp, published a

---

17 Mathias de Grati, Discours de droit moral et politique qui peut servir de remède tant contre la peste des villes et états que contre celle de l'âme et du corps. Seconde partie, Liège 1676, 13. Mathias de Grati was a Liège administrator and diplomat. He was born in the first half of the seventeenth century and dies in Liège after 1685. See Alphonse Le Roy, De Grati, Mathias, in: Biographie nationale de Belgique (hereafter: BNB) 8 (1885), 211–214.

18 Isaac Quatroux, Traité de la peste contenant sa définition, ses espèces, et différences, ses causes, ses signes, ses accidens, sa cure, et les moyens de s'en garantir, Paris 1671, 125.

19 Although contagion was mentioned along with animals as contaminating agents, it was unclear how contagion took place. See Jean-Noël Biraben, Les hommes et la peste en France et dans les pays européens et méditerranéens, vol. 2, Paris/La Haye 1976, 25, 27; Jacques Revel, Autour d'une épidémie ancienne. La peste de 1666 à 1670, in: Revue d'histoire moderne et contemporaine 17 (1970), 953–983, 965.

20 Jean-François Bresmal, Parallèle des eaux minérales actuellement chaudes et actuellement froides du diocèse et pays de Liège, divisé en deux parties avec un avis au public pour se préserver de la peste, des fièvres pestilentielles et malignes, et d'autres maladies de pareilles natures, Liège 1721, 27. Jean-François Bresmal was a physician practising in Liège in the eighteenth century.

21 Bertrand, Contribution à l'étude de la peste (note 14), 46.

22 Ibid., 45.

23 Edme de la Poix de Fréminville, Dictionnaire ou traité de la police générale des villes, bourgs, paroisses, et seigneuries de la campagne, Paris 1769, 247.

24 Peste, in: Antoine Furetière, Dictionnaire universel, contenant généralement tous les mots françois tant vieux que modernes, et les termes de toutes les sciences et des arts, The Hague 1690.

pamphlet in 1604 in which he advised keeping dogs and cats tied up, as they were likely to "contract" the disease.[25]

In this context, the confinement and exclusion of animals were precautions aimed, naturally, at preventing the spread of the disease, but can also be interpreted as a desire to protect certain animals from it. However, there is no explicit mention in the legislative sources of the mortality rate of animals during the epidemic. The fact that some contemporaries refer to mortality is strange, since we now know that dogs, horses, and birds are not usually affected by it. However, as Henri Mollaret and Jacqueline Brossollet suggest, an increased animal mortality may have been caused by the lack of care given to them during the epidemic.[26]

2. The Removal and Elimination of Pests

In times of plague, police edicts usually prohibited town residents from keeping or feeding animals in the enclosure. After publication of the regulation, residents usually had around three days to drive the animals out. In Namur and Huy, pigs were sent to the common herd.[27] However, in some places, those "who have the convenience of keeping them locked in their house, without inconvenience to their neighbours" were allowed to keep their pigs, goats, and rabbits.[28] The possibility of keeping such animals in a garden, a stable, or a "convenient place" was nevertheless far from general or guaranteed. Moreover, it did not always apply in walled towns, but only in outlying districts.[29] In some cases, certain species, such as dogs, cats, and chickens, were allowed to be kept in towns, but had to be locked and tied up, and were not allowed out unrestrained.[30]

25 Bertrand, Contribution à l'étude de la peste (note 14), 46.

26 Henri H. Mollaret/Jacqueline Brossollet, La peste, source méconnue d'inspiration artistique, in: Jaarboek, Antwerp 1965, 3–112, 30.

27 AEN, City of Namur, 370, 31 July 1635, article 16, [n.f.]; Cri du péron prescrivant aux habitants de Huy certaines mesures à prendre pour se préserver de la peste, 7 July 1606, in: Polain (ed.), ROPL, 2nd series, vol. 2, 279–281, article 6; Édits de police, 31 July 1622, in: Jules Borgnet/Stanislas Bormans/Dieudonné Brouwers (ed.), Cartulaire de la commune de Namur, vol. 5, Namur 1922, 4–23, 17. See also Alain Croix, Le familier et le sauvage. Hommes et animaux au XVIIe siècle, in: Robert Durand (ed.), L'homme, l'animal domestique et l'environnement, Nantes 1993, 373–385, 381.

28 "Cri du péron prescrivant aux habitants de Huy certaines mesures à prendre pour se préserver de la peste", 7 July 1606, in: Polain (ed.), ROPL, 2nd series, vol. 2, 279–281.

29 Liège State Archives (hereafter: AEL), Conseil privé, no. 108, 18 August 1615, fol. 118v–119v; BUL, manuscripts, no. 238C, 18 October 1607, fol. 141r–142 r.

30 AEN, City of Namur, 48 bis, 8 December 1636, fol. 36v.

The authorities' main objective was to prevent animals from roaming in the public space. Therefore, they had to be driven out, "tied up" or "locked up" inside homes.[31] Animals that had no owner or moved freely were seen as a real danger, being exposed to all kinds of contamination and possibly spreading the disease. The parallel between the removal of animals and the exclusion of foreigners, beggars, and social dropouts is evident. This has already been observed for the Middle Ages, when health regulations ordered the ejection of certain animals along with the population of wanderers, lepers, and prostitutes.[32] Stray animals cannot therefore be separated from other figures in urban wandering, namely the vagrant – hence the terms "vagrant animal" and "vagrant dog" that are associated with stray animals.[33]

For those with no land or space to keep their animals in town, the only options were to keep them secretly, abandon them, or kill them. Some residents of Huy left animals in the street or drowned them in wells and public fountains.[34] If town dwellers had nowhere to put their animals, slaughtering them may also have been a legal obligation. In Liège, "all members of the infected places shall peremptorily kill their dogs and cats, or have them killed, within 24 hours".[35] Similar requirements were laid down in Hainaut and in Brussels.[36] "Getting rid" of and "disposing of" one's animals could therefore be synonymous with execution.

Nevertheless, it is legitimate to doubt the compliance of town dwellers with these orders to kill their animals. The issue of non-compliance frequently arises when such rules were reinstated during new outbreaks of the plague.[37] In Namur, the plague regulations of 8 December 1634 were updated in the same terms on 5 July 1636 due to a resurgence of the epidemic.[38] Indeed, the magistrate noted that the inhabitants appeared

31 Cri du péron prescrivant aux habitants de Huy certaines mesures à prendre pour se préserver de la peste, 7 July 1606, in: Polain (ed.), ROPL, 2nd series, vol. 2, 279–281.

32 Annie Fourcaut, Peurs dans la ville, peurs de la ville, in: Histoire Urbaine 2 (2000), 5–7, 6; François-Olivier Touati, Un mal qui répand la terreur? Espace urbain, maladie et épidémies au Moyen Âge, in: Histoire Urbaine 2 (2000), 9–38, 21.

33 Arnaud Exbalin, Le grand massacre des chiens, in: Histoire Urbaine 44 (2015), 107–124, 121.

34 Ordonnance prescrivant les mesures à prendre pour se préserver de la maladie contagieuse régnant à Huy, 18 October 1668, in: Polain (ed.), ROPL, 2nd series, vol. 3, 337–338. This practice risked "contaminating" the town's waters, which is why the authorities banned the dumping of any kind of waste into water supply points. On this subject, see Ordonnance touchant le nettoiement des rues et l'enlèvement des immondices, à Liège, 14 May 1689, in: Polain (ed.), ROPL, 3rd series, vol. 1, 142–143.

35 AEL, Placards, 002579A, 27 October 1668.

36 Jean Dugnoille, La peste à Ath et en Hainaut du XIVe au XVIIe siècle, in: Épidémies et endémies à Ath et en Hainaut du Moyen Âge au XIXe siècle, Chièvres 1998, 77–87; Charlier, La peste à Bruxelles (note 4), 62.

37 In Liège, similar decrees with identical content were repeated throughout the seventeenth century: in 1602, 1603, 1617, 1624 and 1666, the legislator reiterated in the same terms the measures that had to be taken to protect oneself from the "contagious disease".

38 AEN, City of Namur, 48 bis, 5 July 1636, fol. 30v.

to have "little fondness for observing the promulgated edicts".[39] In spite of the rules, the local authorities in Namur still suspected some townspeople of "holding" pigs, rabbits, or pigeons in their houses the following year.[40] In view of the essential contribution of some animals, particularly in terms of food, it was difficult to intervene against them without arousing resistance in the urban population. However, the return of the rules did not necessarily lead to categorical disobedience or mean that the regulations were ineffective. It was rather a sign that the police were doing their job, and had to reissue edicts to refresh the community's memory.[41] Similar redundancy was seen in different waves of the epidemic throughout the seventeenth century, which were sufficiently spaced out in time to justify reviving the legislation.

Animals that were found guilty of roaming the public roads in spite of the rules were confiscated.[42] However, there is little information indicating the scope of this rule and what happened to the confiscated livestock. In some circumstances, the seized animal was handed over to the person who had reported the unlawful behaviour.[43] There were also instances of pigs being "redistributed" to charitable institutions, among the poor or to hospitals, which also occurred in France.[44] Yet, there is no evidence for the existence of a pound or a possible enclosure for captured animals.

In addition to bans imposed by legislative means, the authorities occasionally took more drastic measures to combat stray animals. Sometimes they mobilized town residents by allowing them to kill with impunity any vagrant animal they found in the streets, irrespective of what it was – pig, rabbit, cat, dog, etc. (Fig. 1) In Namur, as in Sint-Truiden, Liège, and Verviers, all dogs and "vagrant animals" found abandoned and roaming the city could be slaughtered.[45] Dogs were the authorities' main target, as they

39 Ibid., 20 September 1635, fol. 34r.

40 Ibid., 8 December 1636, fol. 37r.

41 Catherine Denys, La police du nettoiement au XVIIIe siècle, in: Ethnologie française 153 (2015), 411–420, 414–416; ead., 'Afin que nul n'en prétexte cause d'ignorance'. Quelques éléments de réflexion sur la diffusion et la réception du droit dans les villes au XVIIIe siècle, in: Christophe Leduc (ed.), Droit et communication. Dire, enseigner, publier, Arras 2000, 99–117; Nicolas Toussaint Lemoyne des Essarts, Dictionnaire universel de Police, vol. 1, Paris 1786, 311.

42 The owner was also fined.

43 Cri du péron prescrivant aux habitants de Huy certaines mesures à prendre pour se préserver de la peste, 7 July 1606, in: Polain (ed.), ROPL, 2nd series, vol. 2, 279–281.

44 Cri du péron prescrivant les mesures à prendre pour préserver de la peste, 8 October 1554, in: Polain (ed.), ROPL, 2nd series, vol. 1, 247; Croix, Le familier et le sauvage (note 27), 381. The proven usefulness of pigs as food during periods of plague contrasts with their image as pests.

45 AEN, City of Namur, 48 bis, 8 December 1636, fol. 36v.; Pol Bouche, Contribution à l'étude des épidémies dans la principauté de Liège. La peste à Dinant, Liège et Saint-Trond aux XVIe et XVIIe siècles, unpublished Degree Dissertation, University of Liège, academic year 2003–2004, 54; Ordonnance de police pour la ville de Verviers, 20 January 1780, in: Polain (ed.), ROPL, 3rd series, vol. 2, 845–847; Ordonnance approuvant un règlement du conseil de la cité, du 17 mai 1666, renouvelant et amplifiant les mandements antérieurs touchant les incendies et la peste, 19 July 1666, in: Polain (ed.), ROPL, 2nd series, vol. 3, 317–324, article 11.

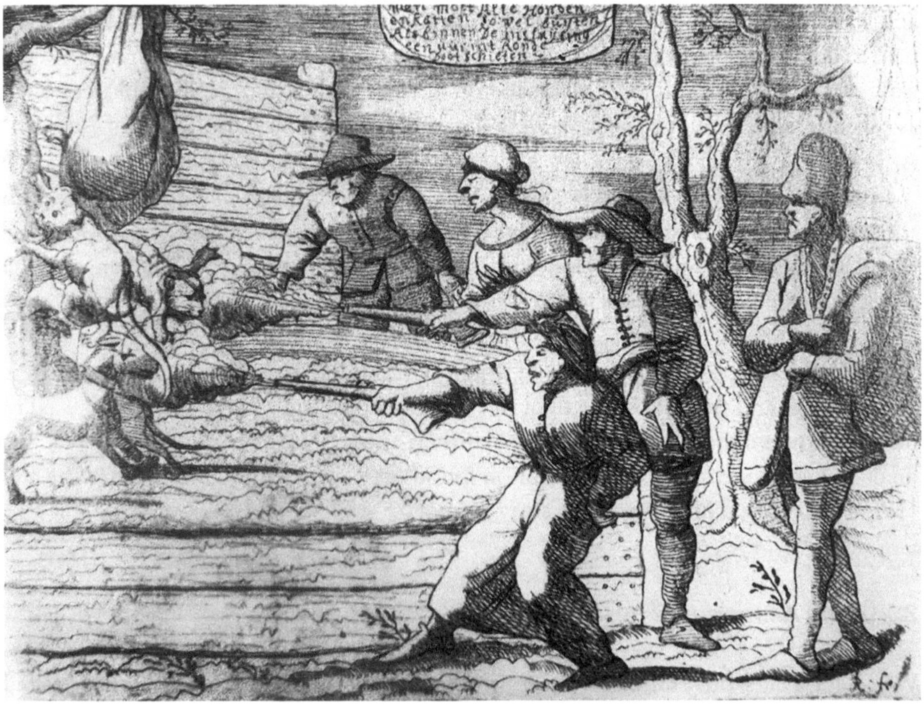

Fig. 1 People shooting on dogs and cats, etching by Jean De Ridder, c. 1720. The text above the illustration recommends killing "all dogs and all cats in and within an hour's walk of the common enclosure". However, the place depicted is not known.

roamed spontaneously in search of food and were a visible source of disorder. As they lived close to humans, they were in contact with the miasma. The English author Daniel Defoe referred to this practice in his famous *Journal of the Plague Year*:

> Wherefore were we ordered to kill all the dogs and cats, but because as they were domestic animals, and are apt to run from house to house and from street to street, so they are capable of carrying the effluvia or infectious streams of bodies infected even in their furs and hair?[46]

The same author states that 40,000 dogs and five times as many cats were destroyed in London in 1665.[47] This practice was carried out by specially appointed individuals

---

46 Daniel Defoe, Journal of the Plague Year, London 1722, 144. This essay by Daniel Defoe was written between 1665 and 1772. Dogs are also the focus of the words of Jean-François Bresmal. See Bresmal, Parallèle des eaux minérales (note 20), 27. See also Mark Jenner, The Great Dog Massacre, in: William Naphy, Penny Roberts (ed.), Fear in Early Modern Society, Manchester 1997, 44–61.

47 Cited by Delumeau, La peur en Occident (note 13), 150.

and was also adopted in several Dutch cities. In Ath, Mons, and Douai, the magistrate paid a "dog killer" from as early as the Middle Ages.[48] The practice continued into the early modern period, although it was then assigned to other municipal employees, such as executioners. Similar massacres were organized, particularly in the city of Antwerp:

> In order to remove the bad smells and filth coming in part from the multitude of dogs which have often brought pestilential and contagious diseases [...] the burgomaster, the Aldermen, and the Council of the City of Antwerp, have designated 3 persons who are authorised to kill dogs encountered in the street [...].[49]

The "*Hondenslaegers*" (dog slayers) of the city of Antwerp used specific weapons, such as the cudgel and the baldric, to fight the straying dogs (fig. 2 and 3). The club used to hit the animals is studded, whereas the baldric is a sign of its owner's official status. The quality of the baldric and the inscription found on it revealed the importance the city of Antwerp placed on eliminating stray animals.

3. Useful Animals and Pests

While dogs, cats, pigs, and, to a lesser extent, rabbits and pigeons[50] are regularly listed as pests during periods of plague, slaughter or draught animals – such as horses – were never targeted.[51] Preventive measures were therefore selective and aimed at stopping the devastating effects of the disease without completely halting business activities and

48 William Riguelle, Le chien dans la rue aux XVIIe et XVIIIe siècles. Le cas des villes du sud de la Belgique, in: Histoire Urbaine 47 (2016), 69–86; Robert Delort, Les animaux dans la ville occidentale à la fin du Moyen Âge, in: Villes, bonnes villes, cités et capitales, Caen 1993, 343–350, 345. For the situation in the late Middle Ages, see Mathieu Béghin, Entre le cœur de ville et les faubourgs. La place de l'animal en milieu urbain dans le nord de la France aux XIVe et XVe siècles, in: Corinne Beck/Fabrice Guizard (ed.), Les animaux sont dans la place. La longue histoire d'une cohabitation, Amiens (forthcoming).

49 "Afin de supprimer les mauvaises odeurs et les saletés provenant en partie de la multitude des chiens qui ont souvent occasionné des maladies pestilentielles et contagieuses […] le bourgmestre, les Échevins, et le Conseil de la Ville d'Anvers, ont désigné 3 personnes qui sont autorisées à abattre les chiens rencontrés dans la rue […]". Order dated 1657. Huyghebaert, Saint Hubert (note 4), 145.

50 AEN, City of Namur, 48 bis, 8 December 1636, fol. 37r; Cri du péron prescrivant aux habitants de Huy certaines mesures à prendre pour se préserver de la peste, 7 July 1606, in: Polain (ed.), ROPL, 2nd series, vol. 2, 279–281, article 6.

51 These are the animals that only very rarely contract the plague. Horses, oxen, goats and sheep do not have fleas, which are repelled by their smell. See Biraben, Les hommes et la peste (note 19), vol. 1, 15. Goats and sheep were nonetheless sometimes targeted and referred to as dirty animals. See Ordonnance prescrivant les mesures à prendre pour se préserver de la maladie contagieuse régnant à Huy, 18 October 1668, in: Polain (ed.), ROPL, 2nd series, vol. 3, 337–338, article 4.

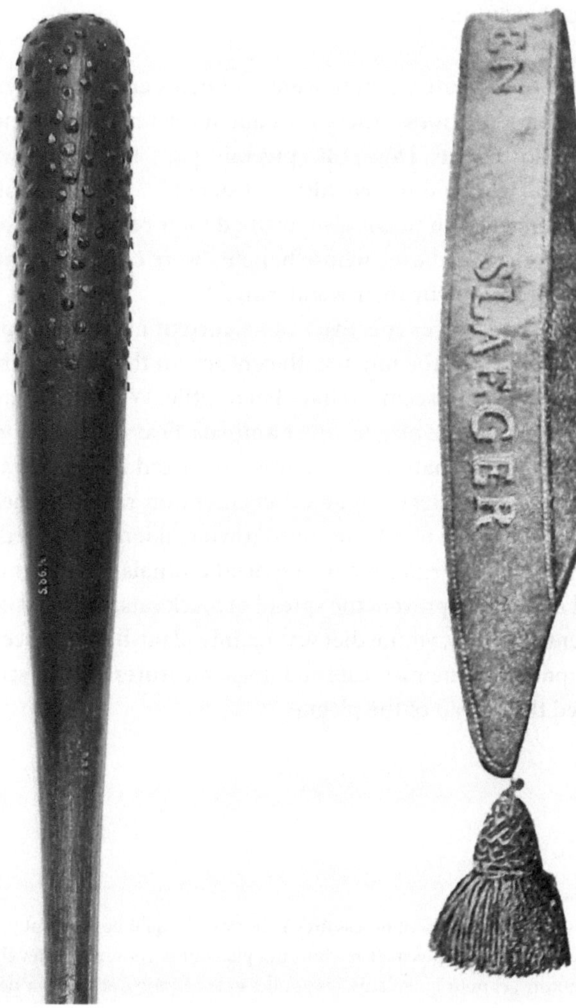

Fig. 2 and 3 Cudgel and baldric of the "Hondenslagers" of the city of Antwerp, eighteenth century.

disrupting supplies to towns.[52] Isaac Quatroux's 1671 *Traité de la peste* is enlightening in this respect:

> As animals are necessary to man, and it is not appropriate to keep them all at a time of plague, it is right to choose the most useful ones, such as horses, oxen, cows and sheep, and chickens

52 Alain Croix, La Bretagne aux XVIe et XVIIe siècles. La vie, la mort, la foi, vol. 1, Paris 1981, 474.

> and pigeons among fowl, and to remove all others from the Cities, as they are very dirty and filthy and of little use [...].[53]

According to the author, there were two main criteria for removing certain animals: uselessness and dirtiness. There is frequent reference to dirtiness and bad smells in the legislative documents. Dogs, cats, pigeons, pigs, and rabbits were described as animals from which "we could receive filth and stench".[54] The fact that some animals provided no visible benefit to humans also justified their removal or execution. This was mainly the case for dogs and cats, whose benefits were considered minimal compared to the health hazard posed by their wandering.[55]

Were these measures effective from a current medical perspective? Given the knowledge acquired since the nineteenth century on the plague's mechanisms, the removal or killing of animals seems to have been futile. While the Oriental rat flea (*Xenopsylla cheopis*) transmits the plague, other animals' fleas do so only very rarely, or not at all.[56] Moreover, no elimination of rats was organized in the cities of the Netherlands and the Principality of Liège – regulations mention rats extremely rarely – and the near-systematic exclusion of cats deprived town residents of a predator that would have got rid of them. Even if rules regarding dead animals were part of the hygiene measures, they did not help to prevent the spread of black rats, the most common type of rat in the seventeenth century, whose diet was mainly plant-based. Since regulations also targeted the rats' potential enemies, cats and dogs, measures against stray animals possibly even facilitated the spread of the plague.

53 "Comme les animaux sont nécessaires à l'homme, et qu'il ne convient pas dans le temps de peste de les tenir tous, il est à propos de faire choix des plus utiles, comme sont les chevaux, les bœufs, les vaches et les moutons, et pour les volatils, les poulles et les pigeons, et éloigner des Villes tous les autres comme estant très sales et immondes et peu utiles [...]." Quatroux, Traité de la peste (note 18), 34–35.

54 Ordonnance prescrivant les mesures à prendre pour se préserver de la maladie contagieuse régnant à Huy, 18 October 1668, in: Polain (ed.), ROPL, 2nd series, vol. 3, 337–338, article 4.

55 The issue of the usefulness of urban animals, within the theme of pests, needs further examination by broader investigations. There are numerous nuances, both in terms of different tolerance thresholds during an epidemic and also in terms of the specific details within the same species. For example, some dogs were considered more of a pest than others because of their breed or health condition.

56 Indeed, although fleas are undoubtedly the disease's vectors, entomologists have identified more than 2000 species that are generally dependent on one, or sometimes several, species of mammals or birds. Thus, with a few exceptions, the cat flea only lives on cats, the rabbit flea on rabbits, etc. For example, the cat flea and the dog flea, respectively the *Ctenocephalides felis* and the *Ctenocephalides canis*, bite humans, but do not usually transmit the disease. See Vitaux, Histoire de la peste (note 6), 109, 113, 115, 117; Biraben, Les hommes et la peste (note 19), 13.

4. Conclusion

Urban animals are part of the fabric of society.[57] They are part of a community whose place in towns and cities may be called into question under certain circumstances. The plague of the seventeenth century was one such circumstance. In a context where the miasmas carried by animals or produced by their excrement or carcasses were considered harmful, the epidemic transformed some of them into pests. This status was bestowed on them by their inclusion in the preventive measures adopted by the authorities. The stigmatization of stray animals and their classification as pests during the plague was an important step in the regulation and gradual elimination of animals from towns and cities.

Legislation in the Netherlands and the Principality of Liège was similar to what was enacted in France and England[58]. The aim was to prevent the vagrancy of several species and to restrict their movements by expelling them from towns or destroying them. An analysis of the rules laid down in modern-day Belgium has nevertheless revealed several nuances. First of all, the presence of animals was not always entirely banned for residents who had enough space or who kept their dogs, cats, or chickens locked or tied up. The rules were also selective, ignoring horses and cattle – although the latter's status was more ambiguous – and targeting dogs in particular. Finally, it should be noted that the killing of several species was likely to have been carried out informally by town dwellers themselves, who, in some places, were authorized to kill with impunity any stray animal they found in the streets.

Photo credits

Fig. 1 Jean De Ridder, etching, c. 1720, Atlas Van Stolk Museum, Rotterdam. Taken from Henri H. Mollaret/Jacqueline Brossollet, La peste, source méconnue d'inspiration artistique, in: Jaarboek, Antwerp 1965, 3–112, 30.

Fig. 2 and 3 Cudgel and baldric of the "Hondenslagers" of the city of Antwerp, eighteenth century, Antwerp, Museum aan de Stroom, Vleeshuis collection, AV.2491.1-2; AV.2491.2-2.

Abstract:

When studying the legislative measures adopted by the authorities during the plague, historians have placed relatively little emphasis on the role of animals. Yet they are

57 Nathalie Blanc, Les animaux et la ville, Paris 2000, 43.

58 See Mollaret/Brossollet, La peste, source méconnue d'inspiration artistique (note 26), 30; Frank Percy Wilson, La peste à Londres au temps de Shakespeare, Paris 1987; Lucien Bély, Animaux, in: Lucien Bély (ed.), Dictionnaire de l'Ancien Régime, Paris 1996, 62-63, 62; Biraben, Les hommes et la peste (note 19).

central in the regulations implemented to protect cities from the "contagious disease". According to the miasmatic theory, animals were considered to have rotten vapour in their entrails and in their hair or feathers, which could rise into the air and corrupt it. Under the threat of epidemics, the urban animal thus becomes a "harmful", undesirable being, whose breeding or circulation must be limited for health reasons. Using mainly legislative sources, this chapter analyses the plague regulations issued by central and local authorities in the Southern Netherlands and Principality of Liège from the beginning of the seventeenth century to the final outbreak in 1668. It shows that especially freely moving animals such as stray dogs, cats, or pigs were primary targets in the fight against the spread of the disease, while "useful" cattle and horses, but also rats and their fleas, largely escaped both regulation and mass killings.

Keywords:
plague | dogs | urban history | Netherlands | Principality of Liège | seventeenth century

Dominik Hünniger

Bugs, Worms, and Dying Cattle

Multispecies Histories of Cattle Plague Outbreaks in the Long Eighteenth Century

Throughout the eighteenth century, cattle epizootics occurred repeatedly across Europe with varying degrees of severity and expansion.[1] As a consequence, hundreds of thousands of cattle died or were culled.[2] Despite the immense impact of these epizootics, historians have been slow in studying them. Only since the late 1990s has interest in Rinderpest and other cattle diseases grown, especially in the context of colonial history, environmental history, and the history of one health.[3] An interest in the roles of animals

1 The specific disease was probably Rinderpest, which the FAO declared eradicated in May 2011. However, retrospective diagnosis is suspect. Therefore I will use the modern term *epizootic* or contemporary terms like "livestock disease" or "(horned) cattle plague" throughout this chapter. See Lise Wilkinson, Animals and Disease. An Introduction to the History of Comparative Medicine, Cambridge (Ma) 1992, 37. In addition, diseases themselves are subject to historical changes and could have had different manifestations in earlier times, see Wilhelm Dieckerhoff, Geschichte der Rinderpest und ihrer Literatur. Beitrag zur Geschichte der vergleichenden Pathologie, Berlin 1890, 2. Historical research on bubonic plague argues accordingly, see e. g. Stefan Kroll, Die „Pest" im Ostseeraum zu Beginn des 18. Jahrhunderts. Stand und Perspektiven der Forschung, in: id./Kersten Krüger (eds.), Städtesystem und Urbanisierung im Ostseeraum in der Frühen Neuzeit. Urbane Lebensräume und Historische Informationssysteme, Berlin 2006, 124–148, 130.

2 For a detailed description of the different outbreaks see Bernhard Laubender, Das Ganze der Rindviehpest. Oder vollständiger Unterricht die Rindviehpest genau zu erkennen, sicher zu heilen, und das gesunde Vieh vor Ansteckung zu bewahren; nebst einer allgemeinen und ganz neuen Theorie, alle Krankheiten der Thiere überhaupt, richtig zu beurtheilen und glücklich zu behandeln, Leipzig 1801, esp. 35–46, and Clive Alfred Spinage, Cattle Plague. A History, New York 2003. The exact duration varied in individual European territories of course and not all countries were affected to the same extent.

3 For colonial and environmental history, see e. g. Klemens Wedekind, Impfe und herrsche. Veterinärmedizinisches Wissen und Herrschaft im kolonialen Namibia 1887–1929, Göttingen 2021, or Karen Brown/ Daniel Gilfoyle (eds.) Healing the Herds. Disease, Livestock Economies, and the Globalization of Veterinary Medicine, Athens (Oh) 2010. For one health history, see e. g. Abigail Woods, Michael Bresalier/ Angela Cassidy/Rachel Mason Dentinger, Animals and the Shaping of Modern Medicine. One Health and its Histories, London 2018. For early modern Europe, see e. g. Dominik Hünniger, Die Viehseuche von 1744–52. Deutungen und Herrschaftspraxis in Krisenzeiten, Neumünster 2011; Carsten Stühring, Der Seuche begegnen. Deutung und Bewältigung von Rinderseuchen im Kurfürstentum Bayern des 18. Jahrhunderts, Frankfurt/Main 2011; Adam Sundberg, Natural Disaster at the Closing of the Dutch Golden Age, Cambridge 2022; Filip Van Roosbroeck, Caring for Cows in a Time of Rinderpest. Non-academic Veterinary Practitioners in the County of Flanders, 1769–1785, in: Social History of Medicine 32/3 (2019), 502–522, or Johanna Widenberg, Cattle Plague and Society. Rinderpest, Anthrax and Epizootic Control in

as both victims and causes of cattle diseases is even more recent. In this chapter, I will analyse eighteenth-century scholarly debates in Germany on the origins of and responses to cattle plagues from a more-than-human perspective. It will be shown that some authors considered "insects" and "worms" both as causes and/or effects of the "cattle plague". However, as there was still no distinct veterinary expert community that could monopolize the discourse, conceptions of the animals' roles varied significantly. How did physicians, economists, and theologians conceptualise "disease vectors"? What was the role of comparative anatomy, autopsies, and experiments in establishing certain hypotheses? And how did assumptions about contagion and/or environmental factors influence conjectures about the cause of diseases? This essay's focus on the animals' roles in the epizootic discourse of eighteenth-century Germany hopes to provide new insights into the conceptions of a multispecies world in the Age of Enlightenment.[4]

1. Social Status and the Diagnosis of Animal Diseases

The study of diseases in non-human animals proved problematic for the social status of physicians well into the eighteenth century. Before the first veterinary schools were established in the 1760s, many physicians felt themselves obligated to justify their interest in the diseases of "lower creatures". In the prefaces of their treatises, they stressed the importance of cattle for Man – and underlined its special position in the hierarchy of animals. The Breslau polymath Johann Kanold (1679–1729) argued that he might well deal with cattle if other renowned scholars like Girolamo Fracastoro had dealt with hunting dogs, since, in his opinion, cattle occupied a higher step on the great scale of beings.[5]

Kanold's statement is interesting because it contradicts several hegemonic contemporary assessments. Hunting dogs were usually considered special and prestigious among domesticated animals because of their proximity to the nobility.[6] Kanold, however,

the Eighteenth Century Kingdom of Sweden, in: 1700-tal. Nordic Journal for Eighteenth-Century Studies 17 (2020), 8–33.

4 This chapter takes inspiration from recent work in historical animal studies and more-than-human histories, like Chris Pearson, Beyond 'Resistance'. Rethinking Nonhuman Agency for a 'More-Than-Human' World, in: European Review of History 22, 5 (2015), 709–725, Erica Fudge, Quick Cattle and Dying Wishes. People and their Animals in Early Modern England, Ithaca 2018, and Emily O'Gorman/ Andrea Gaynor, More-Than-Human Histories, in: Environmental History 25,4 (2020), 711–735.

5 Johann Kanold, Historische Relation von der Pestilentz des Horn-Viehes, welche anno 1711 und 1712 in Schlesien, wie nicht weniger diese, und das vorhergegangene 1710. Jahr in Moscau, Polen, Ungarn, Oesterreich, Siebenbürgen, Italien, und andern Ländern starck grassiret, Breslau 1713, VII.

6 On the perception and classification of animals in the early modern period in general, see Keith Thomas, Man and the Natural World. Changing Attitudes in England 1500–1800, London 1983, 92–191. On the environmental history of hunting, see Martin Knoll, Umwelt – Herrschaft – Gesellschaft. Die landesherrliche

seems suggested that cattle should be valued even more than noble canines because of their utility to human society. While Kanold and other enlightened veterinary scholars were embedded in a strictly hierarchical early modern worldview, they put forward new principles to "ennoble" their field of study. Thus, medical treatises on cattle diseases not only examined the causes and treatment of the plague, but also served to distinguish their authors from other animal and health experts.[7]

In this context, correctly diagnosing the disease was depicted as a refined art. The physicians attributed their difficulties in diagnosing non-human animal diseases first and foremost to the difficulties of communication. According to the physician Rudolph August Behrens (c. 1700–1748) from Braunschweig, for instance, animal patients were unable to make discernible the first signs of their sickness.[8] These shortcomings point to the difficulties that human physicians encountered in the treatment and diagnosis of non-human animal diseases. It is remarkable how medical professionals used the undebatable difference in how species communicate as an excuse for their own lack of experience, knowledge, and ability to cure their "patients."

Regarding the animals' abilities to feel and think, physicians expressed different opinions. In describing shivering, Johann Nicolaus Textor (1703–1765) noted that some other physicians attributed these chills "not without reason" to the animal's "fearful and anxious sensation". Textor's assumption that sick animals are sensitive was not unique – statements of this kind became even more frequent in later writings. In contrast to these remarks, other physicians, like Johann Hermann Fürstenau (1688–1756), still put forward a Cartesian position, arguing that animals definitely lacked reason. Everything that seemed like memory or affect in animals was, according to him, merely the result of imitation and breeding. These differences notwithstanding, it is also striking that all

---

Jagd Kurbayerns im 18. Jahrhundert, St. Katharinen 2004. For an overview on recent work in historical animal studies see Mieke Roscher/André Krebber/Brett Mizelle (eds.), Handbook of Historical Animal Studies, Berlin/Boston 2021.

7 See Oliver Stenzel, Medikale Differenzierung. Der Konflikt zwischen akademischer Medizin und Laienheilkunde im 18. Jahrhundert, Heidelberg 2005, for these demarcations in human medicine and how those tendencies even gained further momentum in the course of the eighteenth century. For the history of veterinary schools see Kit Heintzman, A Cabinet of the Ordinary. Domesticating Veterinary Education, 1766–1799, in: The British Journal for the History of Science 51/2 (2018), 239–260.

8 Rudolph August Behrens, Gutachten, die Abwendung und Cur der schlimmen grassirenden Vieh-Seuche betreffend, Wolfenbüttel 1745, 4: "tierischen Patienten [...] die ersten Regungen ihrer Kranckheit nie können zu erkennen geben, sondern solche alsdann erst mercken lassen, wenn dieselbige völlig überhand genommen hat, und die endlich keine Nachricht von denen äußerlich nicht zu bemerckenden Wirkungen derer ihnen gebrauchten Mittel geben können." This sentence would merit a much deeper linguistic analysis as the use of passive voice reveals a lot about the struggle of ealry modern scholars to fathom human-animal distinctions or, for that matter, similarities. Laubender, Rindviehpest (note 2), 47 also spoke of the lack of reason and speech in non-human animals. In general on this topic see Sarah D. P. Cockram, History of Emotions, and André Krebber, History of Ideas, both in: Roscher/Krebber/Mizelle, Handbook (note 6).

sources analysed here remained rather vague on another much-debated issue of the time: the question of the cattle's ability to suffer or express emotions.[9]

In any case, looking at how eighteenth-century medical professionals described observed symptoms and tried to make sense of the disease reveals a great deal about how humans grappled with non-human agency.

2. Symptoms, Disease Description, and the Question of Causes

Recent medical history emphasizes that the idea that one pathogen causes a particular disease is a development of the nineteenth century and the emergence of microbiology.[10] In contrast, in the premodern era there were several explanatory models for epidemics or diseases and their pathogens.[11] However, most physicians who commented on epizootics in the eighteenth century emphasized the importance of accurately diagnosing the disease. This was seen as crucial to determining the necessary precautions and finding effective remedies. Although there were various debates about the nature and type of certain diseases throughout the century, most authors assumed that the "cattle plague" was one and the same across Europe.

In addition to detailed observation of external symptoms, autopsy had been a widespread diagnostic tool since the beginning of the eighteenth century. Although not all medical treatises discuss internal organs, many physicians emphasized the need for autopsy to establish the type of disease and its control. For scholars of multispecies histories, these dissections and the reports on them are vital, as here, non-human animals – worms and insects – take centre stage. For example, the Wismar doctor Johann Carl Brun (1711–1775) reported that a large number of worms had been found in the stomachs of diseased animals, namely in the rumen (*ventriculus primus*) and the second stomach (*reticulum*). These worms were the size of wheat grains and the colour

9 Johann Hermann Fürstenau, Kurze Einleitung zur Haußhaltungs-Vieh-Artzeneykunst. Oder vernünftige Gedanken von unvernünftigen Haußaltungs-Thieren, deroselben Mängel, Gebrechen und Hülffsmittel überhaupt, Wolffenbüttel 1747, 7. Generally on the connection between illness and feeling in the early modern period see Michael Stolberg, „Zorn, Wein und Weiber verderben unsere Leiber." Krankheit und Affekt in der frühneuzeitlichen Medizin, in: Johann Anselm Steiger (ed.), Passion, Affekt und Leidenschaft in der Frühen Neuzeit, Wolfenbüttel 2005, 1033–1059.

10 See Karl-Heinz Leven, Von Ratten und Menschen. Pest, Geschichte und das Problem der retrospektiven Diagnose, in: Mischa Meier (ed.), Pest. Die Geschichte eines Menschheitstraumas, Stuttgart 2005, 11–32, 16, and Martin Dinges, Bedrohliche Fremdkörper in der Medizingeschichte, in: Ruth Mayer and Brigitte Weingart (eds.), Virus! Mutationen einer Metapher, Bielefeld 2004, 79–95, here 80–81.

11 See also Robert H. Dunlop and David J. Williams, Veterinary Medicine. An Illustrated History, St. Louis 1996, 277–283, and Wilkinson, Animals (note 1), 44–50, for a brief overview of Italian and English language publiations on the cattle plague of the early eighteenth century and their statements on transmission and disease causes.

of ripe rosehips: "with the thick ends, presumably their head, they sat firmly [...] with the thin end of the body they hung almost all together in pairs, in the same way as the earthworms when they copulate."[12] According to Brun, the worms could be found in all autopsies, in some animals even "10,000" in number.[13] He argued that by their rapid reproduction – a property he attributed to all insects – they soon colonized the whole stomach and destroyed its functioning.

In his Latin university dissertation from 1730, however, Johann Otto Brückner, rejected this assumption in a very polemical way. Those who claimed such a thing "put worms in their heads with Kircher", and revive an opinion that has long been out of fashion." The reference to an older theory, here that of the seventeenth-century polymath Athanasius Kircher (1602–1680), which was by 1730 considered backward and outdated, is typical of Enlightenment scholarship. In this sense, like many contemporary authors of treatises on cattle epidemics, Brückner presented his writing as new and modern.[14] He himself favoured a model of disease transfer via contagion, and thus rejected the "worm hypothesis."

As an alternative to the "worms", the remarkably unstable, rather fluid category of "insects" was also considered to be the cause of the disease. One author who subscribed to this explanation was Ludvig Holberg (1684–1754), who, however, was not a physician. He referred to "Hartsöcker's hypothesis [...], which assumes that the plague is caused by small poisonous insects in the air, which kill by their poisonous stinging."[15] Holberg vividly described how he imagined the process of infection: the insects are invisible to the naked eye and, after being inhaled by the cattle, very quickly attack their intestines. Like "flying armies in the air" or a "gang of predatory birds", insects thus moved from territory to territory, but spared certain areas.[16] With this argument, Holberg also claimed to have found an explanation for the fog or "blue clouds" that were frequently

---

12 Johann Carl Brun, Unvorgreifliches Gutachten über das an einigen Orten im Hertzogthum Mecklenburg eingerissene Viehsterben, mit eilfertiger Feder entworfen von einem Medico in Wismar, Wismar 1745, 16.

13 This was also stated by Georg Hannaeus, Historische Beschreibung der Vieh-Seuche welche seit dem Jahre 1745 in den hiesigen Gegenden grassiret, Hamburg 1746, 24. However, he specified that this was only the case in cows, while the gallbladder in oxen was "supernaturally small."

14 Johann Otto Brückner, Ausführliche Beschreibung von einer Hornviehseuche, in: Magazin der Vieharzneykunst, 1 (1784), 74–144, 114. This text was a German translation of a Latin dissertation defended at the University of Frankfurt an der Oder in 1730, http://resolver.sub.uni-goettingen.de/purl?PPN719218071 (21 January 2023), p. 26: "qui verminosam in sanguine putredinem sibi imaginantur, ii verminosam Kircheri hypothesin dudum antiquatam inaniter tantum recoquunt." Athanasius Kircher published his well-known plague treatise in 1658 in Rome as *Scrutinium Physico-Medicum Contagiosae Luis, Quae Pestis Dicitur*. See Johann Werfring, Der Ursprung der Pestilenz. Zur Ätiologie der Pest im loimographischen Diskurs der Frühen Neuzeit, Wien 1999, 135.

15 Ludvig Holberg, Kurtzes Bedencken über die jetziger Zeit regierende Vieh-Seuche mit einigen Oeconomischen Anmerckungen, Wismar 1746, 9. The reference is to Nicolaas Hartsoeker's work on microscopy.

16 Ibid., 14.

associated with livestock epidemics. According to Holberg, these mists were nothing more than a swarm of insects.[17]

By the middle of the eighteenth century, the "insect theory" associated with Antoni van Leeuwenhoeck (1632–1723) and Nicolaas Hartsoeker (1656–1725) and their microscopy of small organisms and cells had become one of the most influential explanatory models for the outbreak of cattle diseases. The Copenhagen professor of medicine Johann Balthasar von Buchwald (1697–1763) advocated this theory in his treatise on the cattle epidemic, which appeared in the writings of the Copenhagen Science Society in 1745.[18] In 1747, another treatise promoting the "insect theory" appeared anonymously in the *Hamburgisches Magazin*.[19] Claudius Peter Ellius opposed these assumptions in another publication from Hamburg in 1756,[20] while the famous Dutch physician Petrus Camper (1722–1789) would take up ideas on insects as disease propagators in a prize-winning essay in 1779.[21]

3. Transmissibility to Other Human and Non-Human Animals

Just as the observations and conclusions surrounding the causes of cattle plague were controversial, so too were the debates on how the disease spread diverse, especially when it came to possibilities of interspecies exchange. Even though the (supposed) comparability between human and non-human diseases played a major role in the attempts to diagnose cattle plagues, interspecies transmission was rarely discussed in the sources analysed here. Only a few authors considered the issue at all, and explanations and findings varied greatly.

---

17 Ibid., 15. As with most theses on the nature of the cattle epidemic, an explicit counter-opinion could be found here as well. Johann Otto Brückner rejected the view that the matter of the disease was a fog of any kind as a "fairy tale". See Brückner, Beschreibung (note 14), 111.

18 See Hans Rieck, Studien zu Betrachtungen der Kopenhagener Professoren J.B. von Buchwald, Georg Detharding und Ludwig von Holberg zur Rinderpest 1745 in Dänemark, Gießen 1979, 18.

19 See Anonym, Muthmaßung, daß die Viehseuche von Insecten entstehe, welche aus der Tartarey durch die Ostwinde verwehet werden, in: Hamburgisches Magazin, oder gesammlete Schriften, zum Unterricht und Vergnügen 1 (1747), 97–103.

20 Claudius Peter Ellius, Kurzgefaßte doch gründliche Untersuchung der itzt im Schwange gehenden Rindviehseuche, wobey die bishero von der Ursache derselben entstandenen Meynungen durch die Erfahrung widerleget, und die wahre Ursache dieser Seuche mit ihrer Einschleichungs- und Wirkungs-Art bey dem Rindviehe, völlig entdecket werden. Wornach Versuche, eine souveraine Cur derselben betreffend, angestellet werden können, Hamburg 1756, 9.

21 Petrus Camper, Über die wahre und eigentliche Ursache der Krankheiten, die unter dem grossen und kleinen Viehe, als ansteckende Seuchen, wüthen, eine von der Gesellschaft N.F.F. gekrönte Preisschrift, in: Beschäftigungen der Berlinischen Gesellschaft Naturforschender Freunde 4 (1779), 95–166.

A recurring argument relied on humourism. Georg Hannaeus (1705–1750), for example, assumed that each animal species had a specific constitution which provided a necessary condition for infection.[22] Friedrich Hoffmann (1660–1742) described processes in a similar way, and thus was able to explain why the plague usually only affected a single animal species, or only humans: from the rotting bodies of those who died of the disease, the "*contagium*" escaped and spread in the form of miasma. Eventually, only organisms that belonged to the species of the animal from which the *contagium* arose were infected. In Hoffmann's case, this specific (but not uncommon) combination of ideas, focusing on contagion and miasma, served to explain a number of commonly observed phenomena: the spread of the disease, its irregularities, and the sole infection of cattle.

Similar statements, but with different emphases, were also made by Ludvig Holberg. For him, the theory of infection by insects explained the disease's non-transmissibility, as he assumed that different types of plague were caused by different types of insects. Holberg spoke of "migrations" of insects, each consisting of a different population (*Volk*). The insects responsible for the outbreak of cattle plague were "*buphagi*" who would "find the most or exclusive taste in beef meat", and therefore disdain other animals and people.[23] This "theory" was quite unique, but it speaks volumes about ideas on animal cultures and habits that influenced assessments of the epizootics in premodern times.[24]

4. "Magical" Attributions of Causes and Actions

Cultural anthropological and historical studies have observed a close connection between illness and sorcery or witchcraft in the imaginary worlds of the early modern period. Recent studies, however, pointed out that some forms of "magic" were frequently practiced and tolerated whereas witchcraft itself was of course imaginary but prosecuted. In addition, it has been stressed that there could be differences in the perception of

---

22 The notion of species however was of course undergoing changes and debates exactly during this time and is a matter of contestation in philosophy of biology today, too. See Julia D. Sigwart, What Species Mean: A User's Guide to the Units of Biodiversity, Boca Raton 2018, and John S. Wilkins/Frank E. Zachos/Igor Ya. Pavlinov (eds.), Species Problems and Beyond. Contemporary Issues in Philosophy and Practice, Boca Raton 2022.

23 Holberg, Bedencken (note 15), 10. It was precisely this assumption that there were specific insects for specific animals that made Holberg doubt miasma theories.

24 Interstingly, Holberg urged his fellow Danes to change their culinary habits after the outbreak, as milk products, especially butter, had become scarce. He recommended using olive oil instead and connected this to ideas about national food cultures. See Dominik Hünniger, Konsumverzicht als Teuerungsabwehr. Die Debatte um Ausfuhrverbote für Butter während einer Rinderseuche in den Herzogtümern des 18. Jahrhunderts, in: Detlev Kraack/Klaus Joachim Lorenzen-Schmidt (eds.), Essen und Trinken. Zur Ernährungsgeschichte Schleswig-Holsteins, Neumünster 2010, 159–184.

these practices between rural society and the authorities observing them. In general, it has become clear that magic and magical ideas could be exercised and evaluated in very differentiated and specific ways.[25] Nevertheless, "magical thinking" should be taken seriously in the early modern period, especially as a method for coping with crisis. Only by considering the breadth of contemporary statements on this phenomenon can different worldviews be adequately described without necessarily being framed as contradictory. By framing the disease as divine punishment and incorporating the widespread concepts of miasma and contagion, magic and sorcery offered people in the early modern period valid explanations for the development of plagues and diseases as well as measures for combatting them.[26]

A particularly spectacular example of the use of "magic" to contain the plague has become famous through David Sabean's collection of essays on the history of power relations in Württemberg villages.[27] Burying living animals as a means against the cattle plague was not unusual. Other contemporary sources also mention the burial of the community bull or other living animals outside a village threatened or affected by the disease at a crossroads in the presence of a large part of the community.[28] In the case analysed by Sabean, dating from the late eighteenth century, this collective magical act incurred official persecution. However, the fact that there was no obvious sense of wrongdoing among the population indicates that this practice was seen as common and not restricted to Württemberg – at least as a rumour or narrative.[29]

In fact, there was no strict line between the evolving medical discourse and such "popular" magical practices. For instance, Textor, who expresses doubts about magic in his text, nevertheless noted that the burial of a living infected animal had often proven to be effective and was therefore at least worth considering as a remedy. He even

25 However, there is a debate among historians of medicine concerning the importance of magical practices for healing diseases in the early modern period. See Stenzel, Differenzierung (7), 64.

26 See also Angelika Bachmann, „Allerhand gottloses abgöttisches Werckhen." Glaube, Aberglaube, Zauberei. Magie in der dörflichen Gesellschaft Württembergs des 17. und 18. Jahrhunderts, in: Johannes Dillinger (ed.), Zauberer, Selbstmörder, Schatzsucher. Magische Kultur und behördliche Kontrolle im frühneuzeitlichen Württemberg, Trier 2003, 27–112, 91.

27 See David Warren Sabean, The Sins of Belief. A Village Remedy for Hoof and Mouth Disease (1796), in: id. (ed.), Power in the Blood. Popular Culture and Village Discourse in Early Modern Germany, Cambridge 1984, 174–198.

28 Bachmann, Glaube (note 26), 44f. reports on a similar case, but from the beginning of the eighteenth century. Dieckerhoff, Rinderpest (note 1), 67, quoted a story in Columella. In his treatise, he cites the advice of an Egyptian writer named Bolus of Mendesia. Bolus wrote that one should bury an infected sheep alive in a pit in front of the barn and then let the whole herd run over the pit. This would keep the disease away from the herd. Dieckerhoff, however, thought this was a "superstitious procedure."

29 In a contemporary collection of legal and medical case histories, the practice of living burial was also discussed. Here, however, it was about a horse buried alive to ward off a horse epidemic. See Johann Christian Wolff, Ob ein lebendig vergrabenes Pferd wieder die Pferde-Seuche helffe?, in: id. (ed.), Seltsame jedoch wahrhafftige Theologische, Juristische, Medicinische und Physicalische Geschichte. So wohl aus

recommended repeating the procedure if it did not prove to be successful immediately. This recommendation was rooted in his conviction that nothing should be left untried and he had a perfectly instrumental explanation:

> If one was allowed to kill many healthy oxen every day in order to feed humans, why should one not be allowed to kill one or the other infected head of cattle, which suffers without hope of recovery anyway, by burying it alive in order to save a very large amount of the same (species) from similar future suffering (because of a possible infection)?[30]

Since animals would be slaughtered for human food anyway, it made no difference if they were also killed to prevent a disease or halt its progress. In addition, he tried to instrumentalize the suffering of the infected animals, but without addressing their agonizing death by being buried alive. Suffering as a category for non-human animals existed for Textor, like for many of his contemporaries, only in medical terms – i. e., when they were ill. As food, animals were not considered to possess any ability to suffer.

In the Schleswig-Holstein administrative sources, there is a recipe that also made use of this "sympathetic" thinking. The farmer Hans Dircks (no dates known) from Sieversfleth in the Eiderstedt peninsula wrote to a senior official:

> It is very bad with my cattle, Mr. Pfennigmeister. Nicklaus Martens from the state manor gave me this advice: I cut off the head of a sick calf and cut it very finely, put it in the brewing kettle and cooked it – and gave it to the other animals. But it doesn't help at all. This is not the way, gentlemen, it costs so many tears, I wish they all were dead, because unfortunately it gives one so much heartache for the poor cattle that the heart in your body seems to break.[31]

Such documents testify to the farmers' tangible frustration and sadness over their helplessness, loss of income, and concern for their animals. It is important however, to acknowledge that these "magical" methods were relatively inexpensive in comparison to pharmacy drugs, and for this reason alone certainly gained attractiveness in times of

---

alten als neuen Zeiten, worüber der Theologus, Jure-Consultus und Medico-Physicus sein Urtheil eröffnet. Aus den Original-Acten mit Fleiß extrahiret, zu mehreren Erleuterung mit kurtzen Anmerckungen versehen und eines jeden vernünfftigen Gedancken überlassen. Sechster Theil, Leipzig 1740, 351–566. A Swedish legends exisit includes the live burial of two wandering children during the plague. See Bodil E. B. Persson, The Boy with the Rake and the Girl with the Broom. Pestilences in Early Eighteenth Century Southern Sweden, in: Stefan Kroll/Kersten Krüger (eds.), Städtesystem und Urbanisierung im Ostseeraum in der Frühen Neuzeit. Urbane Lebensräume und Historische Informationssysteme, Berlin 2006, 172–204.

30 Johann Nicolaus Textor, Vernunft- und Erfahrungs-mäßiger Versuch, wie die gifftig-ansteckende Vieh-Seuchen unter dem Horn-Vieh und Pferdten wohl erkannt, praeserviret und curiret werden können, nebst einer kurtzen Abhandlung von Pferds- und anderen Vieh-Kranckheiten, Karlsruhe 1739, 83.

31 Kreisarchiv Nordfriesland, A2 Parish of Tetenbüll, No. 95.

crisis.[32] At the same time, they were also alternatives to prayers, offering "alternative means of access to efficacious sacred power."[33] Thus, both metaphysical and medical disease management were of great importance in the eighteenth century, and often they cannot be strictly separated from each other. The way magical, religious, or medical interpretations and perceptions of the plague were dealt with was strongly influenced by how their assumptions could be integrated into everyday life. In any case, they reveal the high value that was attributed to the cattle as both a useful resource and a companion species. The appearance of a multitude of non-human animals in both the discourse and practice of epizootics management also reveals the decidedly multispecies world of early modern Europe. Furthermore, the debates show that different species occupied different spaces and importance in these diverse worldviews. As historians of disease, we need to pay close attention to these multi-species world(view)s in order to fully understand humans' roles and actions in past environments.

Abstract:
Before disease-causing organisms became identifiable through microbiological analysis in the late nineteenth century, scholars and lay people alike considered multiple disease vectors for epizootics. In fact, what we now know as specific diseases and pandemics were rarely considered as individual entities, but rather within a continuum of health hazards. This chapter analyses the eighteenth-century scholarly debates on cattle plague from a more-than-human history perspective. It shows that smaller "animals", such as "insects" and "worms", were considered both as causes and/or effects of the "cattle plague." The ways in which German physicians, economists, and theologians conceptualized such animal "disease vectors" reveal important elements of an eighteenth-century multispecies worldview.

Keywords:
more-than-human histories | epizootics | medical thought | insects | cattle

32 See also Bachmann, Glaube (note 26), 83.

33 Robert W. Scribner, Cosmic Order and Daily Life. Sacred and Secular in Pre-Industrial German Society, in: Kaspar von Greyerz (ed.), Religion and Society in Early Modern Europe 1500–1800, London 1984, 17–41, 25.

Lucinda Cole

Cow-Doctors, Cholera, and the "Animal Economy"

British Cattle Politics, 1865–1866

By 1842, when memories of England's eighteenth-century cattle plagues had begun to recede, the British government abolished all prohibitions against the importation of cattle, thereby abandoning disease control in the name of free trade.[1] This *laissez faire* attitude almost immediately resulted in outbreaks of foot-and-mouth disease, pleuropneumonia, and other ailments, although rinderpest – the scourge of the eighteenth century – did not return to Great Britain until June of 1865.[2] Despite repeated warnings by John Gamgee, the noted Scots veterinarian, and others about the dangers of importing cattle, Britain found itself, again, in the throes of a devastating outbreak. The number of cases of infected cattle doubled every four weeks for months. The Privy Council, faced with no operative means to arrest the plague, and without naming it "rinderpest", issued an anemic Order of Council in July, leveling a small fine against cattle owners in the Metropolitan Market who failed to report diseased cattle. This action was followed by a second order on August 11 that employed the more ominous term "Cattle Plague", and then by a host of bills proposed, withdrawn, amended, and consolidated throughout 1865. Yet by the end of the year over 120,000 cases of cattle plague had been reported, almost 74,000 thousand cattle had died of rinderpest, and another 17,000 thousand had been slaughtered to prevent the spread of the disease infection.[3] Finally, in February of 1866, the *Cattle Diseases Prevention Act 1866* made it through both houses of Parliament.[4] Diseased animals were to be slaughtered and buried, cattle owners would be compensated, and local inspectors would be appointed to ensure compliance.

Afterwards, two scientific or epidemiological questions and several policy issues dominated discussions of, and controversies surrounding, the *Cattle Diseases Prevention Act 1866:* whether cattle plague was imported or of "spontaneous generation" – a debate

---

1 J.R. Fisher, The Economic Effects of Cattle Disease in Britain and its Containment, 1850–1900, in: Agricultural History 54 (1980), 278–294.

2 Clive Spinage, Cattle Plague. A History, Dordrecht 2003, 272.

3 Ibid., 179.

4 For the Act in full, see The Statutes of the United Kingdom of Great Britain and Ireland, 29 & 30 Victoria, 1866, London 1866, 29, c. 2, pp. 2–11, "Act to amend the Law relating to Contagious or Infectious Diseases in Cattle and other Animals", 20 February 1866.

often framed as "Contagionism" versus "anti-contagionism" – and whether the cows should be culled or cured.

Most veterinary histories would agree with broad outlines of the above account. In this chapter, however, I want to complicate received stories of the nineteenth-century livestock disease by considering its real and imagined relationship to a nineteenth-century human one: cholera. With major outbreaks in the 1830s, 1840s, and 1860s, Britain lost about 150,000 people to cholera during the nineteenth century; in India, large-scale troop movements associated with colonization and subsequent rebellions, the East Indian railways, and famine killed upwards of 20,000,000, disproportionately among the poor and undernourished.[5] From the beginning of these outbreaks, some physicians and commentators suggested that there might be connections between human contagion – cholera – and outbreaks of diseases in animals. In 1831, London's cholera outbreak, according to Thomas Southwood Smith, physician and sanitary reformer, coincided with "diseases of the lower animals – horses, cows, sheep, and all domestic creatures" possibly with a common cause in a "peculiar epidemic constitution of the air."[6] In the 1850s, when founder of epidemiology John Snow first traced a London cholera outbreak to the Broad Street pump, *The Lancet, The British Medical Journal* and other scientific publications published a series of articles by William Lauder Lindsay and others on the relationships between "steppe disease" and cholera.[7] Like cholera, according to Lindsay, rinderpest is "essentially a fever," both involve "collapse" followed by "excitement of the system," or diarrhea; after nine days, both diseases exhibit "pustules" and possible respiratory difficulties; both are "incurable, intensely contagious, and very fatal, the deaths amounting to from fifty to ninety per cent."[8] Although admitting that there is not yet proof that the diseases are identical, Lindsay points out that the resemblance is so striking that "various authors" describe "*choleraic* diarrhoeah" as the final stage of rinderpest, preceding death.[9] Recounting his own experiments on cholera and dogs, he advocates for more experimentation on "diseases transmissible between man and animals" and of epizootic diseases "occurring coincidently with epidemics in man," such as cholera and steppe disease.[10] Given the similar symptoms of these two diseases, along with their historically destructive power, it is hardly surprising that cholera and

5 David Arnold, Cholera and Colonialism in British India, in: Past and Present 113 (1986), 118–151.

6 Thomas Southwood Smith, The Common Nature of Epidemics and Their Relation to Climate and Civilization, Philadelphia 1866, 2.

7 Cf., e. g., Works on Cholera, in: The Dublin Quarterly Journal of Medical Science 42 (1866), 132–162, 137. In this review, the author discusses eight different texts on the disease.

8 William Lauder Lindsay, M.D., The Cattle Murrain in Some of Its Aspects, in: The Lancet 69 (16 May 1857), 496–499.

9 Ibid., 497.

10 Ibid., 499.

cattle disease became linked in the British imagination in ways that provoked panic, controversy, and – eventually – new policies aimed at controlling outbreaks.

Underpinning discussions of these two great nineteenth-century pandemics was another, both medical and philosophical: how similarities between humans and non-human constitutions could make both vulnerable to the same diseases. Within this context, although smallpox, as we shall see, also was compared to rinderpest, I focus on cholera here for two reasons: first, the diagnosis and treatment implied similarities, rather than differences, between humans and animals; second, even when those similarities were rejected in the name of scientific accuracy, "preventative" practices for cholera – primarily, improved sewage, better ventilation, and piped, filtered water systems – made their way into popular measures for addressing cattle disease. Nineteenth-century cattle plague, in this respect, offers us the opportunity to reimagine some of the major conflicts of nineteenth-century medical science as an overlapping series of provisional and sometimes contradictory representations of disease ecologies, representations forged in the fires of pandemic response. These representations cannot be reduced to a battle between contagionism and import theory, represented by veterinary giants John Gamgee and James B. Simonds, respectively.[11] Instead, as we shall see, they proliferated in and through popular magazines, such as *Punch*, in addition to medical journals and a rash of pamphlets from farmers, doctors, satirists, and politicians. Written within a decade after the publication of Darwin's *On the Origin of Species*, some of these pamphlets promoted policy changes, but also recorded existential fears about similarities between humans and non-human animals, and our shared entanglement in a microbial world whose most powerful and destructive agents are both fatal and, to the naked eye, invisible.

1. Cross-species Cures

For more than fifty years, according to Clive Spinage, German veterinarians had treated rinderpest as the "precise counterpart" of abdominal typhus or enteric fever. Although we now know that typhus is mainly caused by a salmonella typhi, cholera by a bacteria, and rinderpest by a morbillivirus, the relationship between rinderpest and typhus was "so widely supported" at the beginning of the 1865 outbreak "that it was almost a matter of common belief".[12] In 1865, articles on cholera and cattle plague began to appear side-by-side in the *British Medical Journal*; the diseases were treated as related, if not

11 John Gamgee, Cattle Plague; With Official Reports of the International Veterinary Conference Held in Hamburg, 1863, and in Vienna, 1865, London 1866. On responses to Gamgee, see Spinage, Cattle Plague (note 2), 222–233.

12 Spinage, Cattle Plague (note 2), 9.

identical.[13] On September 16, to take only one example, James Gardner, a colonial medical officer, warns that the "spreading of cholera on the continent, the presence of zymotic diseases, the disease amongst cattle, all show that it is not at all unlikely we may yet have a visit from cholera in an epidemic form."[14] By "zymotic diseases", Gardner means acute infectious diseases, a group that includes typhus, smallpox, and cholera, all of which were known to be contagious and characterized by fevers. The term carries with it traces of miasma theory; in the words of the physician Daniel Holt, this "class" of diseases implies that a "morbid principle or miasm" has entered the nervous system, blood, and tissues, eventually affecting "the system generally."[15] By linking cholera, cattle disease, and fevers, Gardner treats them as part of a general pestilential condition against which, "we are told," it will be necessary to "adopt strict hygenic measures," including cleanliness, healthy diets, and improved drainage systems, especially in low-lying areas. "If everyone were to adopt such measures," Gardner maintains, there would be "no such thing as cholera or any other infectious disease known"; people who ignore such strictures "succumb to the disease then propagate it to their neighbors".[16]

As cattle plague and cholera showed up more frequently, if spottily, in the British Isles, so did prayers, pamphlets and monographs.[17] In 1865, James Tucker, a medical officer in Ireland, published his *Essay on the Nature and Treatment of Cholera and Fever, With Medical Remarks on the Treatment of Cattle Plague*, which contained an appendix on "Public Health".[18] He makes explicit what Gardner implied: that "cholera, fevers, and the typhoid fever of cattle – the Siberian plague – [...] are members of one family of zymotic disorders" traceable to "one common fosterer": "We inhale these pestilential germs in foul air, and drink them in foul water."[19] Citing microscopist Dr. Lionel Beale, Tucker calls these entities "particles of living germinal matter" that, once introduced into the body, either may "grow, multiply, give rise to a particular form of disease", or, if introduced into a "healthy organism", may die.[20] He calls on physicians to "extinguish these maladies in the light of sanitary science", which, he argues, largely

13 Cf., e. g., The Treatment of the Cattle Plague, in: The British Medical Journal (31 October 1865), 424–426. The article is followed by two reports of cholera outbreaks, one in Epping, the other in Paris.

14 James Gardner, Cholera, in: The British Medical Journal (16 September 1865), 282–84.

15 Daniel Holt, MD, The Pathology of Zymotic Diseases, in: Boston Medical and Surgical Journal 19 (12 June 1856), 369–376.

16 Gardner, Cholera (note 14), 282.

17 Spinage reports that during 1866 official prayers alternated between those for cholera and for cattle plague; by August 9, a "new prayer for relief from both cattle plague and impending cholera was issued". See Spinage, Cattle Plague (note 2), 393.

18 James Tucker, Essay on the Nature and Treatment of Cholera and Fever, With Medical Remarks on the Treatment of Cattle Plague, London 1865.

19 Ibid., preface.

20 Ibid.

means exposing cattle to saline waters and hot-air baths.[21] In any case, his cattle plague text, like Gardner's, is remarkable less for its proposed solutions than for his confidence in the possibility of curing humans and cattle alike. Pitting himself against continental veterinarians and their British counterpart, John Gamgee, who maintained that culling was the only real option for infected cattle, Tucker represents himself as the voice of scientific modernity: "We are on the threshold of great sanitary science. It is not in this age that surgeons of any class should consign their patients to slaughter."[22]

Although these two pamphlets were written by physicians, a third full-length argument – *The Human Blight and Cattle Blight, Or an Explanation of the Cholera and Cattle Plague* – written apparently by a layperson also appeared in August 1866, at the height of the rinderpest outbreak.[23] Published anonymously, the pamphlet begins by admitting that its author is not a "professor of physic"; although *ne sutor ultra crepidam* ("shoemaker, not beyond thy shoe") is generally an "excellent maxim," he concedes, he argues that because cattle disease is at present "no man's land", he intends to approach the subject with "the common rules of observation and meaning".[24] Like Gardener and Tucker, this writer describes cholera and rinderpest as seemingly curable, but attributes Tucker's "pestilential germs" and Gardener's "zymotic diseases" to "animalculae" – insects or eggs of insects that "come from the regions of the East" then settle on "the mucus of the intestines, and ultimately the intestines" of cattle or men.[25] In the same way that apple and pears trees have their own pests, there is one blight for the "bovine" and one for the "human tribe".[26] In both cases, though, the eggs either "germinate and breed inside the animal," or germinate and spread "from the excrement of the animals; and thus each animal becomes a center of fresh infection".[27] Through expelled fecal matter, the disease "gathers strength from each victim".[28] If cholera is less fatal to humans than rinderpest is to cattle, that is largely, he suggests, because men eat cooked food.

Read from the perspective of germ theory, *The Human Blight and the Cattle Blight* creates some cognitive dissonance. Although the text admits that we know little about the "nature of the insects whose attack causes the diseases", it correctly identifies water as a common medium of infection for both cholera and rinderpest:

---

21 Ibid., 6. Tucker, not coincidentally, was also the author of a treatise on how roman "thermo-electrical baths" are "temples of health" for both humans and cattle. See James Tucker, The Reformed Roman or Oriental Baths, Reviewed as Thermo-electrical Temples of Health. With Medical Remarks on the Nature and Scientific Treatment of Cattle Distempers by the Hot Air Bath, Dublin/London 1860.

22 Ibid., 5.

23 Anonymous, The Human Blight and Cattle Blight, or an Explanation of the Cholera and Cattle Plague, London 1866.

24 Ibid., 2.

25 Ibid., 5.

26 Ibid., 7.

27 Ibid.

28 Ibid., 6.

> The cattle disease has especially been observed to follow the course of streams; the cattle on the stream apparently imbibe the eggs of the blight. When no other means of contagion is discoverable, and in times of the cholera, the outbreak in certain districts is clearly traceable to particular wells.[29]

And without naming John Snow, it mentions how some years ago the "Golden Square" (on Broad Street) in London was devastated by cholera traced to a particular well. On the other hand, the "cures" proscribed by the anonymous author are, at best, dubious: "The true mode of treating the disease in man," the author writes,

> and the only mode of treating it in animals, is to introduce into the stomach of the victim a drug which shall poison and kill the insect blight while yet in the stomach, and thus enable the digestive powers of the man or animal to deal with the dead insect blight as it would any other kind of food.[30]

Having described the infectious agent as a kind of insect, the author offers insecticides as a cure. The one he recommends – also proposed by Mr. Maurice Worms – involves *assafoetida,* often called "devil's dung" in English, a traditional cure for cholera in India and one also highly toxic to mosquito larvae.[31] But, the author continues, any insect poison will do, either as cure or preventative. The "proper remedy" for the treatment of cholera is "the strongest insect poison which is compatible with the preservation of human life", and the "preventative" is "whatever keeps the stomach in such a condition as to destroy the eggs of the insects as soon as they are swallowed."[32] What is good for man, is good for cattle too: "Observe what is ordinarily deadly to insect life, and adapt it to the internal use of animals."[33]

In the context of a global epidemic in which ivermectin, an anti-parasitic commonly used on horses and cows, is deployed by a defiant and deluded segment of the US population as an alternative to the Covid vaccines, one's reading of this anonymous nineteenth-century pamphlet can seem uncanny, as do mixed responses from the scientific community.[34] In October of 1866, the *British Medical Journal* included a short

---

29 Ibid., 23–24.

30 Ibid., 30.

31 See Ephantus J. Muturi, et al., Amylose Inclusion Complexes as Emulsifiers for Garlic and Asafoetida Essential Oils for Mosquito Control, in: Insects 10/10 (11 Oct. 2019), 337.

32 Anonymous, The Human Blight and Cattle Blight (note 23), 14.

33 Ibid.

34 Surprisingly, some studies attest to the value of ivermectin in Covid treatment. The American Journal of Therapeutics published one such study in July-August of 2021, Andrew Bryant et al., Ivermectin for Prevention and Treatment of COVID-19 Infection. A Systematic Review, Meta-analysis, and Trial Sequential Analysis to Inform Clinical Guidelines, in: The American Journal of Therapeutics 28/4 (2021),

notice of *The Human Blight and Cattle Blight*, referring to the preface and the author's description of cattle plague as "no man's land": "As the professional knowledge fails, the anonymous writer concludes that non-professional knowledge may be able to explain the case. The reasoning is curious, and enables one to judge, without reading, the character of his argument, and the value of it."[35] This quick dismissal, while perhaps justified from an experimental perspective, was symptomatic of a growing divide between "official" medical knowledge, generally represented by the *Lancet* and the *British Medical Journal*, and a host of popular publications that sought to promote "general observation" over specialized scientific knowledge.

More immediately, though, the response in the *British Medical Journal* represents a scientific and governmental consensus around the *Cattle Diseases Prevention Act 1866*, a consolidation signaled by *The Lancet* some months earlier. In September of 1865, an article entitled "Cholera and the cattle disease" begins by noting "differences in the remedies recommended for this disease by the profession and by the public."[36] "The profession rely mainly on preventative measures," it continues, while "the public, who are ever so ready to accuse us of drenching them with drugs, still stick to some special panacea."[37] After describing some sanitary measures used to clean up sewers, it ends with a gentle satire about several recommended remedies and cures for cattle disease – charcoal, vinegar, *datura stramonium*, and "inoculating with quassia, whatever that means"[38] – a few examples of the panaceas "with which the daily press teems." The irony, it concludes, is obvious: although "the reputed physic-givers," the medical professionals, "would show how to prevent the disease, or to diminish its violence, by sanitary measures," the public "think it more important to make known some infallible cure."[39] Prior to debates about contagionism and anti-contagionism, then, or at least concurrent with them, medical and popular periodicals were awash with accounts of competing disease ecologies, some emphasizing cures for cross-species, trans-corporeal pathologies; others asserting that cattle disease is spontaneously generated from filthy conditions; still others believing that the time for cures either already has passed or lies in some vaccinated future. Not only does the discourse of interspecies infection in Mid-Victorian Britain help highlight the complex relationships between traditional knowledges and "modern" medical science, and between a pastoral past and a com-

434–60. This article is accompanied by the journal editors' "Expression of Concern": "This decision is based on the evaluation of allegations of inaccurate data collection and/or reporting in at least 2 primary sources of the meta-analysis performed by Mr. Andrew Bryant and his collaborators."

35 The British Medical Journal 301 (6 October 1866), 388.

36 Cholera and cattle disease, in: The British Medical Journal 2/245 (9 September 1965), 263–267, 263.

37 Ibid.

38 Ibid., 264.

39 Ibid., 265.

mercial present, it allows us to understand more about the head-winds professional medicine faced during the Britain's last great outbreak of cattle plague.

2. Punch, Prevention, Playfair

In the weeks both before and after the *Cattle Diseases Prevention Act 1866,* the popular press was deeply invested in public health policy for both livestock and humans – in what Michel Foucault called biopolitics, widespread efforts to "administer, optimize, and multiply" life, subjecting it "to precise controls and comprehensive relations."[40] The biopolitics of cattle disease in 1866 were marked by contentious debates characterized by the resentment of any government regulation, especially regulation that affected profits; a rabid commitment to free trade, even if imported cattle damaged public health; and a growing popular commitment to anti-contagionist views that rejected the basic premises of what, in the eighteenth century, had been acknowledged as contagious infection, and what we now recognize as germ theory. In the popular press – and especially in the conservative press – biopolitics is structured by an endemic distrust of the still-new veterinary profession, unless it contributed to individual profits or imperial ambitions. In February of 1866, *Punch, or the London Charivari* ridiculed government action – or inaction – in a full-page cartoon (fig. 1) featuring a suffering bovine, "The Patient," surrounded by "cow-doctors" who, indifferent to the dying cow, argue among themselves. The cow laments, "Oh, if they'd only leave off quarrelling, and just try "united action," it might be the saving of me!"[41] By displacing blame on to "quarrelling" veterinarians, the cartoon gestures to supporting a strong national plan – the same plan that many of its conservative middle-class readers in particular mostly opposed.

The paradoxical position of *Punch* becomes more explicit in the March 3 issue, which contains a poem called "Bos Locutus" ("The Ox Speaks"). The ox voices frustration with government interference. It begins

> Pity the sorrows of a poor old Cow
> With Rinderpest a-knocking at the door,
> And what's far worse, these Acts that won't allow
> A chance for life, e'en if the plague's got o'er."[42]

40 Michel Foucault, The Will to Knowledge. The History of Sexuality, vol. 1 (1976), trans. Robert Hurley, New York 1998, 157.

41 Punch; or the London Charivari, 17 February 1866.

42 Punch; or the London Charivari (3 March 1866), 87.

PUNCH, OR THE LONDON CHARIVARI.—FEBRUARY 17, 1866

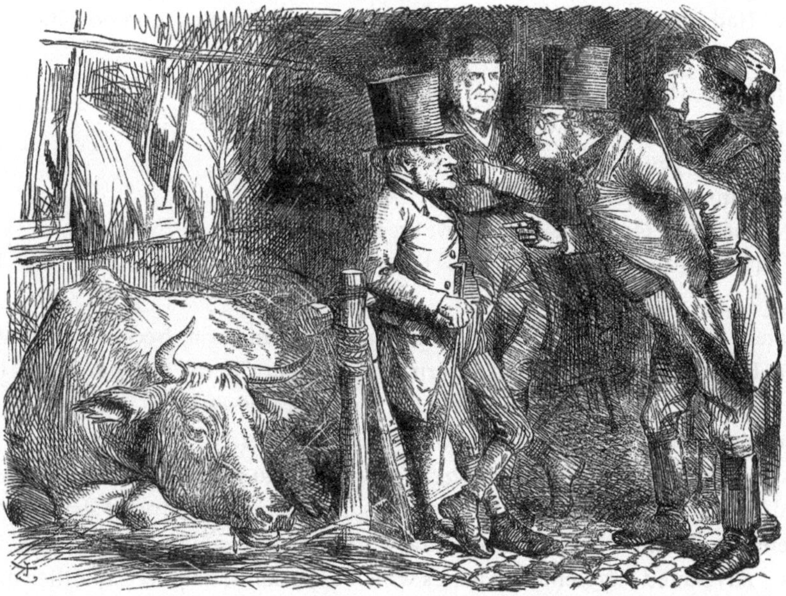

THE POLITICAL COW-DOCTORS.

THE PATIENT. "OH, IF THEY'D ONLY LEAVE OFF QUARRELLING, AND JUST TRY 'UNITED ACTION,' IT MIGHT BE THE SAVING OF ME!"

Fig. 1 The Political Cow Doctors, in: Punch; or the London Charivari, 17 February 1866.

Subsequent stanzas lament the loss of English "self-government" under new Council Orders, which are to "Slay, isolate, stamp out!" – in other words, to employ the traditional methods of culling and quarantine. The ox complains about regulations on movement – "Forbade to change a field, or cross a road, / Fined if we move, and if we linger, slain" – and then about laws regarding import and export:

> If foreigners, doomed where we land, to die;
> If natives, when we're sick, debarr'd from cure;
> No medi'cine but the pole-axe let to try –
> A remedy at once too sharp and sure![43]

Like the cartoon, the poem's humor relies on tensions – even contradictions – in attitudes toward preventative measures against the cattle plague. The first few stanzas lament laws against import ("doomed where we land, to die") and the loss of traditional cures ("No medi'cine but the pole-axe let to try"), even as the poem as a whole blames Parliament

43 Ibid.

for failing to act quickly. “Months since, perhaps,” it continues, “one effort sharp and strong, / Had stamped the plague out,” but Parliament dawdled, and now it’s too late:

> You had halted between “kill or cure” so long,
> The case has grown past cure, howe’er you kill.
> And when the pest, sown broadcast, wide had spread,
> To panic from paralysis you swing;
> And to the Cattle plague the steppes have bred.
> Add all the cattle-plagues your Act must bring.[44]

Ultimately, the government, like the doctors in the cartoon, become promoters of disease. Because the government, alternating between “panic and paralysis,” fails to decide between “kill or cure”, it must now be regarded as a source of infection, as deadly in its own way as the disease bred on the Russian steppes.

It is true that the *Cattle Diseases Prevention Act 1866* offered no plan of treatment. Instead, it restricted imports and movements, required the culling of sick cows (with compensation), and – in line with sanitary principles developed during cholera outbreaks – advocated “hygienic measures which experience acquired in other diseases shows to be important in the spreading of contagion, and in diminishing the intensity of its attack.”[45] “Every farmer”, it read,

> should look to the housing of his cattle in the present emergency, as he would to the housing of his own family, if cholera or other formidable disease were in his neighborhood. Through cleanliness of the houses, good drainage, freedom from evil smells, nourishing diet with pure air and water, cannot give immunity from the disease, but they may offer obstacles to its propagation.[46]

Lyon Playfair – British chemist, Liberal member of Parliament, sanitary movement advocate, and one of the authors of the *Cattle Diseases Prevention Act 1866* – elaborates on the reasoning behind this decision. In his treatise *The Cattle Plague in its Relation to Past Epidemics and to the Present Attack*, he outlines and defends the scientifically mainstream views that “Nothing can be more definite than the contagious virus of the cattle plague”,[47] and that plague is endemic on the Russians steppes, from which it is imported to Eastern Europe: Russia is either the “birthplace” of cattle plague “or its nurs-

44 Ibid.

45 I quote this section of the report from Lyon Playfair’s extended defense, see Lyon Playfair, The Cattle Plague in its Relation to Past Epidemics and to the Present Attack, Edinburgh 1866, 61.

46 Ibid.

47 Ibid., 48.

ery".[48] Much of the text, however, is devoted to why and how sanitary or "preventative" measures must now take the place of efforts to cure infected livestock.

Although he holds open the possibility of effective vaccines for rinderpest (not developed until 1960), Playfair recognizes from the example of vaccination programs in Russia that it sometimes takes thirteen to fifteen generations before a virus is mitigated, or a population reaches what we now call "herd immunity".[49] In 1866, he argues, there is no cure for cattle disease, and therefore the government has no choice but to return – and return quickly – to some version of the regulations that obtained during Britain's last outbreak of cattle plague in the 1740s and 1750s. In advocating these measures, Playfair is deeply aware of their unpopularity, as attested by the popular press. "It is curious", he writes, "to read *The Gentleman's Magazine* from 1745 to 1757, and see how history repeats itself."[50] One finds:

> the same energetic correspondents who now send their lucubrations to the newspapers, protesting against the use of the pole-axe, advocating or opposing the system of compensation for slaughtered cattle, farming insurance societies, fighting against ideas of contagion, and importation of the disease, and describing all kinds of cure. We have not yet seen one method of cure, except homoeopathy, tried in 1865, which was not tried and found wanting in the plague of 1745.[51]

If anything, 1866 England was in a worse position than in 1745, in part because the nation was embedded in a more highly-developed network of commercial exchange:

> The density of her population, the large quantity of her horned stock, and, above all, the enormous facility of communication by railroad, make her peculiarly liable to the ravages of a contagious disorder, and render the prospect of eradicating it, within any reasonable time, either by slaughter or by curative and disinfecting measures, almost hopeless.[52]

Playfair's use of the word "hopeless" is telling: it suggests that the controversy as a whole assumes the overtones of the *Punch* cartoon: while experts argue, the farmers of Britain remain victims of a dedication to free trade over tried and effective measures.

At some level, Playfair's reform efforts, his promotion of local sanitary interventions, derive from this sense of futility. What he calls "preventative" measures in the context of plague are always-already symptoms of scientific, environmental, and public policy

48 Ibid., 18.

49 Ibid., 29.

50 Ibid., 15.

51 Ibid.

52 Ibid., 45.

failures. As he writes toward the end of his treatise, "In our previous remarks we have said very little as to the cure of diseased animals, and in truth, we have little that we can say on this subject."[53] In ways that indirectly recall *Punch's* commentary on the "cow-doctors", he admits:

> Medicine has never shown great powers of sure in cases of great plagues. No curative means were ever found for the human plague which formerly prevailed in Europe, and still lingers in the East. Small-pox and cholera do not subject themselves to specific cures, although their attacks may be repelled by preventative agencies. Perhaps the small diminution of mortality in such diseases is owing more to careful nursing and dieting than to the use of medicinal agents.[54]

If this is the case, then farmers – rather than doctors or veterinarians – carry an unusual share of responsibility for mitigating the disease.

Consequently, much of Playfair's treatise chastises farmers for failing to follow what he hopes to establish as sanitary "laws". The cattle "are looked upon by the farmer in the double-light of flesh-making and manure-producing beasts", and although this is "right and natural", to house manure and cattle in the same stall is both unnatural and potentially pestilential.[55] Resurrecting the idea of a shared "animal economy much the same in men and beasts", he argues that when men were "stalled like oxen on rush-covered floors" during the Middle Ages, they became susceptible to disease, and ultimately were "ravaged" by the Black Death.[56] Extending this analogy, he claims that much like cattle "made glutton by their mode of fattening" become "prone to disease", "the upper classes in the thirteenth century", equally "gluttonous and unruly" were met by the Black Death, "a scythe quite as keen for cutting down the well-conditioned members of society as it had used for the poorer classes."[57] If most people in the nineteenth century "no longer dread" the import of plague seed – "even in the porous cotton which comes to us from plague-infected Egypt" – that is not because medicine has developed an effective cure, but because of improved sanitation.[58]

In traditional histories of medicine, Playfair usually is described as a moderate contagionist, an advocate of germ theory who tended to contextualize moral questions in terms of germ theory and environmental factors. He "denounced as 'fanatics' those who thought the cattle plague a punishment for whatever sins they most despised", writes for example Mark Harrison, "but believed that God had made laws governing creaturely

---

53 Ibid., 53.

54 Ibid.

55 Ibid., 58.

56 Ibid.

57 Ibid., 59.

58 Ibid., 58.

welfare" and "that transgression of those would necessarily bring penalties."[59] These laws, I would emphasize, turn on the analogy between humans and cattle, with which he ends his treatise. "The God of the human race", Playfair declares, "who are the 'cattle on a thousand hills', governs this world by wise and beneficent laws, which are sufficient, when obeyed, to insure the wellbeing of his creatures".[60] The phrase "cattle on a thousand hills" comes from Psalm 50, which commends the Israelites for following divine laws; these include animal sacrifice, but the Psalmist reminds readers that, in contrast to the pagan gods, God does not *need* these animal offerings: "For every beast of the forest *is* mine / *and* the cattle on a thousand hills. / I know all the fowls of the mountains / And the wild beasts of the fields *are* mine."[61] Playfair reads the passage analogically, conflating men and beasts in ways that sublimate the laws of sacrifice into a different kind of law – physical law, or laws of nature: "The violation of these laws inflicts on us the penalties attached to their transgression" – notably, illness and suffering – "and it is our duty to discover, understand, and obey them."[62] Similarities between human and animal disease also seem to engender a kind of cross-species empathy, especially apparent in his lengthy comments on crowded railway cars. Noting a probable relationship between crowded, filthy conditions and rinderpest, he advocates for larger compartments with water troughs: "But such a simple device," he complains, "is much beyond the humanity of railway officials, who, as long as they can obtain cattle according to the present system of transport, choose to consider them as inanimate objects, to be treated with as little consideration as bales of merchandise."[63] Although *The Cattle Plague in its Relation to Past Epidemics and to the Present Attack* mentions cholera only four times, the sanitary "laws" Playfair hopes to establish for cattle are derived from the practical knowledge clearly associated with cholera, plague, and other human epidemics.[64] For Playfair, as for many other members of the Commission, the methods developed in Victorian England to combat rinderpest did not differ substantially from those used to confront cholera. To ameliorate the multi-generational failures of public and animal health policy that have been exacerbated by global commerce, he turns to an updated version of eighteenth-century quarantine measures by defining "sanitary conditions" in terms of space, light, and implicit visions of a less populated and pastoral Britain.

59 Mark Harrison, Contagion. How Commerce Spread Disease, New Haven 2013, 218.

60 Playfair, The Cattle Plague (note 45), 62.

61 Psalm 50, 10–11.

62 Playfair, The Cattle Plague (note 45), 62.

63 Ibid., 62.

64 Ibid., 23, 33, 53, 61.

3. "Veterinary delusion"

One of the longest and most revealing satirical texts to emerge during the rinderpest outbreak was Henry Strickland Constable's *Observations Suggested by the Cattle Plague, about Witchcraft, Credulity, Superstition, Parliamentary Reform and Other Matters* (1866).[65] The main objects of Strickland Constable's ire are the regulations passed in the 1866 Cattle Bill, displaced onto the person of the Scottish veterinarian John Gamgee. Although Gamgee, unlike Playfair, was neither in Parliament nor on the Commission that produced and amended acts pertaining to cattle plague, he was an outspoken and deeply political contagionist who repeatedly had warned the British against the unsanitary perils of free trade. After 1865, as Spinage points out, Gamgee delivered a series of public lectures in which he excoriated cattlemen, dairy farmers, and other "obstructionists" and maintained their "selfishness and greed" for the current outbreak.[66] In 1866, arguing on the side of contagionism and culling, he published a lengthy account of two international veterinary conferences, 1863 in Hamburg, 1865 in Vienna, devoted to cattle plague; his preface chastised the British government for ignoring his warnings and failing to act quickly when cattle disease appeared in July1865. Strickland Constable mimics and misrepresents both the Cattle Plague Commission report and Gamgee's "exceedingly entertaining"[67] international proceedings:

> I laughed a little at the report of our own Commissioners on the Cattle Plague, in consequence of its inconclusiveness, want of unanimity and strong veterinary flavour, but it was the wisdom of Solomon in comparison with these strong German enunciations.[68]

From the perspective of germ theory, Spinage is probably correct that Strickland Constable's treatise "contributes nothing of value," except to illustrate "the kind of perverse opinion Gamgee was confronted with, opinion held by educated and wealthy people."[69] But this kind of illustration is crucial for cultural historians, and especially for those of us who, 160 years later, are still battling the pick-and-choose-your-science strategies of pandemic disinformation.

Like the treatise writers I have so far discussed, Strickland Constable often compares rinderpest to cholera. Indeed, he accuses Gamgee of failing to see "the unity of principle between typhus in a man, and rinderpest in a cow, because he only has an eye for

65 Henry Strickland Constable, Observations Suggested by the Cattle Plague, about Witchcraft, Credulity, Superstition, Parliamentary Reform and Other Matters, London 1866.

66 Spinage, Cattle Plague (note 2), 236.

67 Strickland Constable, Observations (note 65), 11.

68 Ibid.

69 Spinage, Cattle Plague (note 2), 235.

the differences".[70] But unlike Gardner, Tucker, Playfair, the *Punch* writers, and the anonymous purveyor of internal insecticides, Strickland Constable is aggressively anti-contagionist: "It seems generally thought that the question of contagion or non contagion is in any case very easy of proof; but it is on the contrary almost impossible to prove it one way or the other."[71] In his mind, the spontaneous generation of disease is a given and "the *onus probandi* rests with those who assert it cannot be so taken."[72] This position offers him the security to make light of every policy and strategy intended to confront every contagious disease, including cholera and rinderpest. "In the newspapers printed in the winter of the year 1866," Strickland Constable writes,

> we read of a vast destruction amongst cattle, caused by poisonous influences which exist without beginning in, and flow without cessation from, some remote but unknown corner of the Russian deserts. We read of mysterious emanations that were carried by the winds for miles, and left death wherever they lighted. We read that this subtle power was conveyed by the birds of the air, by insects, by mice, by cats, by dogs, by rats; and that it was even carried and imparted by the very men who were appointed by the Government to stop its spreading.[73]

For Strickland Constable, theories of contagion have the same truth value as witchcraft and other forms of superstition because the actual means of transmission remain, he claims, obscure. No one "in the present state of science", he argues can say, why "one village is attacked and the next escapes, any more than they can say in the case of cholera, or any other epidemic."[74] Without being able to identify causal agents, then, contagionists, like their superstitious and ill-informed ancestors, make up "idle theories", such as Jews poisoning the wells to account for Black Death, or "subterranean vapours issuing from the clefts in the earth's surface" as a reason for epidemics.[75] His contemporaries' explanations for rinderpest as the product of "mysterious contagious emanations" ultimately derive from unconvincing attempts to hide their ignorance: "for to say, 'I don't understand,' is a thing that as a rule the human soul abhors."[76]

Through a series of pretend summaries mirroring *Punch*'s "The Essence of Parliament", weekly and often humorous reports on Parliamentary discussion, Strickland Constable accuses the veterinarians at Gamgee's conference of being self-interested quacks influenced by premodern pseudo-science and incapable of arriving at any consensus about how to manage the present plague, other than mass culling. Ignoring

70 Strickland Constable, Observations (note 65), 48.

71 Ibid., 28.

72 Ibid., 30.

73 Ibid., 9.

74 Ibid., 30.

75 Ibid.

76 Ibid., 26.

the consensus among them that rinderpest is contagious and transmitted through the international cattle trade, Strickland Constable pushes hard to align himself with the modern sanitary movement, in part by casting Gamgee and fellow scientists as "half-cultivated"[77] throwbacks to the eighteenth century and to the *cordon sanitaire*. The following quotation is typical:

> About contagion some say the question is of no consequence; that all we want is to get rid of the plague, and that the question of how it came no matter. I say it is of great consequence. I say that disease in cattle, if right notions prevailed, might in future be almost entirely prevented. My moral in all I have said, is, that good food, cleanliness, light, and open field management, would save us from a repetition of the disease for all time. The moral of Mr. Gamgee's book is, 'They that are filthy, let them be filthy still;' for that all the diseases mentioned there in are inevitable dispensations of Providence. I preach food and air. Mr. Gamgee preaches slaughter.[78]

In such passages, he tethers Gamgee and his contemporaries to a history of religious superstition and aligns himself with "modern" systems of sanitation. In this respect, Strickland Constable tries to represent himself and his anti-contagionist, anti-regulatory views as humane, pious, and progressive, even identifying his position with Playfair's. Glossing over Playfair's contagionism by dismissing it as a "veterinary delusion", he recommends "the latter part of Dr. Lyon Playfair's little book about the Plague"[79] which then he subsequently misrepresents. Playfair, according to Strickland Constable, says,

> that the rapid growth of the disease, is owing to our gross neglect of sanitary laws; and that what is wanted, is by good management to make our animals proof against it as we have already done with men in the case of Oriental [bubonic] plague.[80]

Apparently, Strickland Constable refers to the passage I discussed earlier, Playfair's comparison between the Black Death infecting men "stalled like oxen on rush-covered floors"[81] and rinderpest attacking cattle packed in manure-ridden stalls. But, as we have seen, Playfair never argued that "good management" makes animals immune to ("proof against") disease, only that such measures "may offer obstacles to its propagation"[82] and slow its spread. Elsewhere in the treatise, Playfair defines "contagious" explicitly in ways that Strickland Constable ignores or marginalizes: "there is a specific entity which causes the disease, and has the power of propagating its own species rapidly under favouring

77 Ibid., 30.
78 Ibid., 53.
79 Ibid., 53.
80 Ibid.
81 Playfair, The Cattle Plague (note 45), 58.
82 Ibid., 61.

circumstances."[83] By dismissing such clear statements as "veterinary delusions" even as he promotes Playfair's sanitary recommendations, *Observations Suggested by the Cattle Plague* offers a master-class in the rhetorical maneuvers of anti-scientific discourse in the name of a simplistic common sense.

Strickland Constable's representation of his position as "modern" may seem jarring to twenty-first century readers, but as Erwin Ackerknecht has argued, anti-contagionism peaked during the second half of the nineteenth century in the aftermath of Darwin's *Origin of the Species*. Accoording to Ackerknecht, contagionism never was – and still isn't – "a mere theoretical or even medical problem" because it "found its material expression in the quarantines and their bureaucracy."[84] Insofar as contagionism was associated with "old bureaucratic powers", Victorians who tried to reduce "state interference to a minimum" in the name of free trade found anti-contagionism (like anti-masking or anti-vaccination) both congenial and strategic; it allowed them to position themselves as reformers, "fighting for the freedom of the individual and commerce against the shackles of despotism and reaction."[85] Clearly, Strickland Constable casts himself in that liberatory tradition. "A time may come," he pronounces, sarcastically, "when it will not be illegal for a man to cure his cow when she catches a cold."[86] He whines about a "tenant" who had forty animals infected "after the Act for the prevention of recovery had come into force", so [instead of being allowed to heal], "they were of course shot."[87] Strickland Constable appeals to economic interest rather than most of his contemporaries' understanding of "sanitary" science. By the end of his treatise, having expressed his "opinion about the doctrines of Mr. Gamgee and his fraternity, clearly and decidedly," he justifies his rhetoric on mercenary grounds:

> When I consider, that by their ignorant treatment, and blood-thirsty counsels, they have caused a loss to the community of a very great many thousand pounds, I do not think I have spoken too strongly.[88]

But even as he condemns this "loss", he ignores the arguments made by contagionists that short term quarantines and culling will prevent endemic cattle plague and long term economic pain.

83 Ibid., 23.

84 Erwin H. Ackernecht, Anticontagionism between 1821 and 1867, in: International Journal of Epidemiology 38 (2009), 7–21, 9. For a nuanced critique of "anticontagionism", see Christopher Hamlin, Commentary. Ackerknecht and "Anticontagionism". A Tale of Two Dichotomies, in: *International Journal of Epidemiology* 38/1 (2009), 22–27.

85 Ackernecht, Anticontagionism (note 84), 9.

86 Strickland Constable, Observations (note 65), 37.

87 Ibid., 39.

88 Ibid., 54.

4. Conclusion: The Slow Cull?

Lyon Playfair's cognizance of a shared "animal economy" – constitutional similarities between humans and animals – helped direct him into progressive social causes, including sponsorship of the second version of the 1876 Cruelty to Animals Act, that came to be known as the Vivisection Act, which required the use of anesthesia on vertebrate experimental subjects. In his texts, even in the midst of a global zoonotic pandemic, one finds glimmers of animal welfare concerns; in his complaint about "filthy" stalls, one hears echoes of Jeremy Bentham's lament that, thanks to ignorance and the biases of ancient philosophy, many animals "stand degraded into the class of things."[89] Strickland Constable, in contrast, is remembered now mostly for his increasingly eugenicist writings about race, and for manifestos with such titles as *Equality: A Socialist-radical Fallacy*.[90] His texts from the 1880s and 1890s invariably raise questions about occult relationships between anti-contagionism and racist pseudo-science. As Christopher Hamlin has noted, in the familiar binary of contagionism/anti-contagionism, anti-contagionism functions primarily as an act of negation, a rhetorical maneuver designed to shift the burden of proof onto scientists working at the forefront of germ theory.[91] In the hands of Strickland Constable and other eugenicists, the belief that epidemics are inevitable slips too easily into the chilling position that epidemics are therefore a desirable means of population control. In the animal world, he claims, almost "the only natural evil is famine and its consequent diseases."[92] If food were plentiful enough, "animals would no longer have to work for their living," which would bring about

> a state of things [...] so awful and destructive, that animal life would shortly cease to exist upon the globe. So with men, if they are not kept in some degree of order by plagues and diseases, following vice, dirt, and indolence, the race would soon become extinct.[93]

For Strickland Constable, then, both cholera and rinderpest become litmus tests for healthy "races", or forms of natural selection; the origin and mode of transmission of these diseases is less important than their effects: to "cull" the human and animal worlds of their presumably inferior members. Strickland Constable rejects the pole-axe on mercenary grounds, even while his rhetoric works to build a society in which food and hygiene, rather than medicine, have an outsized role in heath. And since food

89 Jeremy Bentham, Introduction to the Principle of Morals and Legislation (1789), Chapter XVII, Section 1, quoted from: http://www.animal-rights-library.com/texts-c/bentham01.htm (12 September 2022).

90 Henry Strickland Constable, Equality A Socialist-Radical Fallacy, London 1897; Id., Ireland from One or Two Neglected Points of View, London 1888.

91 Hamlin, Commentary (note 89), 24.

92 Strickland Constable, Observations (note 65), 51.

93 Ibid.

and hygiene are largely dependent on imperial wealth and colonizers' power, these socioeconomic factors determine who will be exposed to, treated for, and thus better positioned to survive a global pandemic.

Photo credit

Fig. 1 The Political Cow Doctors, in: Punch; or the London Charivari, 17 February 1866. Wellcome Collection, Public domain.

Abstract:
When cattle plague returned to Great Britain in 1865, there were active debates about its mode of transmission. Focusing mostly on the years 1865 and 1866, when new government policies were being developed and implemented, this chapter examines "cattle politics" in the popular press, or how medical journals and popular magazines (such as *Punch*) joined veterinarians in trying to shape a public response. A repeated theme in this material, both medical and popular, is a surprising connection between cattle plague and cholera, which, in the mid-nineteenth century, was epidemic throughout the world. Although the association between cattle disease and cholera was based on a shared set of symptoms, rather than (as we now know) on a shared etiology, the *possibility* of cross-species infection probably influenced policy in ways that are yet to be appreciated fully.

Keywords:
cholera | rinderpest | Lyon Playfair | H. Strickland Constable | medical posthumanities

Delphine Berdah, Camille Noûs

Veterinary Expertise, Public Health, and Animal Contagion

The Control of Bovine Tuberculosis in France and Britain, 1860–1960

1. Introduction

Animal diseases have not always been viewed as a health concern to humans.[1] In France and Britain, as in many countries in nineteenth-century Western Europe, hygienists who proposed reforms, transformations of towns, and sanitary norms to control and protect the health of populations mainly focused on climate, waste, fumes, smells, quality of water, or diet. Of course, some animal diseases were known to affect humans (rabies, cow pox). But the French ate the flesh of diseased animals until the last quarter of the nineteenth century,[2] as did the British, since trading in diseased meat was a common practice in Britain, despite the first veterinary and medical alarms following the debates about food adulteration in the 1850s.[3] Nevertheless, animal epidemics (epizootics) were a problem as they could jeopardize farm labour and the production of food. With industrialization and the opening up of the markets for free trade, increasing food supply and ensuring its quality became a major concern. In 1866, in order to fight rinderpest and sheep pox – two diseases harmless to humans but extremely contagious and fatal to animals – the governments of France and Britain passed new acts inspired by measures established in Italy in the eighteenth century against "cattle plague":[4] the suspension of fairs, markets, and animal movements, as well as the disinfection of the premises and the culling of sick animals and their contacts. Passed at about the same period as a set of laws against food adulterations, these acts expressed the same desire to allow animals to move across borders without limitations, even if the two countries had

1 Lise Wilkinson, Animals and Diseases. An Introduction to the History of Comparative Medicine, Cambridge 1992; Anne Hardy, Animals, Disease, and Man. Making connections, in: Perspectives in Biology and Medicine 46/2 (2003), 200–215.

2 Except for pork, which, since the Middle Ages, has been examined for trichinosis (roundworm larvae removal) and rabies. See Madeleine Ferrières, Histoire des peurs alimentaires, du Moyen Âge à l'aube du XXe siècle, Paris 2002; Alessandro Stanziani, Histoire de la Qualité Alimentaire XIXe – XXe siècles, Paris 2005.

3 Anne Hardy, Animals, Disease, and Man, (note 1); Keir Waddington, The Bovine Scourge, Meat, Tuberculosis and Public Health. 1850–1950, Woodbridge 2006.

4 In England, two Sheep Pox Acts in 1848 and the Cattle Diseases Act of 1866. In France, the law of 30 June 1866.

neither the same kind of farms (a multiplicity of very small farms with no specialization in France versus large farms, some of them already specialized in cattle breeding, in Britain) nor the same export trade.

This chapter aims to analyse how certain contagious animal diseases were considered an issue – or not – by French and British governments from the mid-nineteenth century onward. It will clarify how, depending on socio-cultural imaginaries and knowledge, as well as on the pressure of different stakeholders (economic, political, industrial, or professional), the repertoire of actions available to combat these diseases in the two countries differed significantly. In this, this chapter follows sociologist Pierre Lascoumes and his study of the application of public policies. Lascoumes analyses legislations not as steady measures, but as systems of potentialities that enable more than one concrete application. He calls these systems *secondary application norms*, i. e., "standards for the application of reference rights" that result from "direct or indirect negotiations amongst the stakeholders involved in their application."[5] Indeed, although the two countries passed the very same set of laws, closer analysis shows how these regulations left open the possibility of negotiating alternative means of control with other actors involved in the trade and maintenance of "production animals." The example of the fight against bovine tuberculosis (BTB) – a zoonosis asymptomatic for bovines (except at the end of life, when the animal appears gaunt, see fig. 1, part 1) that caused significant infant mortality through the consumption of milk – allows for a finer analysis of this legislative regulation.

This chapter is based on a cross-analysis of parliamentary sources, archives from the French and British Ministries of Health and of Agriculture, the Veterinary Services, and the Pasteur Institute, as well as on a survey of scientific and professional veterinary literature.

2. In Britain: Repelling the Contagion[6]

In the mid-nineteenth century, Britain was involved in an important livestock exchange based on Adam Smith's economic principles: cheap meat from South America (mainly Argentina) and Europe (Netherlands and France) was imported, while expensive pedigree livestock was exported to the British colonies, the Commonwealth, and the USA.[7] This pedigree trade was very lucrative, both for stockbreeders and the British sea transport companies. In 1866, to maintain this trade in spite of the rinderpest epizootic, the government decided to slaughter contaminated livestock. In parallel, the Board

5 Pierre Lascoumes, Normes juridiques et mise en œuvre des politiques publiques, in: L'année Sociologique 40 (1990), 43–71, 61.

6 This part is mainly based on the historical literature. Any errors in interpretation are our own.

7 Abigail Woods, A Manufactured Plague? The History of Foot-and-Mouth Disease in Britain, London 2004.

of Agriculture – the former Ministry of Agriculture and Fisheries, or MAF – set up the State Veterinary Department, charging it with the collection of data and initial statistics on the incidence of the disease, with the purpose of evaluating the efficiency of the regulations. (The nineteenth century saw the emergence of vital statistics as a government tool.[8]) The statistics showed not only the efficiency of the sanitary policy, but also, unexpectedly, that border control had reduced the incidence of other diseases that had been thought to be due to the climate, such as foot-and-mouth disease (FMD) and pleuro-pneumonia. Contagious animal diseases suddenly appeared to be "imported diseases" that could be controlled through sanitary measures: strict control at the borders, and a drastic eradication of germs through the slaughtering of sick animals.[9] The idea was to "cleanse" areas, from small zones to the entire country.

This way of thinking was deeply linked with an environmental conception of contagion, which associated infectious bodies with their environment. Thus, fighting contagion meant acting not only on individuals, but also on their surroundings.[10] Veterinarians actively defended this "stamping out" policy and its accompanying "keeping out" practice (rejection of imports of suspicious animals), which relied on their diagnoses of contagious diseases. For them, the control of contagion seemed a perfect *market shelter*, in Eliot Friedson's sense[11], of a monopoly that could be secured through the adoption of new regulations that excluded their rivals: the numerous empirical practitioners (farriers, gelders, and country wardens) who were still free to heal animals.[12] The Board of Agriculture shared this view, not only because it supported the interests of the pedigree stockbreeders, but also because it fitted well with the cultural representation of Britain as a strong nation, able to challenge its enemies with "virile" assets such as strength, energy, and efficiency.[13]

---

8 Gérard Jorland/Annick Opinel/George Weisz (eds.), Body counts. Medical quantification in historical and sociological perspectives, Montréal 2005; Eileen Magnello/Anne Hardy (eds.), The Road to Medical Statistics, Amsterdam/New York 2002.

9 Woods, A Manufactured Plague? (note 7), 11.

10 Susan D. Jones, Mapping a Zoonotic Disease. Anglo-American efforts to control Bovine Tuberculosis before World War I, in: Osiris 19 (2004), 133–148.

11 Eliot Friedson, Professional Powers. A Study of the Institutionalization of Formal Knowledge, Chicago 1986.

12 See Michael Worboys, Spreading Germs. Disease Theories and Medical Practice in Britain, 1865–1900, Cambridge 2000; id., Killing and Curing. Veterinarians, Medicine and Germs in Britain, 1860–1900, in: Veterinary History 7 (1992), 53–71; id., Germ Theories of Disease and British Veterinary Medicine, 1860–1890, in: Medical History 35 (1991), 308–327; John Fisher, To Kill or Not to Kill. The Eradication of Contagious Bovine Pleuro-Pneumonia in Western Europe, in: Medical History 47 (2003), 314–331; id., Not Quite a Profession. The Aspirations of Veterinary Surgeons in England in the Mid-Nineteenth Century, in: Historical Research 66/161 (1993), 284–302.

13 Woods, A Manufactured Plague? (note 7), 100.

As a result, the State Veterinary Department proposed to expand the legislation to other contagious diseases and to hire a larger number of inspectors of livestock both at disembarkation ports and within the territory. However, though the 1869 Contagious Diseases (Animal) Act widened the provisions of the 1866 Act to include FMD, sheep-scab, and glanders, it maintained isolation without imposing slaughter. This was the result of both a conjunction of interests and of empirical experience with these diseases: the most liberal government ministers preferred animal inspection and isolation in ports over quarantine, as this limited state intervention in the private realm of stockbreeders. The Treasury was determined to avoid the expense that compensation for a mass slaughter would have entailed. Most farmers and stockbreeders were also satisfied, as they supported a no-slaughter policy for FMD, which they considered a more benign disease that only temporarily disrupted agricultural production. Moreover, they did not hide their hostility to the free-trade measures, which they blamed for falling prices and stagnation in their sales. They therefore supported the expansion of the list of contagious diseases as a good means for imposing additional restrictions on livestock-exporting countries, thereby limiting competition without excessively constraining their own activities.[14]

These protectionist ideas gradually became dominant in many countries, even as free trade officially remained the general rule, and at the end of the nineteenth century, the USA prohibited the importation of British pedigree cattle because of FMD.[15] As shown by Abigail Woods, pedigree livestock breeders belonged to the aristocratic elite and were highly influential in the House of Lords. To maintain their profitable exports, these stockbreeders needed FMD to be eradicated, and they put pressure on the government. They supported their claims with the statistical evidence collected by the State Veterinary Department, which had been able to calculate the exact number of direct and indirect losses inflicted on the rural economy by contagious diseases.[16] This, in turn, allowed for cost/profit analyses of the different sanitary policies, as vital statistics were the cornerstone of sanitary reforms in the late nineteenth century. These economic concerns coincided with those of the stockbreeders' associations, such as the Central and Associated Chambers of Agriculture, which, according to John Fisher, worked actively to restrict the import of animals suspected of introducing "foreign" diseases.[17] Supported by conservative members of government, these stockbreeders' associations introduced a bill in 1878 aiming to ban meat and livestock imports from countries

14 Fisher, To Kill or Not to Kill (note 12).

15 Patrick Zylberman, Making Food Safety an Issue. Internationalized Food Politics and French Public Health from the 1870s to the Present, in: Medical History 48 (2004), 1–28; Stanziani, Histoire de la qualité (note 2).

16 Woods, A Manufactured Plague? (note 7), 8.

17 Fisher, To Kill or Not to Kill (note 12).

considered "infected."[18] This climate of hostility to imports gradually increased: in 1884, an amendment banned livestock imports from infected countries (amongst them France), and slaughter became mandatory for all instances of contagious diseases in 1894.[19]

In the course of these events, veterinarians' diagnostic competences were solicited, and the conditions of their professional practice improved, since the new 1878 Act consecrated their knowledge on contagion and distinguished them from practitioners who did not hold a degree and were not members of the Royal College of Veterinary Surgeons. In 1881, the Veterinary Surgeons Act protected their title and status, conferring a mandate from the state to deal with contagion by controls at ports, fairs, and markets wherever possible. British veterinarians, hired by the state each time there was an epizootic outbreak, were then taught at their schools to diagnose contagious animal diseases.[20] Thanks to this conjunction of interests, stamping out became the standard approach to animal diseases in Britain.

3. In France: Controlling the Contagion Within

In France, most of these animal diseases were more or less endemic. Farmers were used to dealing with them and had developed empirical knowledge to limit their negative effects on the local economy. For example, they knew how to treat mild diseases or lesions using folk remedies, most often made with thyme or vinegar.[21] Dealing with contagion was a problem that farmers could manage without any state intervention. Diseases were, therefore, not really perceived as a national problem, as animal products were mainly consumed locally and did not jeopardise trade.

However, for a small part of its trade, France was also involved in exporting and importing feeder cattle, mainly from Algeria and Italy, and to Britain. This production was in fact uneven, depending on the agricultural region: certain north-western regions produced enough for export, while others suffered from shortages. A lack of centralization contributed to these disparities, as did flaws in road networks and means of transportation.[22] When a rinderpest epizootic broke out in France in 1871, the government revived the law of 1866. In theory, this should have entailed the slaughter of all sick animals and their contacts in exchange for compensation, but a circular from the Ministry of

---

18 Abigail Woods, The Construction of an Animal Plague. Foot and Mouth Disease in Nineteenth Century Britain, in: Social History of Medicine 17/1 (2004), 23–39, 36.

19 The 1894 Diseases of Animals Act.

20 Ian Pattison, The British Veterinary Profession, 1791–1948, London 1984.

21 Luigi Morandi, Rapport sur l'emploi du thym et du serpolet, d'après le procédé de Luigi Morandi, contre la fièvre aphteuse, Milan, nd.

22 Stanziani, Histoire de la qualité (note 2), 194.

Agriculture recommended a certain "reservation as regards the slaughter orders," as too many animals were affected.[23] Slaughtering would have strongly jeopardized farm labour (harvests relied on animal force[24]) and agricultural production. Moreover, the cost of compensation would have been heavy. In practice, therefore, local authorities let the disease run its course, limiting their intervention to isolation and the suspension of livestock movements, fairs, and markets. As a consequence, secondary norms multiplied (from simple isolation to the use of various remedies, religious prayers, or magical incantations) as various actors (local authorities, farmers, animal practitioners, or even priests) helped to control the disease or its symptoms.

In parallel, mirroring the British discussions, the French government set up a commission in 1876, the Consultative Committee on Epizootics (*Comité Consultatif des Épizooties*, or CCE) to find the most appropriate measures to control contagious animal diseases.[25] The CCE included government officials, members of the Ministry of Agriculture and Trade as well as other agricultural associations, and veterinarians. This was an important moment of recognition for veterinarians, as animal medicine was still freely performed by numerous "empirical" practitioners who had favourable rural social foundations. The veterinary elite, most often professors at the national schools, believed that this competition damaged their social legitimacy, lowering their diploma-sanctioned theoretical and practical training to the level of an apprenticeship.[26] By implementing what Andrew Abbott calls *cultural work* to mark the boundaries of an area of expertise – that is, the redefinition of contagious animal disease in such a manner that veterinarians were the only ones able to deal with it – veterinarians then developed new knowledge that helped to construct infectious diseases not only as a problem for agriculture, but also for human health.[27] For the first time, glanders, farcy, rabies, and anthrax were explicitly described as diseases that could endanger the humans who lived in contact with the sick animals.[28] This affirmation came from veterinary involvement in clinical experiments that followed Claude Bernard's style, as vivisections were often performed by the veterinary schools' professors with the collaboration of certain physicians.[29] As early as the mid-nineteenth century, some veterinarians had started to experiment with the blood of contaminated animals to determine whether these diseases could be

23 Circular from the ministry of agriculture to all mayors of 10 April 1871, Journal Officiel, 21 June 1874, 4218.

24 Jean-Luc Mayaud, La petite exploitation rurale triomphante, France XIXe siècle, Paris 1999.

25 Decree of 24 May 1876.

26 Ronald Hubscher, Les Maîtres des Bêtes. Les vétérinaires dans la société française, 18ème-20ème siècle, Paris 1999.

27 Andrew Abbott, The System of Professions. An Essay on the Division of Expert Labor, Chicago 1988, 9, 59.

28 Journal Officiel, 18 December 1878, Senate, session of 4 November 1878, Rapport sur le Projet de Loi relatif à la Police Sanitaire des Animaux, 12051–12056.

29 Hardy, Animals, Disease and Man (note 1).

transmitted by ingestion or inoculation and if it was possible to protect animals from contagion via inoculation with citrated or heated blood.[30] They inspired and contributed to the development of French bacteriology, helping Louis Pasteur and his collaborators to test their new vaccines.[31]

Veterinarians thus redefined contagious animal diseases as a public health problem that they were able to manage by diagnosing contagion, controlling the germs within the animal organisms, and preventing transmission to humans through animal food products. Linking animal and human health became characteristic of French veterinarians, who said that humans were animals first, and that the two branches of medicines had to learn from each other. Their influence in the CCE was significant. Indeed, its report concluded that the failure of the sanitary policy was due to a lack of qualified veterinarians. The veterinary members of the CCE belonged to the elite of their profession. They drafted a bill that entrusted certified veterinarians with the inspection of livestock at all fairs and markets, proscribing any intrusion by non-certified practitioners in the management of contagious diseases. Nevertheless, although they favoured the slaughter of the sick animals, the veterinary elites refused to endorse the responsibility to "restrict the property rights" of the farmers by taking the decision to impose slaughter.[32] According to them, only the state had that power.

The committee's report stressed the difficulty of enforcing these measures. Following the 1789 Revolution, France remained politically unstable throughout the nineteenth century, with many revolts and revolutions inspired by an ideal of freedom that may have frightened the Committee. The bill was thus hotly debated before being eventually adopted "in an emergency,"[33] as Britain had imposed a ban on French livestock because of FMD.[34] To restore the trade, a deputy suggested that France should adopt the British regulation "in the terms and conditions set up by the English in their country"[35] and

---

30 Gerald Geison, The Private Science of Louis Pasteur, Princeton 1995; Henri Toussaint, Vaccinations charbonneuses. Séance du 19 août 1880, in: Association française pour l'avancement des sciences 9 (1881), 1021–1025.

31 Delphine Berdah, Entre scientifisation et travail de frontières. Les transformations des savoirs vétérinaires en France, XIXe – XIXe siècles, in: Revue d'Histoire Moderne et Contemporaine 4 (2012), 51–96; Maurice Cassier, Appropriation and commercialization of the Pasteur Anthrax Vaccine, in: Studies in History and Philosophy of Science Part C. Studies in History and Philosophy of Biological and Biomedical Sciences 36/4 (2005), 722–742.

32 Journal Officiel, 19 December 1878, Sénat séance du 4 novembre 1878, Rapport sur le Projet de Loi relatif à la Police Sanitaire des Animaux, 12101.

33 Journal Officiel, Débats parlementaires, 4 November 1878, 12051–12056; Journal Officiel (JO) 19 December 1878, 12097–12107; JO 22 December 1878, 12208–12212; JO 9 May 1879, 3788–3793; JO 10 May 1879, 3815–3826; JO 12 May 1879, 3875–3878, JO 13 May 1879, 3895–3900; JO 9 March 1881, 454–463; and JO 31 May 1881, 1065–1068.

34 Woods, A Manufactured Plague? (note 7), 17.

35 JO 9 March 1881, 454–463, 455.

delegate the decision to slaughter to prefects[36] rather than the Ministry of Agriculture in order to accelerate administrative decisions, but also to enable local negotiations. Passed in July 1881, the law was similar to the British act, except that where the British used a local tax in slaughterhouses to fund the compensations for the animals' destruction, the French used credits from the Ministry of Agriculture.

This legislation aimed at maintaining international trade, but the economic stakes were low. The share of exports in national revenues was quite small, owing in particular to the colonies, which made it possible to maintain an outlet for French products. While Britain had given top priority to its pedigree export market by applying strong sanitary policies, France did not significantly invest in putting its new legislation into practice, either financially (no significant compensations) or in terms of labour (no massive hiring of veterinary inspectors). Replacing slaughtered animals would have required other healthy animals or machines, but both were lacking. Moreover, farmers were unwilling to accept a total eradication of their indispensable – and often multitasking – animals. Veterinarians were the only ones interested in the application of the law. This gave them a practising monopoly over contagious diseases, and thus delimited their first market shelter. But without the real involvement of the government, too few veterinarians were recruited, and the law remained a façade, effective only at borders, while a multitude of secondary application norms emerged to deal locally with the consequences of contagion.

The example of the fight against bovine tuberculosis (BTB) will help to clarify how these secondary application norms favoured the development of different repertoires of veterinary knowledge and action in the two countries, leading to different forms of control of animal commodities.

4. In Britain: A Repertoire of Actions to Eradicate the Source of Infection[37]

In 1882, the German bacteriologist Robert Koch announced that the bacilli of bovine and human tuberculosis belonged to the same species. According to Keir Waddington, this declaration prompted many debates, and in the 1890s, the bovine disease seemed a

36 The prefects represent the State vis-à-vis the local authorities.

37 About BTB in Britain, see Peter Atkins, White Poison. The Health Consequences of Milk Consumption, 1850–1930, in: Social History of Medicine 5/2 (1992), 207–227; id., The Pasteurization of England. The Science, Culture, and Health Implications of Milk Processing, 1900–1950, in: David F. Smith /Jim Phillips (eds.), Food, Science, Policy and Regulation in the Twentieth Century. International and Comparative Perspectives, London 2000, 37–51; id., A History of Uncertainty. Bovine Tuberculosis in Britain, 1850 to the present, Winchester 2016; Keir Waddington, The Science of Cows. Tuberculosis, Research and the State in the United Kingdom, 1890–1914, in: History of Science 39/3 (2001), 1–27; id., Unfit for Human Consumption. Tuberculosis and the Problem of Infected Meat in Late Victorian Britain, in: Bulletin of the History of Medicine 77 (2003), 636–661; id., The Bovine Scourge (note 3).

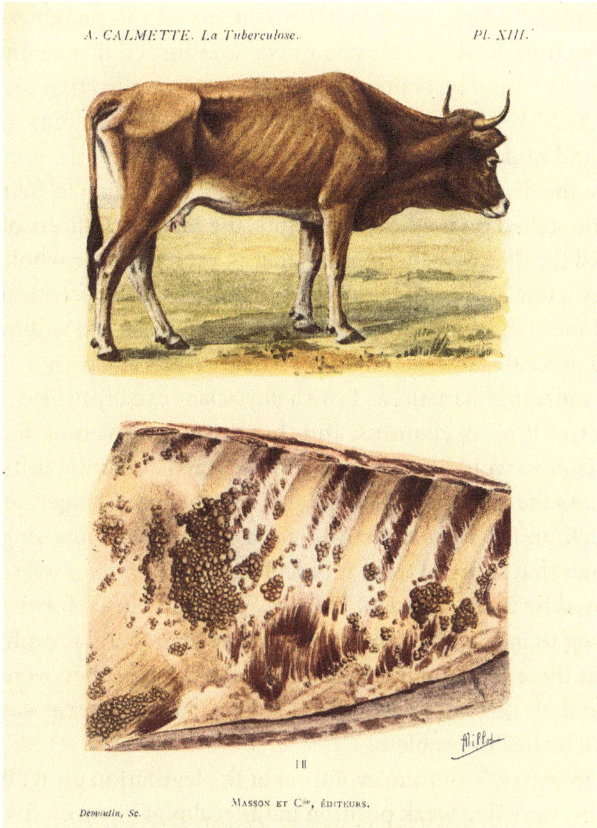

Fig. 1 Albert Calmette, L'infection bacillaire et la tuberculose chez l'homme et chez les animaux, Paris 1920, plate XIII, p. 272. Part 1: Tarentaise cow with tuberculosis, Part 2: Tuberculosis of the pleura in cows.

clear threat for the human population, which demanded new regulations.[38] In response, the British government set up three royal commissions, which eventually agreed on the dangerousness of milk and meat.[39] But although it was possible to diagnose BTB through an injection of tuberculin,[40] no compulsory elimination of contaminated animals was

---

38 Waddington, Unfit for Human Consumption (note 37).

39 Waddington, The Bovine Scourge (note 3), 13; House of Commons, Report of the Departmental Committee Appointed to Inquire into Pleuro-pneumonia and Tuberculosis in United Kingdom, Parliamentary Papers, London, HMSO, 1888, Vol. 32.

40 Tuberculin is a substance extracted from a culture of tuberculosis bacilli. First thought of as a remedy, it was then used as a diagnostic substance both for humans and bovines (it elevates the temperature of

enacted.[41] Under the "pleuro-orders," a large portion of the animals sent to slaughterhouses were found to be suffering from BTB, and the commissions estimated that nearly one-fourth of the national livestock might be contaminated, rendering eradication too expensive for the Treasury.[42] The MAF shared this view and favoured other actions to get rid of contaminated meat and milk. The examination of meat in slaughterhouses varied greatly in the country, to the disadvantage of veterinarians.[43] According to Keir Waddington, most municipalities relied on medical inspectors, the Medical Officers of Health (MOH), who considered the disease generalized – that is, present in the whole body of the animal, even if only a few localised lesions were visible.[44] This conception of contagion – an adaptation of the environmental conception of the disease, but within the animal body – let the MOH order the destruction of the whole carcass at any sign of infection. The case of milk was more problematic, as British physicians usually believed that pasteurization would deprive it of its vitamins, and thus favoured raw milk for children.[45] Moreover, pasteurization would have required investments that the milk industry did not want to make. As the veterinarians estimated that the most dangerous animals were those clinically sick, an incentive directive was passed in 1909 proposing that farmers slaughter all bovines that suffered from tuberculosis of the udder or were emaciated, after being diagnosed by a veterinarian. This was not mandatory, for the Treasury wanted to avoid having to indemnify too many stockbreeders.[46] As a result, the animals were eliminated at the end of their agricultural career, when they were taken to the slaughterhouse and their carcasses destroyed, showing that the disease was not really perceived a major public health problem.

Only veterinarians seemed to worry.[47] But the evolution of the legislation on BTB showed that British veterinarians were in a weak position in the realm of livestock diseases, despite their ability to diagnose contagion (1878 Act).[48] According to Waddington, the veterinarians who represented the elite of their profession were sensitive to the ideas

---

contaminated animals). Adopted in France as early as 1892, it had also been used by certain veterinarians in the UK since 1893. See Waddington, The Bovine Scourge (note 3), 13; Edmond Nocard, La tuberculine, nouveaux faits prouvant sa haute valeur diagnostique, application à la prophylaxie de la tuberculose bovine, Paris 1892. For the history of tuberculin, see Christoph Gradmann, Robert Koch and the Pressures of Scientific Research. Tuberculosis and Tuberculin, in: Medical History 45 (2001), 1–32.

41 Keir Waddington, To Stamp Out 'So Terrible a Malady.' Bovine Tuberculosis and Tuberculin Testing in Britain, 1890–1939, in: Medical History 48 (2004), 29–48.

42 Waddington, Unfit for Human Consumption (note 37).

43 Anne Hardy, John Bull's Beef. Meat Hygiene and Veterinary Public Health in England in the Twentieth Century, in: Review of Agricultural and Environmental Studies 91/4 (2010), 369–392.

44 Waddington, The Bovine Scourge (note 3).

45 Atkins, The Pasteurization of England (note 37).

46 Waddington, The Bovine Scourge (note 3).

47 Pattison, The British Veterinary Profession (note 20), 103.

48 Hardy, John Bull's Beef (note 43).

of France's and Germany's budding field of bacteriology.[49] But according to Worboys, they were far from committing to the application of these theories, which had fervent defenders amongst British physicians. For the veterinarian elite, securing their professional status implied defining their own sphere of knowledge and practice relative to livestock diseases, for which physicians could not be qualified.[50] Slaughter-related sanitary policies were thus defended as the most efficient means to fight livestock diseases.

A second interpretation could also explain British veterinarians' poor involvement in bacteriological prophylactic techniques. In a country where the slaughter and isolation of sick livestock were rigorously implemented, there was not much room for prophylactic alternatives. Veterinary schools developed bacteriological laboratories in the late nineteenth century, but they were used to produce diagnostic substances such as tuberculin or mallein (used to diagnose glanders), which they also marketed.[51] No attempt was made to develop vaccines or sera, since they would not have been used in veterinarians' liberal practice. Moreover, using vaccines would have meant that there was a general acceptation of the presence of the germs in the country as, culturally, it was difficult to separate the sick body from its environment. France was thus represented as a dirty, disorganized nation, which was unable to get rid of any disease.[52]

When a vaccine against tuberculosis (the BCG) started to be used on the Continent on both humans and animals in the 1920s, both the Medical Research Council (MRC) and the MAF seemed interested, but were suspicious of the quality of the French results, as France seemed unable to eradicate contagion and appeared more prone to live with it.[53] The MRC and the MAF wanted to obtain a proper statistical analysis of the effects of the BCG. Together, they set up laboratory and large-scale experiments with the vaccine in a few farms eager to get rid of BTB. Gradually, the calves born on the farms were vaccinated and the older animals replaced, so that the whole herd would eventually be vaccinated.[54] But the rationale was not to introduce a new tool for the control of animal diseases. Indeed, only two veterinarians working on behalf of the MAF performed the inoculations, and no liberal practitioners could master the technique. The objective was to reduce the incidence of the infection before slaughtering all the animals, as the MAF suspected vaccinated animals could remain a source of infection for the non-vaccinated,

49 Waddington, To Stamp Out 'So Terrible a Malady' (note 41).

50 Worboys, Germ Theories of Disease. (note 12).

51 Pattison, The British Veterinary Profession (note 20), 149.

52 Woods, A Manufactured Plague? (note 7), 100.

53 On the same epistemological difference see John Andrew Mendelsohn, Cultures of Bacteriology. Formation and Transformation of a Science in France and Germany, 1870–1914, Ph.D. thesis, Princeton 1996.

54 National Archives: MAF 189/418: ARC "Field Trials with BCG for the immunisation of calves against tuberculosis" Final Report, 1953. For the complete story with the BCG vaccine, see Delphine Berdah, Abattre ou vacciner? Histoires croisées de la lutte contre la fièvre aphteuse et la tuberculose bovine en France et au Royaume-Uni, 1900–1960, Paris 2018.

even if they were asymptomatic. The strategy of using vaccines as complementary tools had also been used against brucellosis with the cooperation of both farmers and veterinarians.[55] However, the adoption of this two-time eradication policy was only possible because the spread of BTB and brucellosis was very slow, and because there was no risk of the diseases becoming endemic. This was not the case with epizootics such as FMD, for example, which spreads so fast that outbreaks had to be stamped out as quickly as possible. Indeed, even once vaccines against FMD were developed in the 1930s and used in mainland Europe, the MAF refused to introduce them in farms, either preventively or in "ring vaccinations" around an outbreak. The argument was that vaccines were not one hundred per cent efficient, that is, able to *eradicate* the disease.[56]

5. In France: A Repertoire of Actions to Control the Effects of Infection

In the late nineteenth century, the contagiousness of human and bovine tuberculosis remained largely ignored. Lion Murard and Patrick Zylberman describe the French population's feelings about inter-human contagion as a "non-disentangled knot of fear and of unconcern."[57] Many veterinarians also complained of farmers' lack of concern about BTB in both the general and professional press.[58] Despite this situation, the veterinarians chose BTB as the battleground for obtaining their monopoly on animal medicine.

After fierce debates in Parliament and the Chamber of Deputies, they managed to have BTB added to the list of contagious diseases in 1888,[59] meaning that any case found at the slaughterhouse mandated the isolation and slaughter of the entire herd. But like the law of 1881, that of 1888 was not enforced. Consequently, French veterinarians enlarged their repertoire of actions to control the effects of infection.

First, veterinarians acquired new skills to control food salubrity. They developed new competences in the inspection of carcasses as well as in the bacteriological examination of milk. Both were taught in the national veterinary schools. These courses were very thorough; they associated physiological studies (using various samples from slaughterhouses) with bacteriological analysis in the laboratories, where students were taught all

55 Abigail Woods, A Historical Synopsis of Farm Animal Disease and Public Policy in Twentieth-Century Britain, in: Philosophical transactions of the Royal Society of London. Series B, Biological sciences 366/1573 (2011), 1943–54; Abigail Woods, "Partnership" in Action. Contagious Abortion and the Governance of Livestock Disease in Britain, 1885–1921, in: Minerva 47/2 (2009), 195–216.

56 Delphine Berdah, forthcoming publication.

57 Lion Murard/Patrick Zylberman, L'Hygiène dans la République. La Santé Publique en France ou l'utopie contrariée, 1870–1918, Paris 1996, 418.

58 René Bissauge, Notions pratiques sur la tuberculose bovine, Orléans 1896; see also various papers in the Bulletin Vétérinaire.

59 Decree of 28 July 1888.

the colouring, culturing, and "revealing" inoculation techniques.[60] When it came to meat, they learned to identify the various aspects of the BTB lesions and how to remove the contaminated parts (see fig. 1, part. 2). This expertise was appreciated by farmers since it limited the seizure of meat, and veterinarians progressively displaced butchers and rural policemen, who had had control over meat until then.[61] In 1909, veterinarians obtained a mandate from the state to supervise slaughterhouse inspections and bacteriological analysis of milk with the institutionalization of the Veterinary Services, a body of inspectors dispatched by the Ministry of Agriculture to all French *départments*.[62]

Second, veterinarians experimented with new prophylactic techniques to protect animals from infection, such as the vaccine against anthrax, developed at the Pasteur Institute with the collaboration of veterinarians,[63] and the serum therapy against FMD.[64] As most of the farms at the beginning of the 1930s possessed fewer than ten cows,[65] one can imagine how important the preservation of an animal instead of its slaughter was. Cows provided milk, but also manure for the fields. They birthed calves, some of whom became the oxen used for farm labour. Animal warmth was also an advantage in dwellings heated only by the fireplace in the main room. Indeed, on most of the small farms, humans and large animals were often housed under the same roof, with the stable adjoining the bedroom (fig. 2).

The proximity between humans and animals was important, as the animals shared the everyday life of the farm with their owners, and were often named and known by their behaviour. The slaughter of all animals was thus often impossible to imagine, even if compensation could be provided, not only because of this proximity and relationship, but also because the training of an ox took time and required the presence of an older animal to guide the young. The concrete reality of French farmers, their necessity of coping with the everyday life they shared with their animals, far outweighed any fear

60 Alcide Railliet, Léon Moulé, Histoire de l'Ecole d'Alfort, Paris 1908, 371.

61 Séverin Muller, Les abattoirs sous haute surveillance. Politiques et normalisation sanitaires à Saint-Maixent-l'Ecole, du 19ème au milieu du 20ème siècle, in: Revue d'Histoire Moderne et Contemporaine 51/3 (2004), 104–120.

62 The 12 January 1909 Act imposes to the departments the financial burden to appoint veterinary inspectors.

63 Cassier, Appropriation and Commercialization (note 31).

64 Delphine Berdah, Serum Therapy Against FMD and the Development of the French Veterinary Profession in the 1930s, in: Review of Agricultural, Food and Environmental Studies 102/2 (2020), 151–169.

65 Centre Historique des Archives Nationales, Série F 10 Agriculture: cote F 10–5431. Production Laitière: Rapports pour l'Assemblée Nationale sur les produits des Chambres d'Agriculture, par Robineau, secrétaire de la Chambre d'Agriculture de l'Yonne et Achard, secrétaire de la Confédération Générale des Producteurs de Lait, 15 et 16 mars 1932.

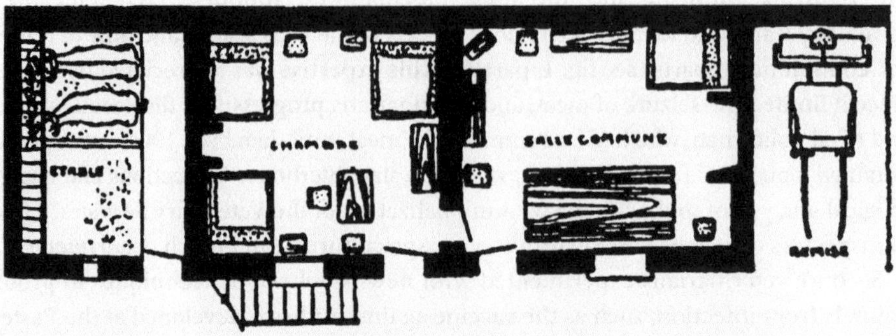

Plan de maison traditionnelle -Manuel de la Maison Rurale (1950).

Fig. 2 A French Traditional House Plan – Rural House Manual, 1950.

of a long-term disease. Veterinarians knew this. They were well aware of the social recognition of empirical practitioners who offered cures for farm animals.

Trained in microbiology[66] in their schools and sometimes at the Pasteur Institute, many veterinarians tried to produce vaccines against BTB, and trials were organized with more or less success.[67] At the beginning of the 1920s, Albert Calmette, a physician, and Camille Guérin, a veterinarian, both from the Pasteur Institute, produced and tested a vaccine against human and bovine tuberculosis, the BCG (Bacille Calmette-Guérin).

The Pastorians were convinced that only a vaccine could get rid of the disease, as the tuberculous bacilli were everywhere in the environment: in houses, stables, and human and animal bodies, whether wild or domestic. According to Calmette and Guérin, the only means to stop the infections was to introduce safe germs (the vaccines) inside healthy bodies in their infancy before the tuberculous bacilli could infect them.[68] The animal trials, including post-mortems on vaccinated animals, were very useful for the two Pastorians, as they provided data impossible to obtain from human experiments. For them, bovines became epistemic models, essential to apprehend the evolution of BCG within vaccinated human bodies.[69] The veterinary vaccine, delivered only to qualified practitioners by the Pasteur Institute, was perceived a professional asset. It was also an asset to farmers, as it impeded the development of BTB within the animal

66 In French, microbiology means the study of both viruses and bacteria.

67 For example, experiments with Joseph Lignières's vaccine (with an avian bacillus), Saturnin Arloing's "homogenous bacillus" and Henri Vallée's "equine bacillus."

68 Berdah, Abattre ou vacciner (note 54).

69 Delphine Berdah, La vaccination des bovidés contre la tuberculose en France, 1921–1963. Entre modèle épistémique et alternative à l'abattage, in: Review of Agricultural and Environmental Studies 91/4 (2010), 393–415.

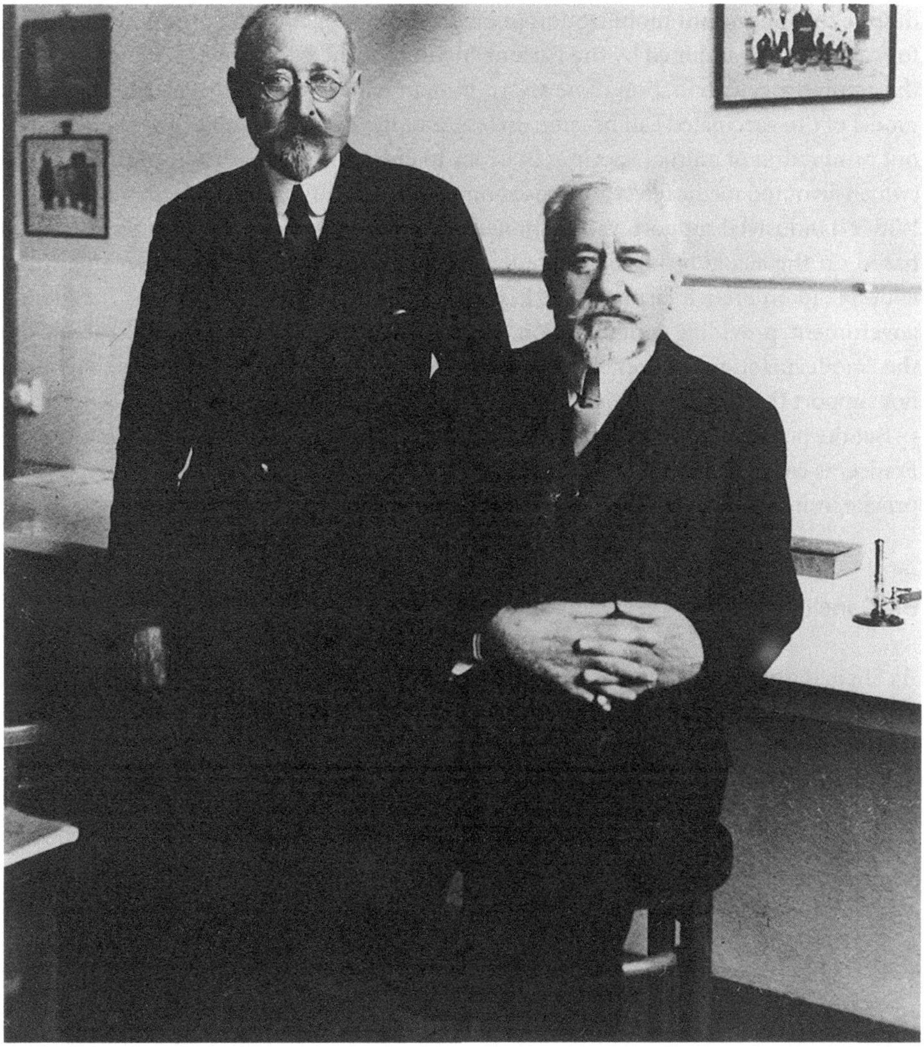

Fig. 3 Camille Guerin and Albert Calmette in the laboratory of the BCG at the Pasteur Institute in 1931.

body, thus maintaining all farm activities and preventing meat seizures. The numerous letters written by veterinarians to the Pasteur Institute show how the BCG was seen a reliable tool, and many veterinarians, including members of scientific societies and those in political roles, advocated for a general national vaccine campaign.[70] However,

70 Archives of the Pasteur Institute, GUE 5: Camille Guérin's correspondence; Compte-rendu des Séances de l'Académie d'Agriculture, séance du 8 février 1950, "Tuberculose bovine" note de M. J.B. Martin, p. 117–119, p. 118; M. Rufin et J.-R. Verdier, "Vaccinations par le BCG dans le département du Cher. Une

despite this important mobilization in favour of the vaccine, the production of BCG for calves was abandoned by the Pasteur Institute at the beginning of the 1960s. With the compulsory vaccination of newborn human babies passed in 1951, the epistemic model of the vaccinated calf became useless, and the Pasteur Institute gradually phased out production of animal vaccines in order to enter the biomedical turn of the 1960s (which favoured medical research based on the new techniques of molecular biology).[71] With no industrial support, vaccination against BTB disappeared, and other initiatives based on the slaughtering of reactant animals prevailed. As tractors became more widespread on French farms, it also became possible to eradicate bovines. The French government, providing compensation, backed this policy, believing it would accelerate the "modernization" of French agriculture by eliminating the small farms that could not support the costs and reorganization imposed by such a policy.[72]

But the popularity of vaccines in the management of diseases remained significant in France, as can be inferred by the success of the FMD vaccine, which was produced by a private industry and widely used as a veterinary tool at the same time.[73]

6. Conclusion

As Sheila Jasanoff and Sang-Hyun Kim have argued, "sociotechnical imaginaries are collectively imagined forms of social life and social order reflected in the design and fulfilment of nation-specific scientific and/or technological projects."[74] Historical comparative analyses are powerful tools for understanding how these imaginaries act as

expérience sur le plan départemental", Bulletin de l'Académie Vétérinaire de France, 6 juillet 1950, p. 399–401; Académie d'Agriculture: "La vaccination des bovidés par le BCG ", Communication de M. Desoulter; Comptes-rendus des séances de l'Académie d'Agriculture, séance du 28 avril 1948, p. 598–603, p. 599; Centre des Archives Contemporaines, Ministère de l'Agriculture, Fonds des Services Vétérinaires, cote 19880158: article 80: Section permanente du Comité Consultatif des Épizooties, séance du 10 février 1949, Vœu du conseil Général de la Savoie; JO du 21 juillet 1950, p. 1584–1585, p. 1585. Documents parlementaires, Assemblée Nationale, "Proposition de résolution tendant à inviter le gouvernement à modifier la réglementation sanitaire en ce qui concerne les étables où la vaccination antituberculeuse des bovidés par le BCG est instituée, présentée par M. Cordonnier et les membres du groupe socialiste, députés".

71 Berdah, La vaccination des bovidés (note 69); on biomedicine, see, for example, Vivian Quirke/Jean-Paul Gaudillière, The Era of Biomedicine. Science, Medicine, and Public Health in Britain and France after the Second World War, in: Medical History 52/4 (2008), 441–452.

72 Delphine Berdah, Suivre la norme sanitaire ou 'périr'. La loi de 1954 sur la prophylaxie collective de la tuberculose bovine, in: Christophe Bonneuil/Gilles Denis/Jean-Luc Mayaud (eds.), Science, Chercheurs et Agriculture, Pour une histoire de la recherche agronomique, Paris 2008, 203–222.

73 Berdah, Abattre ou vacciner (note 54).

74 Sheila Jasanoff/Sang-Hyun Kim, Containing the Atom: Sociotechnical Imaginaries and Nuclear Power in the United States and South Korea, in: Minerva 47/2 (2009), 119–146.

essential components in the shaping of public policies. Indeed, they can explain why, despite the adoption of the same legislations against animal diseases, France and Britain adopted secondary application norms that engaged public authorities, veterinarians, and farmers differently. In Britain, the defence and selection of selected breeds – an activity developed by farmers who were often members of the House of Lords – was linked with an aristocratic vision of pure blood that had to be preserved.[75] This preservation of the blood was the result of inbreeding, but also of the rejection of animal diseases from outside of the country's borders, and thus outside its bodies. As Ludwik Fleck had noted, the idea that the causal agents of diseases are contained in the blood of sick organisms dates back to antiquity, and persisted in the styles of thoughts and imaginaries of physicians and biologists throughout the nineteenth and the beginning of the twentieth centuries.[76] This view certainly influenced the generalized image of tuberculosis, whose appearance at the slaughterhouses prompted the destruction of the carcasses. The destruction of contaminated bodies and "cleansing" of entire areas was perceived to be the only solution for eradicating the source of contagion. A similar idea is expressed with the metaphor of the barrier to prevent intrusion by germ invaders, or the disinfection of surrounding areas to protect bodies that were formulated when the principles of antisepsis and asepsis were introduced to reform surgical procedures in the operating room.[77] The nineteenth century in Britain saw the acculturation of populations to hygienic principles and a corresponding moralization of individuals who felt responsible for not letting the contagion circulate.[78] Pedigree livestock breeders, along with members of the MAF, defended the stamping out policy, not only in order to maintain their lucrative trade, but also because they believed in the image of a strong and civilized nation, able to make sacrifices in order to free the country from disease. It seems other farmers also shared this view, as they used vaccines to reduce the incidence of infection before willingly employing eradication schemes. The vaccinated body could not represent a healthy body, as the BCG vaccine was made from living bacteria. Uncertainty about the future of these bacteria within a living organism, as well as the fact that most vaccines do not prevent the animals from encountering the deadly germs, but simply inhibit the development of symptoms, fuelled the fear of multiplying healthy carriers who were able to spread disease. The fear of hidden healthy carriers certainly

75 The first mention of the word "race" was for the pedigree of dogs that accompanied aristocrats in their hunting expeditions. Thus, according to Zelinger, discourses about race "were part of a social ideology that connected dog 'races' to symbols of nobility and aristocratic supremacy and facilitated the production of class hierarchies." Amir Zelinger, Race and Animal-Breeding. A Hybridized Historiography, in: History and Theory 58/3 (2019), 360–384, 363; See also Mary Bouquet, Reclaiming English Kinship. Portuguese Refractions of British Kinship Theory, Manchester 1993.

76 Ludwik Fleck, Genèse et développement d'un fait scientifique, Paris 2005.

77 Anne Marie Moulin, The Defended Body, in: Roger Cooter/John Pickstone (eds.), Companion to Medicine in the 20th century 2003, 385–398, 388.

78 Peter Baldwin, Contagion and the State in Europe, 1830–1930, Cambridge 1999.

spurred the hunt for dangerous microbes that affected either humans or animals.[79] BCG vaccines had thus no future in the long-term management of tuberculosis. Veterinarians could not include them in their repertoire or develop new competences that might have modified the national application of the legislation – in the direction of prophylaxis, for example.

In France, there were no imaginaries about a national pedigree herd trade that must be protected by any means. Farms were usually quite small, with few animals. Experiences of endemic animal diseases normalized the circulation of diseases within bodies and territories, in a sort of revival of "prebacteriological" conceptions where "the body was regarded as a microcosm reflecting the macrocosm and poised in an unstable equilibrium."[80] The sanitary policy imposed for most of animal diseases thus seemed extreme in comparison to the everyday consequences of these diseases. This paved the way for secondary norms of application of the law, where the main idea was to preserve the lives of the animals, maintain farm labour and milk production, and prevent meat seizures. Veterinarians developed a complete repertoire of actions thanks to their expertise acquired in laboratories of microbiology: cultivated and coloured, bacteria were rendered visible and could be isolated or attenuated. A complete analysis of the milk was possible, and tuberculous lesions could be removed from carcasses. Vaccines and sera could be produced and animals inoculated to prevent the development of diseases. Their vaccinated bodies were thus healthy bodies: active and able to produce work and food. In the end, the BCG was abandoned at the beginning of the 1960s, not because the slaughtering of the reactant animals was considered a better alternative, but because its producer, the Pasteur Institute, entered the biomedical turn. The slaughtering of the reactants then remained the only option for controlling tuberculosis.

Photo credits

Fig. 1 Albert Calmette, L'infection bacillaire et la tuberculose chez l'homme et chez les animaux, Paris 1920, plate XIII, p. 272. Institut Pasteur / Musée Pasteur.

Fig. 2 A French Traditional House Plan – Rural House Manual, 1950. Taken from: G.R.E.A, Paroles et Parcours de Paysans. Nous avons cru au progrès, Paris 1996, 43.

Fig. 3 Camille Guerin and Albert Calmette in the laboratory of the BCG at the Pasteur Institute in 1931. Institut Pasteur / Musée Pasteur.

79 J. Andrew Mendelsohn, 'Typhoid Mary' Strikes Again. The Social and the Scientific in the Making of Modern Public Health, in: Isis 86/2 (1995), 268–277.

80 Moulin, The Defended Body (note 77), 387.

Abstract:
This chapter aims to show how certain contagious animal diseases were considered an issue – or not – by French and British governments from the mid-nineteenth century onward. It analyses the repertoire of actions available against these diseases in the two countries, which varied depending on socio-cultural imaginaries and knowledge, as well as on the pressure exerted by different interests (economic, political, industrial, or professional). Using Pierre Lascoumes's frame of analysis, it demonstrates how public policies were applied through secondary norms that enabled alternative means of controlling these diseases. The fight against bovine tuberculosis (a zoonosis that caused significant infant mortality) offers an opportunity for a finer analysis of this legislative regulation. This work is based on a cross-analysis of parliamentary sources, archives from the French and British Ministries of Health and of Agriculture, the Veterinary Services, and the Pasteur Institute, as well as a survey of scientific and professional veterinary literature.

Keywords:
veterinary expertise | animal diseases | bovine tuberculosis | sanitary policy | vaccination

Axel C. Hüntelmann

"The Beast in the Mosquito"

The Changing Role of Mosquitos in Malaria Research and Control in the Decades around 1900

The relationship between human scientists and animals changed fundamentally with the laboratory revolution in the nineteenth century[1] and again at the end of the century. With the emergence of bacteriology, microorganisms became the smallest but most dangerous enemies of mankind[2] – and animals. Although epizootics were well-known by then, they were mainly considered an economic threat, not as a danger to human health.[3] Diseased animals suffering from swine erysipelas or bovine tuberculosis died earlier and their meat was regarded as inferior. But with the identification of microorganisms that could – potentially – infect humans and other animals, sick animals became a severe health threat. On the other hand, animals susceptible to pathogens that were also dangerous for humans could be used to investigate the etiology of the disease or the living conditions of the pathogen. But the story became more complicated from the mid-1870s and 1880s, when Patrick Manson, David Bruce, and others observed that pathogens might also be transmitted via flies, mosquitos, or fleas. But exactly what role did mosquitos and flies play in the transmission of tropical diseases like malaria, sleeping sickness, or yellow fever? Were they the causal agent themselves? Or did they transmit pathogens, like rats did? Since the 1890s, bacteriological research, especially in France, Italy, and Britain, shed light on the relations between various insects and their human food source, but how diseases were transmitted remained unclear. That is the point where this story starts.

---

1 See Anita Guerrini, Experimenting with Humans and Animals. From Galen to Animal Rights. Baltimore 2003. For the upcoming laboratory revolution Andrew Cunningham/William Perry (eds.), The Laboratory Revolution in Medicine, Cambridge 1992; and within this context the birth of the laboratory animal Axel C. Hüntelmann, History of Animal Experiments, in: Mieke Roscher et al. (ed.), Handbook of Historical Animal Studies, Berlin 2021, 513–528.

2 With reference to a quote of Robert Koch see Christoph Gradmann, Die kleinsten aber gefährlichsten Feinde der Menschheit. Bakteriologie, Sprache und Politik im Deutschen Kaiserreich, in: Stefanie Samida (ed.), Inszenierte Wissenschaft. Zur Popularisierung von Wissen im 19. Jahrhundert, Bielefeld 2011, 61–82.

3 See the chapter by Delphine Berdah in this volume; and also Lise Wilkinson, Animals and Diseases. An Introduction to the History of Comparative Medicine, Cambridge 1992; Anne Hardy, Animals, Disease, and Man: Making Connections, in: Perspectives in Biology and Medicine 46 (2003), 200–215; Abigail Woods, A Manufactured Plague? The History of Foot-and-Mouth Disease in Britain, London 2004; and Keir Waddington, The Bovine Scourge, Meat, Tuberculosis and Public Health, 1850–1950, Woodbridge 2006.

For quite some time, the frog had been the supreme experimental animal; especially for physiologists, the frog as *ranae exploratae*[4] was the martyr of science.[5] With the emergence of bacteriology, this changed. Bacteriologists needed mammals to model infectious diseases in humans and other mammals, and in the search for "the 'right' organism for the job",[6] rodents such as mice, rats, guinea pigs, and rabbits became the animals of choice. But what if there was no "'right' organism for the job" – yet? What did European scientists do in the face of a relatively unknown disease, one which was uncommon in the Western world? And how did they react if there was an intermediate host whose role and relationship to the pathogen was unclear? And if this host's behavior, biology, and living conditions were not as well understood as those of the domestic mouse or rat? This chapter deals with the birth of a new experimental animal – the mosquito – and its consequences for the human-mosquito relationship and humans' view of flying insects more generally. The chapter analyses the entangled relationship of experimental animals to their human companions; the role and agency of animals before, during, and after an experiment; and, depending on their relationship to humans, how these animals' ontological status changed.[7] In particular, this essay asks how mosquitos shifted from an insect, at worst a nuisance for humans, to an experimental animal, and again into a life-threating hazard.

I will first describe malaria research conducted by Ronald Ross in India and the mosquito's transformation from a nuisance into an experimental animal, from nature into a precious scientific object. A short section links Ross' research to similar studies in Germany and Italy. The last part discusses how this precious object then degraded into a pest, how mosquitos were considered a life-threating hazard to humans that had to be eradicated, for instance in Sierra Leone or in the German Empire, by sanitary measures.

---

4 Karl E. Rothschuh, Laudatio ranae exploratae, in: Sudhoffs Archiv 57 (1973), 231–244.

5 Frederic L. Holmes, The Old Matyr of Science. The Frog in Experimental Physiology, in: Journal of the History of Biology 26 (1993), 311–328.

6 Bonnie T. Clause, The Wistar Rat as a Right Choice. Establishing Mammalian Standards and the Ideal of a Standardized Mammal, in: Journal of the History of Biology 26 (1993), 329–349, esp. 330.

7 Ursula Klein and Wolfgang Lefèvre, for example, have written a historical ontology of chemical substances and their classification in the 17th and 18th centuries by bringing together different conceptual strands in the history and philosophy of science: natural materials are transformed via "practices of making", "material knowledge" and "material science", described as an "ontological shift", into scientific, "multidimensional objects". See Ursula Klein/Wolfgang Lefèvre, Materials in Eighteenth-Century Science. A Historical Ontology, Cambridge 2007, and Ian Hacking, Historical Ontologies. Contributions to the Philosophy and History of Knowledge, Zurich 2006. From the growing number of publications on (historical) ontology in Science and Technology Studies, see Andrew Pickering, New Ontologies, in: id./Keith Guzik (eds.), The Mangle in Practice. Science, Society, and Becoming, Durham 2008, 1–14. For the changing ontological status of mice, see Axel C. Hüntelmann, Mäuse, Menschen, Menagerien. Laborchimären und ihre wechselvolle Beziehung im Königlich Preußischen Institut für Experimentelle Therapie nach 1900, in: Kristian Köchy et al. (eds.), Philosophie der Tierforschung, vol. 3: Milieus und Akteure, Freiburg 2018, 221–262.

1. The State of Malaria Research until the mid-1890s

In early May 1897, Ronald Ross spent several days in the deepest Indian jungle. He "started to Kalhutti again on the 5th [of May]. On the 9th I went to Sigur, the bottom of the ghat, & spent the whole day there hunting for mosquito pools," where he

> examined water of puddles, mud, everything – not a sign of a mosquito. There was not a mosquito in the bungalow either. I then offered a reward for every mosquito alive or death, brought to me [...]. After breakfast on the 10th [of May] an intelligent native brought me 5 very small mosquitos. I jumped with astonishment at sight of them & told him to take me where he had found them. Instead of taking me to the servants' huts he led me into the neighboring jungle. It was then midday. He sat down; in one minute four or five mosquitos had fastened on his black legs & arms, one was on my hand & several were prospecting my trousers. I let the one on my hand bit me [...]. They breed apparently only in the darkest & most secluded woodland pools in dried up water courses & are quite different from the ordinary house mosquitos.[8]

This short report, related in a letter from Ross to Patrick Manson about his trip to the jungle near Ootacamund in the south-west of India, contains various aspects of the making of an experimental animal. Firstly, there is Ross, who describes hunting the insects in muddy pools, then his "discovery" of a "small" type of mosquito "with brindled bellies" and his observation that this type of mosquito, which he initially called *Culex silvestris*,[9] differed from related species.[10] Furthermore, we find the characteristic difficulties of research in the tropics.

In the tropics, everything was different from Europe. Even Ross, who was born and grew up in India, and who had worked as an officer in the Indian Medical Service since 1889,[11] had the culture and mentality of a white British man, superior to every other race in the human (and) animal kingdom, with a "perceived normality of the

---

8 Quotes in Ronald Ross to Patrick Manson, 12 May 1897, in: William F. Bynum/Caroline Overy (eds.), The Beast in the Mosquito. The Correspondence of Ronald Ross & Patrick Manson, Amsterdam 1998, letter no. 69.

9 On the forest as a (hidden) reservoir of pathogens, see also the contribution of Matheus Alves Duarte da Silva in this volume.

10 See also Ronald Ross, Memoirs. With a Full Account of the Great Malaria Problem and its Solution, London 1923, 208–210, on p. 208 he remarks that this was the first *Anopheles* he "had ever observed" – or more precisely: where he and a member of the species *Anopheles* met first.

11 For the biography of Ronald Ross see himself, Memoirs (note 10); and E.F. Dodd, The Story of Sir Ronald Ross and his Fight against Malaria, Madras 1956; John Rowland, The Mosquito Man. The Story of Sir Ronald Ross, London 1958; and lately Edwin R. Nye/Mary E. Gibson, Ronald Ross. Malariologist and Polymath. A Biography, Basingstoke 1997.

temperate lands."[12] David Arnold and recently Julia Engelschalt, have described this predisposition and perception "of northern whites moving into an alien world – alien in climate, vegetation, people and disease" as "tropicality."[13] Moreover, Ross had studied medicine and been trained in bacteriological techniques in England, meaning that beyond climate, vegetation, and people, animals, too, were alien, requiring new methods and techniques to be studied.

The environment of and working conditions in a laboratory – or what was supposed to be a laboratory – in the tropics were much more difficult than in Berlin, Paris, or London. Robert Koch, for instance, found during the cholera expedition in 1883/1884 that his method of cultivating bacteria on a solid gelatin-based culture – as was common practice in German bacteriology – liquified in the warm and humid climate of Egypt. He not only had to travel to regions with a more moderate climate (Calcutta in winter), but also had to develop an alternative method of cultivating bacteria[14] in order to prove (by re-infection)[15] that the comma bacillus was the cause of cholera. Beyond that, it was difficult to procure dyes to tincture tissue, scientific literature, technical and optical instruments, and other laboratory equipment.

While German bacteriologists and French microbiologists investigated pathogens causing anthrax, venereal diseases, tuberculosis, diphtheria, or the more exotic plague and cholera, British colonial medical officers like Patrick Manson, David Bruce, and Ronald Ross dealt with bilharzia, elephantiasis, malaria, sleeping sickness, and other

---

12 David Arnold, The Problem of Nature. Environment, Culture, and European Expansion, Oxford 1996, 142–143.

13 See Arnold, Problem of Nature (note 12); and Julia Engelschalt, Climates, Colonialism, and the Politics of Comparison. The Construction of U.S.-American Tropicality in Colonial Medicine and Public Health, 1898–1912 in: Eleonora Rohland et al. (eds.), Contact, Conquest, and Colonization. How Practices of Comparing Shaped Empires and Colonialism around the World, London 2021, 289–311, esp. 290.

14 See Christoph Gradmann, Das reisende Labor. Robert Koch erforscht die Cholera 1883/84, in: Medizinhistorisches Journal 38 (2003), 35–56.

15 An important step within Koch's postulates, a successive three-step process to identify a microorganism as causal agent of a disease, was the identification of a microorganism that was uncommon and different from those found in the tissue or blood of healthy living beings. The second step was to cultivate these microorganisms in pure form, for instance in a gelatin-based culture medium. And thirdly, these purely bred microorganisms, applicated to a healthy organism, had to trigger the same symptoms as the originally diseased organism. However, it turned out that this three-step prove process was more difficult to implement than assumed by Koch and his colleagues – and as we will see in the case of malaria. For Koch's postulates see Christoph Gradmann, A Harmony of Illusions. Clinical and Experimental Testing of Robert Koch's Tuberculin 1890–1900, in: Studies in History and Philosophy of Biological and Biomedical Sciences 35 (2004), 465–481, and id., Das Maß der Krankheit. Das pathologische Tierexperiment in der medizinischen Bakteriologie Robert Kochs, in: Cornelius Borck/Volker Hess/Henning Schmidgen (eds.), Maß und Eigensinn. Studien im Anschluß an Georges Canguilhem, Munich 2005, 71–90.

diseases common to the warm climate of the tropics.[16] But tropical medicine was more than the mere application of bacteriology to tropical diseases and in tropical regions. In his fundamental textbook *Tropical Diseases*, Patrick Manson explains that he employs the term "tropical" in a metrological sense of high atmospheric temperature.[17] Nearly all diseases are caused by germs demanding "certain physical conditions for their well-being," and in the tropics, one of these conditions was high temperature. Many tropical diseases were caused by parasites that "require for their transmission from one individual to another the services of a third and wholly different animal."[18] The pathogens and transmission of tropical diseases depended on the presence of favorable conditions and "the absence of unfavourable ones. Herein lies a vast field for study, and one which, as yet, has not been touched on by epidemiologists."[19] Therefore Manson suggested that a "student of medicine must be a naturalist before he can hope to become a scientific epidemiologist, or a pathologist […]".[20]

And what effect did the tropical environment and pathogen have on the experimental animal? In continental laboratories, scientists working with Robert Koch in Berlin and Louis Pasteur in Paris were busy constructing animal models in order to investigate the life cycle of bacteria, the transmission paths of diseases, and to prove that a specific pathogen was the cause of a specific disease.[21] The human-animal relationship in the laboratory became more complicated in experimental research on infectious diseases in the tropics. Although detailed knowledge on the life cycle of most tropic pathogens was still lacking, Manson pointed out that some parasites needed the services of third

16 For research on tropical diseases see for example David Arnold (ed.), Imperial Medicine and Indigenous Societies, Manchester 1988; John Farley, Bilharzia. A History of Imperial Tropical Medicine, Cambridge 1991; Randall M. Packard, The Making of a Tropical Disease. A Short History of Malaria, 2nd ed., Baltimore 2021; François Delaporte, The History of Yellow Fever. An Essay on the Birth of Tropical Medicine, Cambridge MA 1991; Ilana Löwy, Virus, moustiques et modernité. La fièvre jaune au Brésil, entre science et politiques, Paris 2001; Mari K. Webel, The Politics of Disease Control. Sleeping Sickness in Eastern Africa, 1890–1920, Athens 2019; Sarah Ehlers, Europa und die Schlafkrankheit. Koloniale Seuchenbekämpfung, europäische Identitäten und moderne Medizin 1890–1950, Göttingen 2019; Christos Lynteris (ed.), Framing Animals as Epidemic Villains. Histories of Non-Human Disease Vectors, Cham 2019, esp. the contributions of Maurits B. Meerwijk on tiger mosquitos; and Gabriel Lopes/Luísa Reis-Castro on *Aedes aegypti*.

17 See Patrick Manson, Tropical Diseases. A Manual of the Diseases of Warm Climates, New York 1898, xi.

18 Ibid., xii–xiii.

19 Ibid., xv.

20 Ibid., xvi.

21 Friedrich Löffler, for instance, a bacteriologist at the Imperial Health Office in Berlin, described extensively how he tested numerous species on their susceptibility on diphtheria, see Friedrich Löffler, Untersuchungen über die Bedeutung der Mikroorganismen für die Entstehung der Diphterie beim Menschen, bei der Taube und beim Kalbe, in: Mittheilungen aus dem Kaiserlichen Gesundheitsamte 2 (1884), 421–499; Axel C. Hüntelmann, Krank machen. Tierkrankheiten im Modell der bakteriologischen Forschung, ca. 1880–1910, in: Tierstudien 14 (2018), 83–95.

animals[22] not only as carriers, but also as a habitat for a certain stage of their life cycle. The interplay between humans and animals therefore became a sine qua non within the life cycle and evolution of the pathogens.

In November 1880, while working in Algeria, C.L. Alphonse Laveran observed a specific microorganism in the blood of patients suffering from malarial fever. In 1884, Laveran proclaimed that this microscopic parasite could also be found in numerous species, including mosquitos, and it was "widely distributed [...] in the blood of man and animals".[23] Some years before, Manson had made a similar observation in China: in blood samples of patients suffering from elephantiasis, a disease named for the enormous swelling it causes in the legs, he found microscopic, wormlike parasites blocking the blood vessels. Manson suspected mosquitos as transmitters because he found the same wormlike parasites in the abdomen of mosquitos that had previously bitten elephantiasis sufferers.[24] Thus, the idea of parasites, transmitted by mosquitos or other flying insects, was widely discussed in the mid-1890s.

While Manson was working on filariasis and Laveran on malaria, Ross was studying medicine in London and working as a ship's doctor. He passed his entrance examinations for the Indian Medical Service, and from 1881 to 1888, he worked as a medical officer in various places in India.[25] In 1888, Ross spent several months in Europe, studying bacteriology in London and acquiring a Diploma of Public Health. Upon his return to India, he became interested in infectious diseases of the tropics and in malaria. But in his laboratory abroad, Ross had difficulties identifying the organisms described by Laveran under the microscope. In April 1894, during another visit to England, he contacted Patrick Manson, who showed him within minutes the microorganism, so-called crescents, in a blood stain from a malaria patient. They remained in touch, discussed issues of tropical medicine, and Manson encouraged Ross to do further research.[26] Too many things were still unclear, and there were numerous theories about the mode and path of infection, as well as the role and interplay between human and mosquito in the parasite's life cycle.[27] Various organisms of different shapes were found in blood samples from malaria patients: pigmented, swarming and moving around,

22 Manson, Tropical Diseases (note 17), xv–xvi.

23 For the quote Richard Jones, Mosquito, London 2012, 90; see also Rubert Boyce, Mosquito or Man? The Conquest of the Tropical World, London 1909, 39; and Ross; Memoirs (note 10), 124–125.

24 See Boyce, Mosquito (note 23), chap. V; Jones, Mosquito (note 23), 87.

25 "[H]e was an ordinary medical officer, playing golf, fishing and shooting, and largely uninterested in his medical duties." See Bynum/Overy, Introduction, in: iid. (eds.), Beast (note 8), v–xxviii. For further information about Ross' life and work see Ross, Memoirs (note 10); Nye and Gibson, Ronald Ross (note 11).

26 Bynum/Overy, Introduction (note 8), xi–xii; and Ross, Memoirs (note 10), 128–129.

27 See, e. g., Ronald Ross, Surgn.-Lieut.-Col. Lawrie and the Parasite of Malaria, in: Indian Medical Gazette 31 (1896), No. 10.

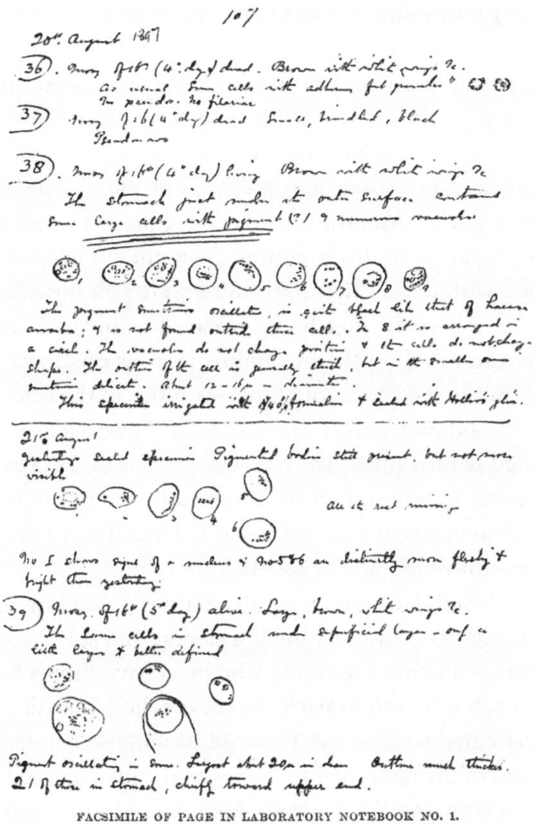

Fig. 1 Sketches from pigmented cells in a notebook of Ronald Ross', 1897.

with semilunar or flagellate bodies. Were these different organisms? How were they related to similar bodies observed in mosquitos?

Ross left London in March 1895 and returned to India, where he continued his research on malaria. We do not want to follow the numerous trials and errors, successes and failures, and the single steps in the epistemological process in the "discovery" of the infectious cycle of malaria transmission, but we want to follow Ross in his provisional laboratory, the clinical wards, into the outskirts of the places where he was stationed, and into the jungle with the mosquitos.

2. Mosquito: The Making of an Experimental Animal in the Tropics

Soon after his return to India, Ross found that one of his research objects resisted him and exerted its own idiosyncratic agency: while he soon located parasite specimens in the blood samples of a woman suffering from tertian fever, it was much more difficult with the mosquito. He caught three and put them into bottles, but they "were too frightened or otherwise un-willing to bite".[28] And the next day he realized that all his "mosquito grubs have been killed owing to my foolishly putting the bottles in the sun".[29] Two weeks later, Ross still struggled with difficulties: mosquitos were still unwilling to bite, and due to the heat, they "died shortly after being released from the bottle. Nothing I could do persuaded them to bite [...] the mosquitos [are] as obstinate as mules and myself nearly frenzied".[30] But in the course of his observations of the insects, Ross became familiar with their habits and preferences. He found out "how to make the insects bite; that is by wetting the bed & mosquito-net with water – this makes them hungry in the moment".[31] But his problems were not over: "I bottled him, smoked him (or rather *her*) and separated the abdomen just as you had described; but it was now so hot & dry again that the blood dried almost as soon as squeezed out".[32]

"Separating the abdomen", as Ross called it, or rather, the dissection of small insects was more difficult than dissecting humans or larger animals and required specialized experience and knowledge of the insect's anatomy. Manson, who must have shown him how to dissect insects, had had to teach this skill himself decades earlier: "I shall not easily forget the first mosquito, I dissected so charged. I tore off its abdomen, and by rolling a pen-holder from the free end of the abdomen to the severed end, I succeeded in expressing the blood the stomach contained."[33] In 1895, Ross could build on this experience when he described the process of dissection in detail.[34]

The context of Ross' research became clear one week and one letter later. He explained to Manson that he hated dry smears. He observed that staining blood samples "with a

28 Ross to Manson, Secunderabad 1 May 1895, in: Bynum/Overy (eds.), Beast (note 8), letter no. 2.

29 Ibid.

30 Ross to Manson, Secunderabad 15 May 1895, in: Bynum/Overy (eds.), Beast (note 8), letter no. 3.

31 Ibid.

32 Ibid.

33 See Boyce, Mosquito (note 23), 35; Jones, Mosquito (note 23), 87.

34 "A mosquito is dissected for examination of the stomach in this manner. A needle, held in the left hand, is passed through the thorax, the legs and wings are pulled off, and, if necessary, the scales of the body brushed off with a camelhair brush. The tail is then lowered into a drop of water, salt solution or weak formalin placed on a glass slide; and with another needle held in the right hand, the last two segments of the tail are partially separated and held down upon the slide. The left hand is then moved in such a manner as to draw away the insect. If done skillfully, the alimentary and generative apparatus will remain on the slide attached to the last two segments of the tail." Ronald Ross, Report on the Cultivation of Proteosoma, Labbé, in Grey Mosquitos, Calcutta 1898, 7.

water solution of methylene without fixing" produced a dry smear, in which the "cellular structure of the spherules was shown more clearly". He instead developed an alternative procedure:

> [I] gave the patient instructions to let the mosquitos fill themselves completely, while I provided myself with a small pair of tweezers with which I could squeeze out the mosquito's stomach with one hand, while I held the cover glass with the other, ready to clap on. The result was my first perfect specimen of mosquito blood.[35]

Malaria patients were put under a mosquito net – not to protect them from getting bitten by mosquitos, but the contrary: previously caught mosquitos were also put under the same net, and the patients were offered as a source of food.[36] As catching mosquitos at twilight was difficult and time-consuming, Ross began to breed his own – though not without setbacks: "Another disaster among my mosquito grubs owing to heat, I suppose. All dead."[37]

Soon, mosquitos transformed from a nuisance (though they still were this for the patients) into scientific objects and experimental animals. Ross learned soon how to breed and take care of them, how to protect them from sun and heat. As they became "laboratory" animals, they acquired individuality: after a few weeks of research, Ross started to number his mosquitos: "on looking through mosquito 19", and "I began with mosquito 20 of yesterday".[38] Additionally, even during the first months of research the borders between humans and animals as scientific object began to blur: in whose body were the round or semilunar parasites discovered, whose blood had been observed? Who was the scientific object: the human guinea pig under the net, or the mosquito in the bottle?

Although Ross had been unsuccessful in discovering the connection between mosquitos and the transmission of malaria (as a precondition to prove that the varying round, lunar-shaped, and flagellated bodies observed in the blood of malaria patients and mosquitos were the causal agents of malaria), he became an expert in breeding, feeding, and dissecting mosquitos, and in observing plasmodiae in the blood of humans and mosquitos.[39] Becoming an expert in the normal structure of the

---

35 Ross to Manson, Secunderabad 22 May 1895, in: Bynum/Overy (eds.), Beast (note 8), letter no. 4.

36 Ibid. Similarly, Manson had done in the 1870s, when he "placed a Chinaman who had the parasites in his blood under a mosquito net with hungry mosquitos", see Boyce, Mosquito (note 23), 35. Bynum/Overy note in their introduction (see note 8, xiii) that Ross and Manson using patients in a colonial setting as human guinea pigs were aware of ethical considerations.

37 Ross to Manson, Secunderabad 22 May 1895, in: Bynum/Overy (eds.), Beast (note 8), letter no. 4.

38 Ibid.

39 Despite his growing experience, new difficulties arose from time to time, for instance because Ross had to change the location or use other mosquito species: "As I suspected, my pots of water all yield brindled

mosquito's digestive system was a sine qua non for differentiating the normal from the pathological.[40] Then suddenly, in September 1895, he was ordered south to investigate a cholera outbreak in Bangalore, which left few opportunities for malaria research and occupied most of his time until the spring of 1897.[41] In April 1897, he was ordered to Ootacamund, where he and some of his servants contracted malaria, and where he stayed until June. After his recovery, he combined the typical leisure activities of an English gentleman like fishing with science examining water of mud and puddles in the jungle around Ootacamund. There, Ross found new types of mosquitos as well as cases of malaria, and he began to understand that mosquitos did not per se transmit malaria, but that the type of mosquito was important in the process of transmission. The "discovery" of this new mosquito species led to further investigations about its living conditions and environment.[42]

In June 1897, he returned to Secunderabad. Although he had been distracted by his work on cholera, he observed and described the varying and developing forms and bodies of the pathogen that was supposed to cause malaria. He now involved the new type of mosquito that he had observed in the jungles of Sigur Gat near Ootacamund and examined them carefully.[43] After Ross had "found some fair cases of crescents" in the mosquitos, he entered the "full tide of work again".[44] Each malariated mosquito had been dissected with utmost care, which took about two hours. Two weeks later, Ross

---

insects […]. I have a fair stock of these grey fellows & my quartan subject [quartan fever] is still going at the rate of 1 parasite to 1000 corpuscles (no quinine & little fever now owing to systemic toleration); but I cannot get the creatures to bite. […]. They sit stupidly on the net & won't touch the patient. I have bathed him, put him in the sun to bring his flavour out, & have kept him in the net for hours during the day & all night." Ross to Manson, Kherwara 8 February 1898, in: Bynum/Overy (eds.), Beast (note 8), letter no. 115.

40 See for instance his reflections on pigmented cells: "I first saw them; but a little reflection showed it to be extremely unlikely. If the cells be such they must be *physiological* cells, that is, *ordinary* cells of the mosquito's stomach capable of such action & should therefore be found in all, or in a large percentage at least, of mosquitoes. Such is distinctly not the case. I have *never* seen them in hundreds of brindled malariated mosquitoes; nor in scores of barred-back mosquitoes fed on crescents or healthy blood; or in numerous small dappled-winged mosquitoes fed on healthy blood." Ross to Manson, Kherwara 10 November 1897, in: Bynum/Overy (eds.), Beast (note 8), letter no. 100, emphasis Ross.

41 Bynum/Overy, Introduction (note 8), xiii–xvii; Ross, Memoirs (note 10); Nye/Gibson, Ronald Ross (note 11).

42 "I must track the habits of Silvestris a little more." Ross to Manson, Ootacamund 12 May 1897, in: Bynum/Overy (eds.), Beast (note 8), letter no. 69; Ross, Memoirs (note 10), 199–213.

43 Ross to Manson, Secunderabad 18 July 1897, in: Bynum/Overy (eds.), Beast (note 8), letter no. 81.

44 His research was guided by questions like: "Do healthy mosquitoes fed on malarial blood contain any parasite which similar mosquitoes fed on normal blood do not contain?" Was it possible to cultivate flagellulae in mosquitos, after they were fed on crescents? Ross to Manson, Secunderabad 27 July 1897, in: Bynum/Overy (eds.), Beast (note 8), letter no. 84; see also Ronald Ross, On some Peculiar Pigmented Cells found in two Mosquitos fed on Malarial Blood, in: British Medical Journal, 18 December 1897, 1786–1788.

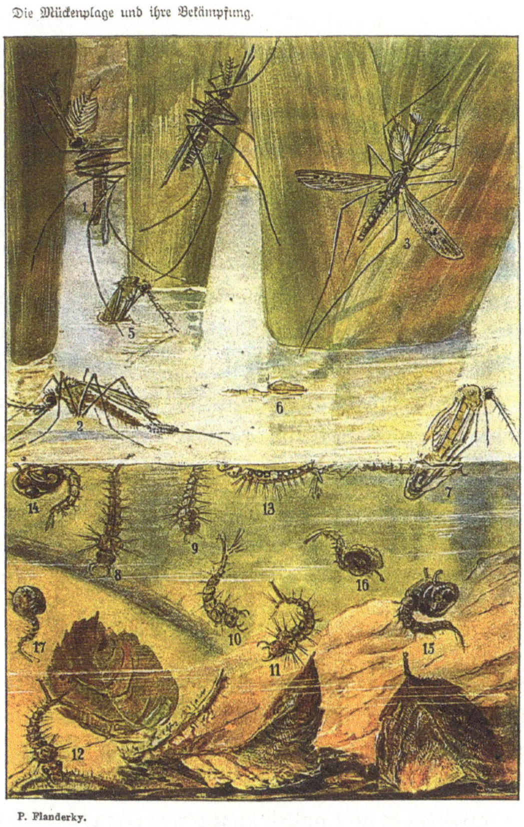

Fig. 2 The evolution and life cycle of a mosquito, contemporary illustration, 1911.

reported to Manson that he had "examined only 20 malariated & 4 non-malariated insects", although he had worked four to five hours a day.[45]

During Ross' intense interaction with the brindled, brown mosquitos, they became more and more valuable to him.[46] Not only did he spent much of his time on them, but they were also rare and hard to catch: "Unfortunately I can't get any more of those brown devils."[47] Due to their rarity, they were well-kept and fed. After they had been nurtured with the blood of malaria patients, they were killed, dissected, and their intestines examined under the microscope. In the stomach of malariated mosquitos, he observed

---

45 Ross to Manson, Secunderabad 4 August 1897, in: Bynum/Overy (eds.), Beast (note 8), letter no. 85.

46 "I have packed & posted the two specimens (worth £ 1000 each) and enclose the registration receipts." Ross to Manson, Bangalore 13 September 1897, in: Bynum/Overy (eds.), Beast (note 8), letter no. 92.

47 Ross to Manson, Secunderabad 18 July 1897, in: Bynum/Overy (eds.), Beast (note 8), letter no. 89.

numerous black cells that were different to "the usual very delicate stomach cells" of mosquitos fed with non-malariated blood.[48] With the two mosquitos left, dissected one day after another, he observed that these black cells had grown in number as well as in size. Previously, he had observed similar pigmented objects in the blood of malaria patients. He concluded that these pigmented bodies had to be the pathogen that caused malaria, in developing stages of evolution, circulating between human and mosquito. But before he was able to prove his hypothesis and investigate further, he was again ordered to different places in India, first to Kherwara, then to Calcutta.[49]

In Kherwara, Ross observed that the pigmented cells he had found in mosquito blood and conserved in formaline had turned "into clusters of black crystals which make it appear different to what it was at first & much more bulky & distinct". It meant that, even if he was able to explain the infectious cycle from mosquito to human, his proof had been falsified and he would be unable to demonstrate his results to a broader public:

> I tell you this to warn you that the pigment of the specimens which I sent you may have undergone a similar change; so don't be surprised if their pigment differs from the description of Smyth & myself & from that of the malaria parasite in man. I fancy formaline has some chemical action on pigment.[50]

And there were further problems ahead: "there is *no fever* here & I cannot go on with the work at present".[51] But the lack of human cases had the positive effect that Ross turned his attention to birds, so that alongside the parasite, the mosquito, and the human, a fourth party entered the "laboratory".

While he combined the leisure time activities of an English gentleman with his scientific research, shooting birds, he found *Halteridium*, a parasite later named *Haemorproteus*, in wild pigeons: "These are persecuted by a horrible kind of black horse-flies which live among their feathers", sucking "large quantities of blood from the poor birds". He suspected the flies of being the carrier of *Halteridium* and examined the blood in the

48 Ibid.

49 See Bynum/Overy, Introduction (note 8), xvi–xix; Ross, Memoirs (note 10), 240–290; Nye and Gibson, Ronald Ross (note 11). Ross first had feared that he would have been ordered to the battle front on active service, Ross to Manson, Bombay 27 September 1897, in: Bynum/Overy (eds.), Beast (note 8), letter no. 94.

50 Ross to Manson, Kherwara 12 October 1897, in: Bynum/Overy (eds.), Beast (note 8), letter no. 97.

51 Ibid., emphasis Ross; another complain in Ross to Manson, Kherwara 10 November 1897, in: Bynum/Overy (eds.), Beast (note 8), letter no. 100; and 14 December 1897 (no. 107): "I get only a very few cases of fever which turned out to be the mildest possible quartans with one or two parasites found with great difficulty in a whole specimen […] it is so cold that there is great difficulty in breeding mosquitoes at all, and, when hatched, they die as soon as they are let out of a bottle, & absolutely refuse to bite under the net […]."

stomach of thirty of them, where he found the parasite.[52] He assumed that the infectious cycle was closely related to that of malaria in humans.[53]

In February 1898, Ross moved to Calcutta, where he continued his research under much better conditions. There, he could use a small laboratory and, as he had been granted six months' research leave, focus on his scientific work.[54] However, it did not start very well. "I am having all sorts of petty difficulties at first," Ross complained to Manson. "It is of course a healthy season."[55] His only scientific "subject", a child, was so sick and anemic and "such a bad subject" that "I sent her away next day". His work as physician had turned upside down: it was not the severely ill child who caught his attention, but the "healthy" mosquitos.[56] While Ross was still struggling to explain the transmission path of malaria, Manson suggested he investigate malaria in birds, reminding him "that mosquitos bite birds and that the plasmodia of birds are just as likely to be conveyed through mosquitoes as are the plasmodia of man".[57] Ross followed his advice, enthusiastically reporting that he had "found active vermicules in mosquitos recently fed on a crow. [...] Numerous sparrows & larks contained no parasites. Got a new lot; also two pigeons & a crow." He "put them all in their cages in a net with a swarm of greys [mosquitos]".[58]

Over the course of several days, Ross fed mosquitos on the blood of various species of birds, but rarely found any suspicious bodies in the mosquitos' blood, except in those who had fed on three larks and one sparrow. On the night of 17–18 March, 1898, ten mosquitos were fed on these larks. Three days later, when Ross "judged these mosquitos to be ready", he killed and dissected them and found pigmented cells or clumps in most of their stomachs.[59] In the following days, he fed mosquitos on infected larks, and established a system of constant infection and re-infection (of fresh larks) to obtain malariated mosquitos in large numbers. These were dissected in increasing intervals (three, four, and five days after "feeding") – "one mosquito lived to 102 hours & was examined just now" – and their stomach and intestines investigated under the microscope.[60] He observed that the pigmented bodies grew in number and size with every additional day after feeding, and for some he "saw signs of sporulation" until they

52 Ross to Manson, Kherwara 21 January 1898, in: Bynum/Overy (eds.), Beast (note 8), letter no. 113.

53 Bynum/Overy, Introduction (note 8), xix.

54 Ross to Manson, Calcutta 2 March 1898, in: Bynum/Overy (eds.), Beast (note 8), letter no. 116.

55 Ross to Manson, Calcutta 9 March 1898, in: Bynum/Overy (eds.), Beast (note 8), letter no. 118.

56 Regarding Ross' and Manson's reflections on ethical considerations see Bynum/Overy, Introduction (note 8), xiii.

57 Still referring to Ross' unsuccessful experiments in Kherwara, Manson to Ross, London 7 February 1898, in: Bynum/Overy (eds.), Beast (note 8), letter no. 117.

58 Ross to Manson, Calcutta 9 and 15 March 1898, in: Bynum/Overy (eds.), Beast (note 8), letters no. 119 f.

59 Ross to Manson, Calcutta 21 March 1898, in: Bynum/Overy (eds.), Beast (note 8), letter no. 120.

60 Ibid.

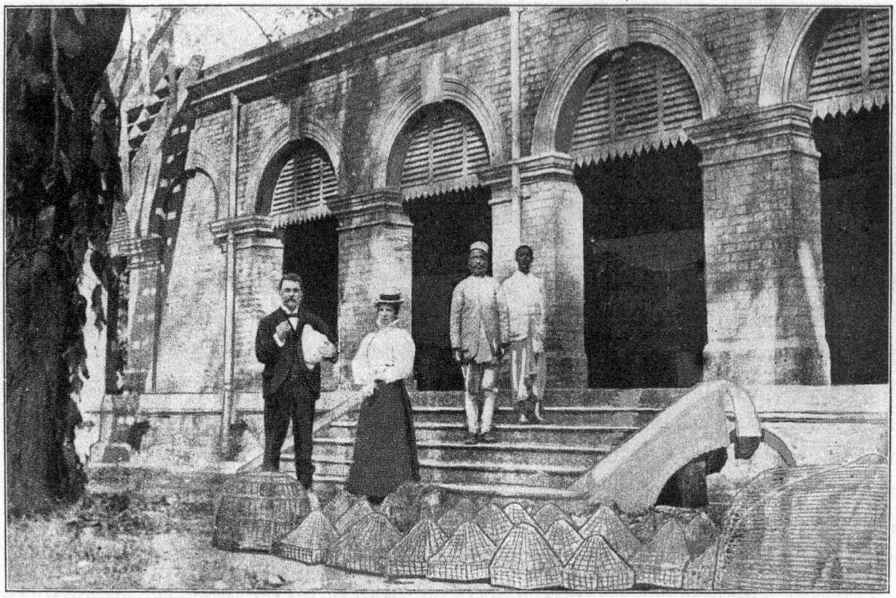

Fig. 3 Ronald Ross and Mrs Ross, together with assistants (one of them Mohamed Bux) outside the laboratory of the Calcutta Hospital, June 1898. The cages on the floor are for birds.

burst out, containing little oat-shaped bodies.[61] The final proof, according to Koch's postulates, that parasites were the causative agent and that infection took place in a complex evolutionary cycle between mosquito and human, was an experiment with a healthy sparrow (or at least free of malaria), and one who suffered severely from bird malaria. They both served as food source for freshly bred, parasite-free mosquitos. In this control experiment, Ross demonstrated that only the mosquitos that had fed on the sick sparrow developed black pigmented bodies – whereas the other group showed neither signs of infection nor any additional parasites. "Well, the theory is proved. Not a shadow of a doubt remains that we have found the alternative form of the gymnosporidia. The mosquito theory is a fact."[62]

But the epistemological process was not quite so simple. At first, Ross' research was interrupted again for some weeks in spring 1898 when he had to travel northwards to Punkarbari and Kurseong. Furthermore, the human-animal – or more concretely, the human-mosquito-bird – relationship ran into difficulties. In Calcutta, Ross had realized

61 Ibid.

62 Ross to Manson, Calcutta 12 April 1898, in: Bynum/Overy (eds.), Beast (note 8), letter no. 124; Ross, Memoirs (note 10), 259–279.

that mosquitos refused to bite, "or, what comes to the same for me, the birds learning some trick to keep them off."[63] And finally, the day before he was to leave Calcutta, most of his birds got ill and died, "carrying off all my proteosoma".[64] So Ross had to build a new stock of mosquitos that were "fed on proteosoma sparrows & another large stock fed on crows with halteridium".[65] But replenishing his supply of birds also proved difficult, so that he even had to ask the local government for help. Ross reported that he

> can't get a single bird with that parasite [protosoma]. I am nearly wild. Sparrows all round and can't catch them. [...] I and my man have practically failed; and now I have set the police and the district magistrate on it. Fancy the whole local Government trying to catch sparrows and failing![66]

Ross' lament continued in the next letter he sent to Manson in mid-May: the birds he was able to catch had no proteosoma, and the larks he received from Calcutta were dead.[67] He was in a "vein of bad luck",[68] and by the end of the month his work was brought to a stop by a plague scare. Medical men became an object of suspicion, especially Ross. One planter begged him not to work again, bird catchers bolted, and there were rumors about "a doctor sahib shooting coolies preparatory to inoculation!"[69] Furthermore, he was unable to examine infected mosquitos because it was too cold and rainy. Thus, Ross returned to Calcutta. There his work made progress. After several weeks, he was able to explain the whole infection cycle, having clarified the question of how the parasites were transferred from mosquito to human. He observed that the motile flagellae moved forward in the mosquito's body, finally settling in the salivary glands. From there, Ross concluded, they were transmitted to a bird or a human while the mosquito was sucking his or her blood.[70]

This detailed and somewhat tedious story of Ross' research on the transmission of malaria from mosquito to human – and vice versa – reflects Ross' own tedious, extended, and often unsuccessful scientific work and epistemological process. When Ross had began his research in 1895, the theory that malaria was transmitted by mosquitos was

---

63 Ross to Manson, Calcutta 12 April 1898, in: Bynum/Overy (eds.), Beast (note 8), letter no. 124.

64 Ross to Manson, Punkarbari 3 May 1898, in: Bynum/Overy (eds.), Beast (note 8), letter no. 126.

65 Ibid.

66 Ross to Manson, Punkarbari 9 May 1898, in: Bynum/Overy (eds.), Beast (note 8), letter no. 128.

67 Ross to Manson, Kurseong 16 May 1898, in: Bynum/Overy (eds.), Beast (note 8), letter no. 129.

68 Ibid.

69 Ross to Manson, Kurseong 30 May 1898; and Calcutta 13 June 1898, in: Bynum/Overy (eds.), Beast (note 8), letters no. 131 f.

70 See further letters of Ross to Manson from April to July 1898 in: Bynum/Overy (eds.), Beast (note 8); and Ross, Memoirs (note 10); id., Report on the Cultivation (note 34). Ross first described the transmission cycles in birds, later in humans.

still speculative. Ross himself knew very little about mosquitos and their life cycle, and realized that they did not behave and react as he expected: they did not bite, or died soon after being caught and housed in a bottle. Over time, Ross became familiar with the mosquitos' habits and preferences. Their life span and willingness to bite and suck patients' blood depended on many factors: time of day, climate, environment, humidity, temperature, and so on. He dealt with a single mosquito for hours: allowing them to get hungry and stimulate them to bite by wetting linen or the net, turning off the lights, and then, after feeding them with human (or later bird) blood, carefully squeezing out the sucked blood with a tweezer, dissecting the mosquito, and observing their stomach, guts, and blood under the microscope. Over time, while Ross was dealing with the mosquitos, they transformed into an experimental animal.

Despite – or because – of his epistemological detours and scientific failures, working day in and day out with mosquitos, Ross collected invaluable experience. During his countless observations of the mosquitos' stomach and guts, often lamented as an unsuccessful waste of time, he learned to see and recognize the normal structure of stomach tissue and was able to differentiate it from pathological structures. He was "so familiar with the mosquito's stomach that these bodies struck me at once". The black or dark brown of the pigmented bodies he eventually found in one mosquito's stomach were conspicuous because they were "not [the normal] blue, or yellow or greenish like the cell granules, debris etc."[71] It took two years, with interruptions, before Ross realized that a certain subspecies of mosquito – a "brown" mosquito (*Anopheles*) – was crucial in the evolutionary transmission process of infection and that this mosquito was at some places difficult to obtain: in his memoirs, Ross describes how he was lying in wait and stalking mosquitos, how specific mosquitos were caught at twilight in canals, puddles, or ponds. An even more delicate relationship was that between Ross and his human patients: they did not receive quinine, and he had to convince (and to pay: "for each bite a penny") them not to swat the mosquitos at night. Ross himself became a mosquito-like pest for these patients by pricking their fingers to obtain blood samples.

In early 1898, another party got involved. In the absence of human malaria cases, Ross had to deal with birds, modeling the human disease. He had to find out what species was (especially) susceptible to *Halteridium* (avian malaria), he had to organize the supply of and learn how to catch and treat birds, how to take blood samples, and how to arrange for mosquitos to feed on the birds within a controlled experimental setting. All these actors – a constantly transforming and reproducing plasmodiae (with different sexes and in different evolutionary states), specific types of mosquitos, human and avian patients – were essential in explaining the transmission of malaria. And all these actors – influenced by environmental factors, differing living conditions in rural

71 Ross to Manson, Secunderabad 22 August 1897, in: Bynum/Overy (eds.), Beast (note 8), letter no. 89.

and urban India, different (monsoon) seasons that affected their life cycles, well-being, and the presence of mosquitoes – had to be adjusted.

But further actors had to be considered as well. More important than the scientific object itself was the objective representation of the scientific proof.[72] This was even more important as the objective representation, the specimen, had to overcome time and space and convince Ross' scientific colleagues in Europe. But difficulties arose in the staining and preservation of the parasites and the production of specimens and their construction as proof: "That beastly formaline has ruined many of my specimens. Hope to have time to work with other preservatives today."[73] Descriptions and sketches of the microorganisms Ross had observed in the blood of humans and animals featured prominently in his correspondence with Manson, and when Ross sent specimen to him, supplementary instructions were meant to ensure that Manson could see what Ross had seen.[74]

3. International Research on Malaria and Mosquitos

Ross struggled not just with parasites, mosquitos, patients, and environmental factors, but also with competition from other scientists. Ross was only one of many members of the scientific community of bacteriologists (or life scientists working on tropical medicine) competing and cooperating with each other, discussing and publishing their

72 Thomas Schlich, „Wichtiger als der Gegenstand selbst". Die Bedeutung des fotografischen Bildes in der Begründung der bakteriologischen Krankheitsauffassung durch Robert Koch, in: Martin Dinges/Thomas Schlich (eds.), Neue Wege in der Seuchengeschichte, Stuttgart 1995, 143–174; id., Die Repräsentation von Krankheitserregern. Wie Robert Koch Bakterien als Krankheitsursache dargestellt hat, in: Hans-Jörg Rheinberger/Michael Hagner/Bettina Wahrig-Schmidt (eds.), Räume des Wissens. Repräsentation, Codierung, Spur, Berlin 1997, 165–190.

73 Ross to Manson, Calcutta 21 March 1898, in: Bynum/Overy (eds.), Beast (note 8), letter no. 120. In another letter to Manson he gave "a word of warning about the specimens [...] that is unsafe to come to conclusions at variance to mine [...]. I still use formalin, though much weaker, because, where it does not fill the specimen with crystals, it preserves the exact shape & look of the coccidia much better than glycerine & water, glyc. jelly etc. etc. But I don't know what it may do by the time the specimens reach England [...]." Ross to Manson, Calcutta 5 April 1898, in: Bynum/Overy (eds.), Beast (note 8), letter no. 122; see also Gradmann, Das reisende Labor (note 14). In Ross, Report on the Cultivation (note 34), 15, he gave detailed instructions on how to stain the parasite.

74 For instance: "I have prepared a number of specimens for you", and earlier in the letter: "Staining shows (a) that the cells take methylene blue [...] With all, when young, I find that each cell contains a number of deeper stained bodies like bullets in a bag", Ross to Manson, 30 March 1898, in: Bynum/Overy (eds.), Beast (note 8), letter no. 121. In general, regarding the process of cognition and learned experience of seeing, see the articles of Ludwik Fleck, Über die wissenschaftliche Beobachtung und die Wahrnehmung im allgemeinen (1935) and Schauen, sehen, wissen (1947) in: id., Erfahrung und Tatsache. Gesammelte Aufsätze, Frankfurt am Main 1983.

results. Moreover, (human) malaria was only one of many diseases transmitted by vectors; scientists studying sleeping sickness in Africa had similar experiences with gadflies.[75] In the late 1890s, for instance, Robert Koch researched malaria in Dar es Salaam (Tanzania), Neu Guinea, the Austrian Empire (Brioni, in present-day Croatia), and Italy.[76] Other important scientists working on malaria included C. L. Alphonse Laveran and especially Battista Grassi, who became a lifelong enemy of Ross as a result of their priority dispute over who was the first to have described the life cycle of the malaria parasite in humans and mosquitos, and the role of *Anopheles claviger* in the transmission of malaria.[77]

The Italian life scientist and zoologist Battista Grassi was, like Patrick Manson, an expert in the life of mosquitos. He had taken a different approach than Ross. Starting from the observation that there were areas with mosquitos, but no malaria, and that there was no area with malaria where mosquitos were absent, Grassi concluded that only a specific type of mosquito was able to transmit malaria. Thus, he systematically began observing malaria areas, mainly swampy areas in Italy. Grassi also visited areas free of malaria and regions where malaria was relatively rare. Mosquitos in these regions seemed to be unsuspicious, and Grassi was able to eliminate those species from his list of potential transmitters. In the end, only few species were left, and *Anopheles claviger* seemed to be the most promising candidate.[78]

Grassi started experimenting, using rural areas in Italy as a field laboratory. He bred *Anopheles claviger* and allowed the freshly hatched mosquitos, free of any plasmodiae, to suck the blood of healthy human animals – including Grassi himself. None of these subjects became infected. But a healthy human, exposed to *Anopheles claviger* that had previously been fed with malarial blood, soon showed clear symptoms of malaria.[79] Finally, Grassi undertook a larger experiment to verify his theory – and to prove the practical benefit of his scientific work. In the swampy area of Capaceio, populated by poor farming families as well as with large swarms of *Anopheles claviger*, and infamous for its high rate of malaria infections, Grassi selected two groups. One group sat outside at twilight as normal. The other group was instructed to cover their bodies properly

75 For research on sleeping sickness in the context of colonial politics and disease control see Wolfgang U. Eckart, Medizin und Kolonialimperialismus. Deutschland 1884–1945, Paderborn 1997; Hiroyuki Isobe, Medizin und Kolonialgesellschaft. Die Bekämpfung der Schlafkrankheit in den deutschen „Schutzgebieten" vor dem Ersten Weltkrieg, Münster 2009; Webel, Politics of Disease Control (note 16); and Ehlers, Europa und die Schlafkrankheit (note 16). Neither of the authors has a focus on the human-animal relationship.

76 See Bernhard Möllers, Robert Koch. Persönlichkeit und Lebenswerk, 1843–1910, Hannover 1950, 657–684.

77 While Ross described in 1898 the transmission cycle of malaria in mosquitos and birds, Grassi concluded in the same year that female *Anopheles claviger* transmitted malaria in humans, see Packard, Making (note 16), 114.

78 See Paul de Kruif, Mikrobenjäger, Zürich 1941, 268–299.

79 See ibid. and Francis E.G. Cox, History of the Discovery of the Malaria Parasites and their Vectors, in: Parasites & Vectors 3 (2010), Article 5.

with clothes (including gloves), not to leave their houses after twilight, and to cover the beds, windows, and doors with mosquito nets. While most of those who had continued their normal life, unprotected from mosquitos, got infected with malaria, in the other group (112 people in total), only five were infected.[80]

In the second half of the 1890s, mosquitos and gadflies became scientific objects and experimental animals. But they only rarely became laboratory animals in the tropics, where proper laboratories with a controlled artificial environment were rare. Ross, for instance, was delighted when he could use a small laboratory – meaning, focus on his scientific work – when he was ordered to Calcutta in February of 1898. Grassi, by contrast, was able to transfer and investigate his scientific objects in the university laboratories in Catania and Rome.[81] Robert Koch had been interested in malaria since his cholera expedition to Egypt and India in 1883/1884. Inspired by Ross' publications, he researched malaria more closely during an expedition to East Africa in 1897/1898, and in August 1898, he traveled to Italy to study malaria. After Koch returned to Berlin in October 1898, malaria work got more complicated. He was distracted by official work and, in the familiar environment of his laboratory, by organizing the supply of mosquitos: "My local sources of mosquitoes are running dry [...] and so I would very much appreciate it if you could send me a large number of living mosquitoes."[82] He wrote similar requests to friendly colleagues, asking for mosquitos from Germany, Italy, and German colonies – either alive or dead in formalin.[83] And while working with their research object, scientists in Europe gradually became familiar with their animal of choice, their preferences and habits,[84] how to keep them alive, how to kill and how to dissect them.[85]

---

80 Cox, History of the discovery (note 79); Kruif, Mikrobenjäger (note 78). Parckard, Making (note 16), highlights that although Malaria had disappeared in most Western European countries at the end of the nineteenth century, it remained a major health problem in Italy, 78–83.

81 G. Battista Grassi was Professor of Comparative Zoology at the University of Catania (Sicily) from 1883 to 1895 before becoming a professor at the University in Rome.

82 Robert Koch to Arnold Libbertz, 19 November 1898, quoted in Möllers, Robert Koch (note 76), 659.

83 See, e. g., letter to military surgeon Weiß, who was on his way to Africa, 10 January 1899; letters to Professor Bartolomeo Gosio in Rome; or letter of appreciation to military surgeon Karl von Vagedes, 19 November 1898, quoted in Möllers, Robert Koch (note 76), 659–663; the human cooperators are mentioned in Robert Koch, Die Bekämpfung der Malaria, in: Zeitschrift für Hygiene und Infektionskrankheiten 43 (1903), 1–4.

84 "Please, let somebody collect mosquitos every 14 days in Naccarese, and also in the hospital of Terracina. They will hardly be found in the wards now, the collector should search for mosquitos in cellars, under dry leaves, or in the grass." Robert Koch to Bartolomeo Gosio, 26 November 1898, quoted in Möllers, Robert Koch (note 76), 660, translation ACH.

85 "The mosquitos had been packed very suitably, only a few died during their journey, and the others were all the more lively; they began to bite only a few days after their arrival, whereas ours always took about 14 days before they got rid of their superfluous fat [sic] and became mobile again." Robert Koch to Arnold Libbertz, 19 November 1898, quoted in Möllers, Robert Koch (note 76), 659, translation ACH.

4. Shifting Value: From Precious Scientific Objects to a Pest and Public Health Threat

Requests for mosquitos were accompanied by information about (human) malaria cases, microscopical observations about parasites, theoretical reflections on transmission paths, and information about the biology, behaviors, and habits of mosquitos. But by the time Robert Koch had begun his experiments, the focus of research had already shifted to controlling and preventing malaria, that is, away from the role of mosquitos in malaria transmission to controlling mosquitos as vectors.

In February of 1899, Ross left India to become a lecturer in tropical medicine at the newly founded Liverpool School of Tropical Medicine. Founded and mainly funded by the ship owner Sir Alfred Lewis Jones, the Liverpool School set itself two major tasks: instructing medical students in tropical medicine and researching tropical diseases with a focus on disease control and prevention. Research expeditions were sent to port cities and coastal regions in the tropics where Jones' shipping company was active. The first expedition, led by Ronald Ross, went to Freetown in Sierra Leone (the capital of the British colony). Sierra Leone, according to the expedition's report, was selected because it was "much more malarious than India taken as a whole".[86] The expedition's aim was to turn the "discovery" of the infectious cycle of malaria into the "practical account for the better prevention of malarial fever".[87] The researchers aimed to get a full account of the living conditions of humans and mosquitos in Freetown – the "bionomics of the Culicidae" and *Anopheles* – and their encounters, including determining the number of malariated persons and the morbidity rate, as well as the efficacy of measures to control vectors and parasites.[88]

Some of these measures were drawn from Ross' own manual on the life and biology of mosquitos, published in 1899 as a summary of the knowledge he had collected in India.[89] After a short description of malaria, parasites and their relation to other organisms – "[m]en, animals, or plants in which parasites live are called their *hosts*" and some parasites employ "*a second species of animal* as a go-between"[90] – and the infectious cycle, Ross gave some "facts about mosquitos": how they develop from a larvae, found commonly in tubs of water, into adult winged insects. Adult mosquitos might live for months, "and have been kept alive in glass tubes for ten weeks". Important was the differentiation between sex and species: the male mosquitos living on fruit, only

86 Ronald Ross/Henry Edward Annett/E. E. Austen, Report of the First Malaria Expedition of the Liverpool School of Medicine and Medical Parasitology, Liverpool 1900, 7.

87 Ibid., 2.

88 Ibid.

89 Ronald Ross, Instructions for the Prevention of Malarial Fever. For the Use of Residents in Malarious Places, Liverpool 1899.

90 Ibid., 2, emphasis Ross.

the females suck blood. And after feeding on a human or animal, the female must fly to a pond or tub of water to lay her eggs – and return to feed again. Then, Ross differentiates and describes the various types of *Culicidae*, because only *Anopheles* carries malaria.[91]

This knowledge was now turned against the mosquitos.[92] In the chapter "How to Destroy Mosquitos", Ross gave detailed advice. "Now in order to kill mosquitoes in wholesale, it is necessary only to destroy their larvae."[93] Thus, the measures based on his knowledge that "[t]he larvae *must* live in water."[94] Consequently, "the first thing to do is to search carefully in and round the house for vessels and pools of water," but also in broken bottles, flower pots, cisterns, drains, or small ditches.[95] For the *Anopheles* larvae one had to search further afield: pools, rain-water puddles by the side of roads and paths, hollows in rocks, small ponds "or even in 'sloppy' ground amongst grass, or round stables or cattle byres". According to Ross, it was easy if one was trained and alert: "To find them we must simply *go and look for them*."[96] One only had to check these hatcheries regularly and empty all pots and vessels containing stagnant water and brush out small puddles.[97]

> As the larvae take about a week to a week to mature, this procedure will generally be enough to keep the insect away; but, at the same time, it is necessary to *prevent water collecting anywhere near the house*. These duties should be attended to by reliable persons, and *should not be left to native servants*. [...] Hence people can generally keep their houses comparatively free of these <u>pests</u> simply *by attending to their own premises*.[98]

Ross acknowledges that these actions might be difficult to execute in towns with crowded houses, where mosquitos might breed on nearby places like drains and water vessels. He laments that "great stupidity is shown in towns in warm countries with regard to the absence of all check to the breeding of mosquitos" and he suggests that "citizens should lay the matter strongly before municipalities; and all municipalities should employ at least one special agent for the destruction and prevention of mosquitos".[99]

91 Ibid., 6–7.

92 This reversal can also be observed in the chapter "How to avoid being bitten" (ibid), in contrast to numerous complaints in his letters to Manson that mosquitos are not willing to bite and his measures to make them bite.

93 Ibid., 12.

94 Ibid., 6, emphasis Ross.

95 Ibid., 11.

96 Ibid., emphasis Ross.

97 Ibid., 12.

98 Ibid., emphasis Ross. Only the term "pests" as a description of mosquitos is highlighted by the author.

99 Ibid., 12.

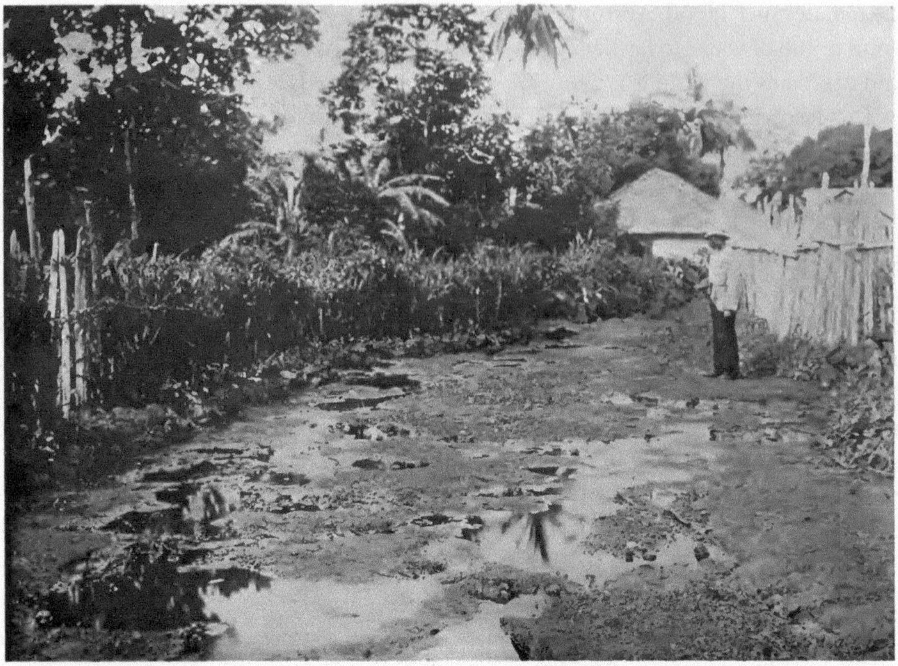

Pools Containing *Anopheles* Larvae.

Fig. 4 Eradication efforts in Sierra Leone. Illustration from Ross' *Instructions for the Prevention of Malarial Fever*, 1899.

But Ross and most experts on public health in the tropics had little confidence in the ability of the local municipalities to execute these measures properly. For this reason, the expedition's long-term aim was "to kill mosquitoes in wholesale". The expedition report presents the results and conclusions of the authors' research and preventative measures. An important aspect of prevention was economic: it was well-known that malaria had often been eradicated by cultivation and drainage of the soil, but these were "generally large and costly measures".[100] Simple measures, such as those suggested by Ross, were much cheaper and, as they relied on individual responsibility, they fit much better into the British liberal political system. In the case of the colonies, restricting public health or broader environmental measures – like the evacuation or drainage of stagnant pools of water, or their filling in with soil, and even the coverage of ponds with kerosine[101] – were also considered as necessary.

100 Ross/Annett/Austen, Report (note 86), 37.
101 Ibid., 40.

The same care that Ross once had devoted to breeding and maintaining mosquitos in India he now spent on chasing and killing them. The expedition to West Africa in 1899 had more the character of a survey, and the measures discussed to control malaria and destroy the vectors were intended as a proposal. This was not the case in another expedition to Sierra Leone in the summer of 1901, which aimed to systematically eradicate mosquitos as transmitters of tropical diseases. In his *First Progress Report of the Campaign against Mosquitoes in Sierra Leone*, Ross describes the campaign and its results.[102] Freetown had been selected "as site of the experiment" because malaria had already been investigated there, and because it was, due to heavy rainfall and the nature of the soil, a difficult environment, and therefore considered a test of the efficacy of Ross' recommended measures. In July 1901, shortly after Ross' arrival, thirty-two men were hired and equipped with carts and tools.[103] One group, mainly focusing on the habitat of *Culex*, collected "broken bottles and buckets, empty tins, old calabashes, and similar unconsidered vessels" from private houses. Another group, concentrating on the habitat of *Anopheles*, started "to drain the pools and puddles in the streets and the backyards" of houses.[104] The first group instructed occupants of houses how to recognize mosquito larvae and how to destroy their habitat by emptying vessels or dropping some oil on the surface of ponds. The second group brushed out small puddles with brooms; filled pools containing rainwater with soil; evacuated the water by building small channels in rocks; and in some cases, where drainage was not possible, pools were treated "with crude petroleum or creosote".[105] These tasks were repeated and, amid the deluge of rain, must have been a Sisyphean task. Nevertheless, Ross reported, that "many of the worst streets were fairly well drained in a few weeks". Altogether, he calculated, during the summer, 6,500 houses and nine-tenths of the town had been cleared, and over a thousand cartloads of rubbish collected. As the dry season started, Ross expressed his hope that the measures had been successful. He declared that the number of mosquitos in the streets was diminishing and that it was "exceedingly difficult to find Anopheles now".[106]

Similar measures were also suggested by the Imperial Health Office in Germany. The brochure *Die Mückenplage und ihre Bekämpfung* (The mosquito plague and its control) advised systematically destroying the breeding sites of mosquito larvae. In addition to filling or draining pools and adding oil and petroleum to open, stagnant water, it also suggested fumigating interior spaces to eradicate adult mosquitos. The authors of the

102 Ronald Ross, First Progress Report of the Campaign against mosquitoes in Sierra Leone, Liverpool 1901.

103 The number of workers had been increased to 53 until the end of summer, and Ross expressed his hope that for future works "a hundred or more men" will be employed, see Ross, First Progress Report (note 102), 5–8, esp. 8.

104 Ibid., 5.

105 Ibid., 6–7.

106 Ibid., 7–9, the quote 9.

brochure stressed that a systematic and long-term approach was necessary to control the outbreak of infectious diseases transmitted by mosquitos or flies.[107]

Aimed at a wider readership, the German brochure explained the need for these measures. According to its authors, in some areas of Germany, mosquitos had become a real annoyance. Swarming in large numbers during the summer, they prevented people from sleeping and exhausted the working population. These swarms had not only been detrimental to individuals, but had also led to economic losses in some areas, such as public baths and recreational forests. Although disease-transmitting mosquitos were rare in Germany, the brochure explained,[108] flies and gnats could also be a source of endemic and tropical illnesses. The common housefly, for instance, was able to transmit typhoid fever, as another brochure issued by the Imperial Health Office later stated.[109] And weren't cholera and plague imported from the tropics? Since malaria cases in the German Empire had been recorded and summarized in medical statistics,[110] public health officials may also have feared the disease's incursion into Western Europe.

Beside information about the habitat, biology, development, and "natural history" of mosquitos and flies, as well as instructions on how to eradicate them and their larvae, brochures by the Liverpool and London Schools of Tropical Medicine or the Imperial Health Office in Germany implicitly contained three further messages. First, there was an economic incentive to control and prevent malaria and other tropical diseases. For shipowners and sponsors like Alfred L. Jones, this correlation must have been clear. Campaigns against mosquitos, even if they involved a large number of men to collect vessels or to build drainage channels, might pay off over the long term and were an investment in public health. Second, investments in public health were necessary to keep the (white) population healthy, especially in the colonies. The role of diseases in war and conflict became obvious during the Second Boer War (1899–1902), when plague and typhoid fever weakened the British troops. Thirdly, controlling and preventing (tropical) diseases was a question of progress and modernization. For example, Ross wrote that in spite of the great stupidity of towns in warm countries[111] and their inability to control and prevent malaria, progress had been in the British colonies, but also in Germany, albeit insufficiently in rural areas.[112]

---

107 Kaiserliches Gesundheitsamt (ed.), Die Mückenplage und ihre Bekämpfung, Berlin 1911.

108 Ibid., 5–6.

109 Reichsgesundheitsamt (ed.), Die Fliegenplage und ihre Bekämpfung, Berlin 1927.

110 A. Schuberg, Das gegenwärtige und frühere Vorkommen der Malaria und die Verbreitung der Anophelesmücken im Gebiete des Deutschen Reiches, in: Arbeiten aus dem Reichsgesundheitsamt 59 (1928), 1–428.

111 See Ross, Instructions (note 89), 12.

112 This is illustrated in a sketch of an old-fashioned-looking farmhouse on the first pages in Kaiserliches Gesundheitsamt (ed.), Fliegenplage (note 109). As national campaigns to eradicate Aedes aegypti became a core political aim to modernize Brazil in the beginning of the twentieth century, see Gabriel Lopez/

5. Conclusion: The Changing Human-Mosquito Relationship in Malaria Research

This chapter has traced the shifting ontological status of mosquitos within the changing relationship between humans and animals: how mosquitos evolved from a nuisance to a valuable research object, and then to a pest, a beast, an epidemic villain, and a threat to public health.

For Ross and other scientist working on malaria, mosquitos became valuable research objects. They took care of them, studied their habits, and after killing them they developed an afterlife as specimen, in notes, tables, and articles. In the theory about the transmission of malaria, they played an indispensable part in the making of a tropical disease. Using the example of Ronald Ross' malaria research, the chapter has focused on the human-animal relationship within this process of knowledge production: how Ross learned to treat mosquitos, how he became familiar with their normal physiological structure before he was able to differentiate the normal from the pathological. Bacteriological research in the tropics also forced Ross to familiarize himself with a different laboratory and research environment: cultivating microorganisms, staining and preserving parasites in formalin, and producing specimen all differed from what he had learned in England. Whereas his colleagues in Europe had difficulties procuring a supply of mosquitos, he had difficulties in procuring formalin, dyes, and scientific literature.

During the process of knowledge production and human-animal entanglement, medical principles were turned upside down in two ways. First, Ross did not focus on human patients, but on the mosquito and the parasite. For the human patients, Ross became a kind of collaborator with the pest. Instead of using mosquito nets to protect them from being bitten, he placed them *together* with mosquitos under the net as a food source, and in addition, he frequently pricked their fingers to draw blood samples. Second, the roles of humans and microorganisms, of colonizers and colonized, were exchanged. The European colonizers were themselves colonized by tropical pathogens and these, in turn, threatened to colonize Europe. Against this backdrop parasites and their vectors were considered a public health threat. In the measures used to control and prevent malaria, the experience and knowledge Ross had acquired about mosquitos during his research – of catching, caring, cultivating – were turned on their head, the aim now being to eradicate them.

But within the human-animal relationship, the role of the human companion and the entire research program also changed. Although in India, Ross enjoyed the leisure time activities of an English gentleman, like playing golf, fishing, and hunting, these

---

Luísa Reis-Castro, A Vector in the (Re)Making: A History of *Aedes aegypti* as Mosquitoes that Transmit Diseases in Brazil, in: Lynteris (ed.), Framing (note 16), 147–175.

activities were not strictly separated from his duties as medical officer and scientific researcher, which had him fishing for mosquito larvae and catching birds that suffered from bird malaria. He became a mosquito and microbe hunter, first in his search for the causal agent of malaria as described by Paul de Kruif, and second when he aimed to kill and destroy them. And the whole endeavor changed: what started as isolated and often interrupted research in India by merely one man, supported only by some servants and faraway correspondence partners, became a global campaign, aiming to eradicate mosquitos in the colonies and in Europe. And the men who organized these campaigns, who went after mosquitos on costly expeditions, fighting the beasts, transformed into, and were described, celebrated, and styled themselves as national and "cultural" heroes in the battle of "Mosquito or Man?"[113]

Photo credits

Fig. 1 Sketches from pigmented cells in a notebook of Ronald Ross 1897. Ronald Ross, Memoirs. With a Full Account of the Great Malaria Problem and its Solution, London 1923. Public domain.

Fig. 2 The evolution and life cycle of a mosquito. Illustration from Kaiserliches Gesundheitsamt (ed.), Die Mückenplage und ihre Bekämpfung, Berlin 1911. Wellcome Library, London/Public domain.

Fig. 3 Ronald Ross and Mrs Ross together with assistants outside the laboratory of the Calcutta Hospital, June 1898. Photograph from Ronald Ross, Memoirs. With a Full Account of the Great Malaria Problem and its Solution, London 1923. Wellcome Library, London/Public domain.

Fig. 4 Eradication efforts in Sierra Leone. Illustration from Ronald Ross, Instructions for the Prevention of Malarial Fever. For the Use of Residents in Malarious Places, Liverpool 1899. Public domain.

Abstract:

The relationship between human scientists and animals changed fundamentally with the laboratory revolution of the nineteenth century. With the birth of bacteriology, microorganisms became the smallest but most dangerous enemies of humans and animals. Since the late 1870s, tropical physicians had suspected that some pathogens might also be transmitted by mosquitos or flies. Until then, mosquitos, gadflies, or

113 See the book titles of Boyce, Mosquito or Man? (note 23); Kruif, Mikrobenjäger (note 78); or Wilhelm von Drigalski, Männer gegen Mikroben. Pest, Cholera, Malaria und ihre Verwandten in Geschichte und Leben, Berlin 1951; and Maurits Bastiaan Meerwijk, Tiger Mosquitoes from Ross to Gates, in: Lynteris (ed.), Framing (note 16), 119–146.

flies had been considered – at worst – a nuisance. As suspicion grew that flying insects carried disease, the relationship between humans and these animals changed. Using the example of Ronald Ross and his research on malaria in India, the chapter analyses the entangled relationship of mosquitos – as laboratory animals – with their human companions; their roles and agency before, during and after an experiment; and how the ontological status of these animals changed as a function of their relationship with humans. The chapter traces the shifting ontological status of mosquitos within the changing human-animal relationship, showing how mosquitos were transformed from a nuisance to a valuable object of research and then to a pest, an epidemic villain, and a threat to public health.

Keywords:
mosquitos | malaria | experimental animals | tropical medicine | Ronald Ross

Jules Skotnes-Brown

Rats, Removals, and Redevelopment

Plague in Port Elizabeth, 1938

On 23 March 1938, bubonic plague re-emerged in Korsten, a freehold multi-racial township on the outskirts of Port Elizabeth (now Gqeberha). Jane Thys, an African woman who lived on Curtis Street took violently ill and was transferred to the Formidable Epidemic Diseases Hospital – an old and dilapidated structure on the outskirts of the city.[1] Later that day, her son George Gama was found "ill with a bubo in the groin".[2] That evening, another African woman called Nonina Toobi was also found to be infected. Over the next few months, this cluster of cases slowly grew and by August, there had been 22 confirmed cases and 16 deaths.[3] Despite this small caseload, the outbreak of bubonic plague – a much dreaded disease – provoked a dramatic state response. Officials feared that plague was endemic in Korsten and that should they need to quarantine Port Elizabeth, commerce would grind to a halt.[4] Terrified white citizens thronged medical doctors with requests for anti-plague vaccines,[5] and demanded that buses be segregated to escape what they described as the "ordeal" of sitting next to "some diseased person".[6]

---

1 D.L. Ferguson, The 1938 Outbreak of Plague in Port Elizabeth, in: South African Journal of Laboratory and Clinical Medicine, 18 (1963), 118–121, 119. – I would like to thank the editors for their extremely helpful feedback on this chapter. I thank also the participants in the "Animals and Epidemics" conference in 2022 for stimulating discussions and conversations. Finally, I am grateful to Christos Lynteris, Oliver French and Matheus Alves Duarte da Silva for their comments on an early version of this draft.
Funding ID: Research leading to this article was funded by the Wellcome Trust (Grant No. ID 217988/Z/19/Z) for the project "The Global War Against the Rat and the Epistemic Emergence of Zoonosis".

2 Louis Fourie to Secretary of Public Health, Plague Port Elizabeth, 28 August 1938, Western Cape Archives and Records Service (WCARS), 3/PEZ, 4/1/1/1326.

3 Ibid.

4 On endemicity of plague in Port Elizabeth: Minutes of Proceedings of Council-in-Committee, Special Meeting Held 11 April 1938, 3/PEZ 4/1/1/1326; Duncan Ferguson to Port Elizabeth Town Clerk, 30 May 1938, 3/PEZ, 4/1/1/1326; Notes of Proceedings of Special Committee re[garding] Outbreak of Plague, Meeting held on 18 July 1938, 3/PEZ, 4/1/1/1326; Extract from Minutes of proceedings of Council; 3 August 1938, 3/PEZ, 4/1/1/1326.

5 Minutes of Proceedings of the Special Committee re[garding] Outbreak of Plague in the City, 12 April 1938, 3/PEZ, 4/1/1/1326; Notes of Proceedings of Special Committee re[garding] Outbreak of Plague in the City, 12 April 1938, 3/PEZ, 4/1/1/1326.

6 Mixed Omnibuses and Public Health, in: Eastern Province Herald, 29 March 1938, 8.

Meanwhile, opponents of segregation condemned the plague scare as little more than a convenient excuse to rid Korsten of its Black residents.[7]

Although Black, Coloured,[8] and some white people challenged the condemnation of their homes and neighbourhood as pathological, the outbreak led to the eviction of 3,145 people and the resettlement of 508 in McNamee Village, an allegedly plague-proof, segregationist "utopia".[9] The removals, however, failed to solve sanitary problems and became a point of great bitterness amongst former residents of Korsten, many of whom were unconvinced that plague had ever existed in the neighbourhood.

The story of plague in Port Elizabeth is an example of how the materiality of plague epidemiology shaped the physical landscape of the city, as well as medical assumptions about rats, fleas, and *Yersinia pestis* (the causative microorganism of plague). Many medical historians of South Africa have been influenced by Maynard Swanson's classic 1977 argument, "The Sanitation Syndrome". Here, Swanson argued in the context of the early twentieth-century Cape Town and Port Elizabeth plague outbreaks that the presence of plague provided a convenient scapegoat for the forced removal of African people from the city centre. In Cape Town, Africans were blamed for the outbreak, their homes destroyed, and contents incinerated under the aegis of the "sanitation syndrome" – the equation of "black urban settlement, labour and living conditions with threats to public health and security".[10] With few exceptions, they were evicted to Uitvlught, a plague quarantine camp, which was later converted into a "native location". Historians of South Africa have subsequently found the "sanitation syndrome" a useful concept to explore the relationship between sanitation and segregation in other parts of the country.[11] It is undoubtable that the sanitation syndrome played a significant role in shaping plague control in Port Elizabeth also, and I do not in any way dispute these

7 See interviews with Korsten residents quoted in Janet Mary Cherry, A Blot on the Landscape and Centre of Resistance. A Social and Economic History of Korsten, BA Hons Thesis, Cape Town, University of Cape Town, 1988, 47–56.

8 A distinct racial identity in South Africa which, although rejected by some, remains in common use. It refers to mixed-race people with a combination of European, Asian, Khoisan, and/or Nguni ancestry. See Mohammad Adhikari, Burdened by Race. Coloured Identities in Southern Africa, Cape Town 2009.

9 Statistical Report on Housing and Slum Elimination in City of Port Elizabeth, 1 July 1934–30 September 1938, City Health Department, Port Elizabeth, 20 October 1938, 3/PEZ, 1/3/2/6/12.

10 Maynard W. Swanson, The Sanitation Syndrome. Bubonic Plague and Urban Native Policy in the Cape Colony, 1900–1909, in: The Journal of African History 18/3 (1977), 410.

11 Elizabeth van Heyningen, Public Health and Society in Cape Town, 1880–1910, PhD Thesis, Cape Town, University of Cape Town, 1989; Sharon Caldwell, Segregation and Plague. King William's Town and the Plague Outbreaks of 1900–1907, in: Contree 29 (1991); Howard Phillips, Epidemics. The Story of South Africa's Five Most Lethal Human Diseases, Athens 2012, 38–67; Gary Fred Baines, New Brighton, Port Elizabeth c.1903–1953. A History of an Urban African Community, PhD Thesis, Cape Town, University of Cape Town, 1994, 30; Cherry, Blot (note 7), 18.

claims.[12] However, additional "pathological" factors that have been understudied such as architecture, infrastructure, and animals also shaped Port Elizabeth's plague control and forced removals.

This article examines how the more-than-human dimensions of Korsten – its architecture, materiality, human residents, animals, and insects – shaped the control of plague.[13] Here, I draw upon two historiographical influences. Firstly, I follow the lead of plague historians who have emphasised the epistemological, material, and environmental aspects of urban plague control.[14] Secondly, I draw upon Jonathan Saha, who has shown how British imperialists in Myanmar were both disgusted and fascinated by the allegedly "excessive intimacies of Burmese encounters with animals".[15] My argument is that colonial sanitarians took both the materiality of Korsten and the alleged presence of disgust-provoking intimacies between rats, humans, and fleas within the neighbourhood as justification for draconian epidemiological interventions. These connections between diseased animals and humans, facilitated by allegedly pathological architecture, in addition to broader concerns about the mixing of races, enabled officials to demolish much of Korsten. This happened despite protests from residents and evidence of infected rats in greater numbers in other parts of the city.

1. Korsten: An Infected and Infective Neighbourhood

Korsten in the 1930s was "home 'for the poor of all races'", and a site of working-class solidarity that posed a challenge to prevailing segregationist sentiments.[16] According to a survey conducted in August 1937, of 1,522 premises in the area, 827 were occupied

12 For example, Medical Officer of Health (MOH) Duncan Ferguson, was pro segregation and explicitly advised that authorities create three new areas for "Europeans", "Coloureds", and "Natives" on the grounds of public health. "The Medical Officer of Health Reports on 2nd August, 1938", 3/PEZ, 1/3/2/6/11.

13 For the term more-than-human see Sarah Whatmore, Materialist Returns. Practising Cultural Geography in and for a More-than-Human World, in: Cultural Geographies 13/4 (2006), 600–609; Donald's gloss of more-than-human geography is helpful for my historical case study. She defines more-than-human geography as "concerned with the multiplicity of agentive actors in space and place". Megan Donald, When Care Is Defined by Science. Exploring Veterinary Medicine through a More-than-human Geography of Empathy, in: Area 51/3 (2019), 470–478.

14 For example, Prashant Kidambi,"An Infection of Locality". Plague, Pythogenesis and the Poor in Bombay, c. 1896–1905, in: Urban History 31/2 (2005), 249–267; Robert Peckham, Hong Kong Junk. Plague and the Economy of Chinese Things, in: Bulletin of the History of Medicine 90/1 (2016), 32–60; Christos Lynteris, A Suitable Soil. Plague's Urban Breeding Grounds at the Dawn of the Third Pandemic, in: Medical History 61/3 (2017), 343–57; Zachary Fleishman, Waste, Reclamation and the Production of Racialised Space in Cape Town, 1882–1913, in: South African Historical Journal 73/1 (2021), 162–186.

15 Jonathan Saha, Among the Beasts of Burma. Animals and the Politics of Colonial Sensibilities, c. 1840–1940, in: Journal of Social History 48/4 (2015), 919.

16 Cherry, Blot, (note 7), 34.

"solely by Natives", 378 "solely by Coloured", 179 "occupied by Coloured and Native", and the remaining 138 were "occupied by others" such as whites, Indians, Chinese people, or were church buildings. Of some 19,571 residents, 13,763 were "Native", 5168 "Coloured", and the remaining 640, "Other".[17] A large portion of its population were victims of a series of forced removals that took place in the context of a previous plague outbreak of 1901. Then, officials quickly correlated Black inner-city "locations" with outbreaks of the disease and evicted their residents without providing alternate accommodation. Many, dependent on work within Port Elizabeth, chose to move to Korsten, rather than the under-construction segregated neighbourhood New Brighton, where officials hoped they might settle. The status of Korsten as a freehold village enabled anyone with sufficient funds – whether white or Black – to purchase property and live in the area. By comparison, New Brighton property could not be purchased, it was under police surveillance (which probably meant constant harassment), and location authorities enforced various restrictions against African movement, economic activity, and alcohol brewing. Moreover, New Brighton was further out of town, had higher rents, and its rail fares into town were more expensive.[18]

Korsten's status as a rapidly growing freehold village without much town-planning or council oversight also meant that slum landlordism was rife. Only a small percentage of Korsten properties were owned by Black and Coloured people: 15.32% and 13.52% respectively. The remainder of the land was owned by a small number of white and Asian residents, organisations, as well as white slumlords like Sidney Wells, who owned some 28% of the land in Korsten.[19] Wells was known for making a fortune out of the 1901 forced removals. In 1902, he purchased "large blocks of erven at Korsten", which he subdivided into small plots, and sold many of these to Africans at a monthly rate with interest of 5%.[20] Many of the homes constructed in this area were built hastily from scrap materials, and without council oversight as the recently evicted Africans scrambled to find new accommodation.[21]

Owing to such conditions, an outbreak of plague had long been feared in Korsten. As early as 1934, Port Elizabeth Medical Officer Duncan Ferguson had already predicted that Korsten would pose a serious menace to the city in the event of a plague outbreak as its "mixture of races" and "very poor" housing conditions would make an "epidemic of

17 Report of Medical Officer of Health to Housing and Slum Elimination Committee, 10 August 1937, 3/PEZ 4/1/1/1326.

18 Baines, New Brighton (note 11), 46–47; Joyce F. Kirk, A "Native" Free State at Korsten. Challenge to Segregation in Port Elizabeth, South Africa, 1901–1905, in: Journal of Southern African Studies 17/2 (1991), 316–324.

19 Report of Medical Officer of Health (note 17).

20 "Housing and Slum Elimination Committee Meeting, 6th May 1938", 3/PEZ, 1/3/2/6/10.

21 Kirk, '"Native" Free State' (note 18), 317–318.

plague or typhus fever" "difficult to control..."[22] Such an outbreak would cause enormous problems because Korsten was connected to the sinews of capital that stretched between the Port Elizabeth docks and the Indian Ocean World. Port Elizabeth was, in this period, a rapidly developing industrial manufacturing centre, and the third largest port of the country, which exported goods across the sub-continent, and internationally via its docks.[23] Many of its dock and factory workers lived in Korsten,[24] and their commutes to and from work provided a route for *Yersinia pestis* to travel across local and international trade networks.

Hence, as early as 1934 Port Elizabeth embarked on a vast slum clearance project, which aimed to redevelop Korsten through categorising properties as unfit for human habitation and flagging them for demolition or serving notices to property owners to repair defective premises.[25] The council aimed to eliminate the supposed health and ideological nuisance posed by Korsten by relocating its Black residents to a new model location, McNamee Village within the suburb of New Brighton, for which the construction of 3,000 houses commenced in November 1937.[26] Ferguson was closely involved in this project and was tasked with inspecting and reporting on the sanitary condition of each property in the area. Although such slum clearance had started before the outbreak of plague, it intensified once the disease was detected. Between 1934 and 1937, some 1,217 rooms were flagged for demolition, and 121 for repair. 525 occupants were "rehomed". By comparison, in January to September 1938 alone, 781 rooms were flagged for demolition and 49 for repair.[27] Ferguson's reports on these properties paint a picture of white middle-class disgust at the conditions in which Korsten tenants supposedly lived. Unfit "for human habitation", these buildings were routinely described as "in a state of collapse", being smeared with "filth and grime", having ceilings of "filthy sacking", walls of "newspaper" and "'Dagga' [cannabis] joints",[28] floors of "earth", and a lack of running water, toilets, or separate kitchens. The only beings that these houses provided an adequate home to, in Ferguson's opinion, were rodents and insects.

Given these allegedly unsanitary conditions, when plague broke out, Korsten was immediately assumed to be widely infected, and the state response was draconian. Firstly, those residents infected with plague and all their recent contacts were lined up,

---

22 Ferguson, 1934, quoted in Louis Fourie to Secretary for Public Health (note 2).

23 Notes of sub-committee appointed to interview representatives of location authorities re[garding] anti-plague measures, 11 June 1937, 3/PEZ, 4/1/1/1326.

24 Sarah Hudleston/George Mnyalaza Milwa Pemba, George Pemba, Against All Odds, Johannesburg 1996, 18.

25 Baines, New Brighton (note 11), 59–60.

26 Ibid.

27 Statistical Report on Housing and Slum Elimination (note 9).

28 Case No. 95. No. 17, Dobson Street and Nos. 17, 19 and 21, Brassel Street, MOH Report 30 May 1938, 3/PEZ, 1/3/2/6/11.

vaccinated, and transferred to the Formidable Epidemic Diseases Hospital.[29] As humans who had been contaminated by the presence of rats, their bodies were treated with the same chemicals used to kill fleas on rats captured for laboratory analysis. Oral histories conducted by Vista University Students in 1987 with elderly former residents of Korsten,[30] attest that suspected or confirmed plague sufferers were vigorously disinfected. Those thought to have been in contact with rats were "dipped in a substance like oil claimed to be an antiseptic".[31] At other times, they were subjected to "great degradation": stripped naked and "greased" with paraffin emulsion[32] in front of their children.[33] At times, authorities also shaved their heads and "hairy parts".[34] At the hospital, a camp was erected to house the victims divided by those diagnosed with or recovering from plague, and those who were contacts of plague sufferers.[35] Patients were held here for a minimum of twelve days,[36] but were at times kept for up to five months.[37]

Secondly, Ferguson's department in collaboration with officials from the national Department of Public Health, sought to modernise Korsten through rat-proofing all houses in the neighbourhood and condemning those that could not be rat-proofed for destruction. Rat-proofing involved retrofitting homes to prevent rodents from entering them through architectural interventions which aimed to block any potential ingress or egress of rats. Virtually all houses in the neighbourhood were also subjected to vigorous fumigation. Those homes that were thought to be too dilapidated to make these alterations or worth less than the cost of rat proofing, were incinerated.[38]

Thirdly, any furnishings or household wares that could not be carried by plague sufferers and their contacts to the hospital were condemned as potential rodent and flea harbourages. Residents of Korsten were advised to "boil all blankets and personal clothing in order to rid them of fleas".[39] Other materials, such as some 1,600 tonnes of

---

29 50,000 people were given two doses of plague vaccine. Ferguson, 1938 Outbreak of Plague (note 1), 120; Louis Fourie to Secretary of Public Health (note 2).

30 Baines notes that these interviews were conducted by Vista University Students. Unfortunately, they have since been lost or destroyed. My thanks to Gary Baines for his assistance in establishing this. Baines, New Brighton (note 11), 116.

31 Cherry, Blot (note 7), 51.

32 Ferguson, 1938 Outbreak of Plague (note 1), 119.

33 Secretary of Korsten Vigilance Committee, 36, Durban Road Writes on 19 July 1938, 3/PEZ, 1/3/2/6/11. See also "one black man", quoted in: Cherry, Blot (note 7), 55.

34 Ferguson, 1938 Outbreak of Plague (note 1), 119.

35 Notes of Proceedings of the Special Committee Appointed in Connection with the Outbreak of Plague, 3 June 1938, 3/PEZ 4/1/1/1326.

36 Ferguson, 1938 Outbreak of Plague (note 1), 120.

37 Charlie Amshaw was detained between 12 April and 12 September. City Engineer to Town Clerk, 22 September 1938, 3/PEZ 4/1/1/1326.

38 See 3/PEZ, 1/3/2/6/10; 1/3/2/6/11; 1/3/2/6/12; WCARS, 4/PEZ 4/1/61; 3/PEZ 4/1/1/1326. In particular: Louis Fourie to Secretary of Public Health (note 2).

39 100 Men Fighting Plague at Port Elizabeth, in: Rand Daily Mail, 19 April 1938, 11.

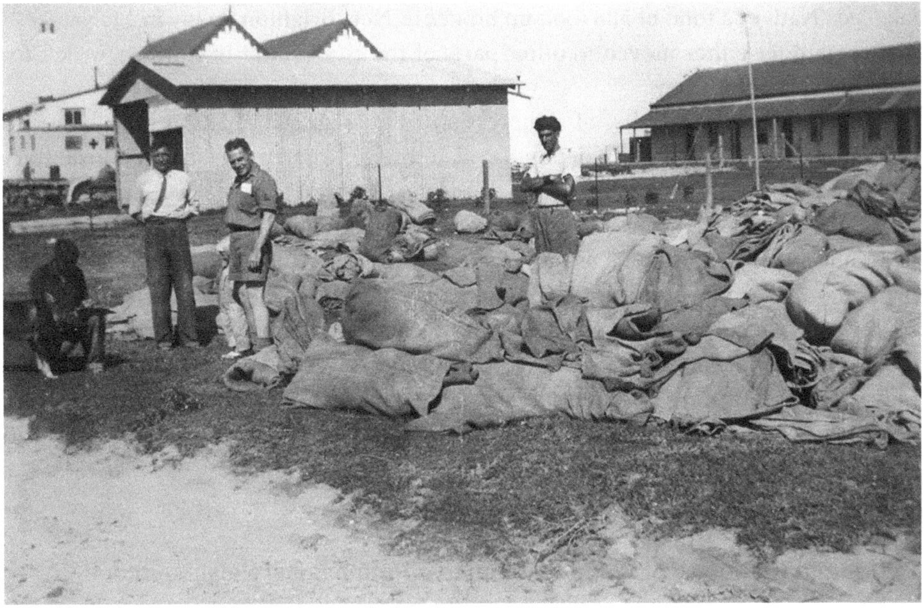

Fig. 1 "Thousands of bags being deverminized at the FED" (Formidable Epidemic Diseases Hospital), Port Elizabeth, 1938. The dog (on the left) was likely trained to detect and kill any rats in the bags.

so-called "scrap" or "junk" material was condemned for destruction, probably because it was thought to offer a cosy, protective habitat for rats.[40] Teams of rodent inspectors appropriated and removed such material from Korsten, or took it out onto the streets and burned it to ash. Requests for compensation for items from money hidden in burned mattresses to pocketknives and crockery were dismissed as fraudulent or frivolous by officials in Ferguson's office.[41] Any possessions that those under quarantine were allowed to take with them to the hospital were subject to close inspection and disinfection. Under suspicion that rats and fleas might have been nesting in such possessions, all were "deverminised" likely through fumigation or washing.[42]

Ultimately, in taking these measures, officials were hopeful that evicted Black residents would settle in McNamee Village, where they could be kept under stringent control, and the agency of rodents could be more easily kept in check. However, these segregationist designs did not entirely come to pass. Of the 3,145 people evicted, 1,974 of whom were

40 Louis Fourie to Secretary of Public Health (note 2).

41 Medical Officer of Health to Town Clerk, 22 July 1938, 3/PEZ, 4/1/1/1326.

42 Port Elizabeth in 1938 – Bubonic Plague collection. A. Schauder Collection, Cory Library, Rhodes University. Available: http://vital.seals.ac.za:8080/vital/access/manager/Collection/vital:26020?site_name=GlobalView. My thanks to Vathiswa Nhanha and Gary Baines for helping me identify the provenance of this album.

labelled "Native", a total of 508 took up homes in New Brighton, many in McNamee.[43] The remainder either moved to other parts of the city, rebuilt in Korsten, or left for other parts of the Union.

This was, then, somewhat of a success story for segregationists: a racially mixed neighbourhood was partially depopulated. Yet here Korsten was deemed insanitary and in need of draconian action not *only* because it posed a problem to segregationist ideologues, or even because of evidence of zoonotic transfers of plague between rats, fleas, and humans. Its status as an infected, and infective neighbourhood, was *also* blamed on its architecture and building materials, which allegedly facilitated multi-species intimacies between rats, fleas, and Black and Coloured people. Attention to these non-human factors through a close examination of Ferguson's home reports not only provides a window onto the epidemiology of plague in 1938, but also reveals how perceived relationships between architecture, objects, and pests could be mobilised in support of segregation and forced removals.

2. From a Pathology of Wood-and-Iron to a Pathological Neighbourhood

From a close study of Duncan Ferguson's hundreds of reports on houses in Korsten over the months of the plague outbreak, one feature is abundantly clear: almost all houses condemned for destruction were "wood-and-iron" buildings. No definition of such a building survives in these files, but it seems that this term referred to the numerous huts in the area, as well as its shacks. Ferguson's descriptions of the interiors of these houses reveal his fixation with the harbourage they allegedly provided to "vermin". One plague-infected "wood and iron" house, inspected on 31 March 1938, he described as "dilapidated and unsightly, unfit for human habitation", "coated with dirt", and "likely to attract and harbour bugs". It was, in his opinion, "so dirty and verminous as to be injurious…to health and liable to favour the spread of infectious disease".[44] This description is so common in Ferguson's reports that it appears to have been cut and pasted over and over.

Maurits Bastiaan Meerwijk has observed that in 1911–1942 Java, when investigating plague-infected houses, medical officers dissected them as if examining the body of a

43 Evicted Coloured people had a choice of "economic" or "sub-economic" housing in seven different suburbs, while whites had a choice of four economic or one sub-economic housing schemes. "Native" people were only offered New Brighton. Statistical Report on Housing and Slum Elimination, 20 October 1938 (note 9).

44 Case No. 83. Lot 58 of ERF 48, Durban Road, Korsten, Port Elizabeth, MOH Report 31 March 1938, 3/PEZ, 1/3/2/6/10.

patient.[45] Ferguson's strategy, both in inspecting properties, and writing his reports, appears to have been similar. His reports broke down "wood and iron" buildings into their pathological elements, emphasising how every architectural aspect of the buildings, and the materials used in their construction, could provide spaces for rats, fleas, or other blood-sucking insects.

The state of flooring in Korsten was particularly repulsive to Ferguson, and his fixation on floorboards and sub-floor space is evident in nearly every report. For example, one slumlord-owned plague-infected building of seven rooms, inhabited by seventeen people, had rooms with floors with "no proper sub-floor ventilation", and its "sub-floor space" allegedly afforded "harbourage to rodents and fleas".[46] Other Korsten properties, however, were in even worse shape, having floors of "earth".[47] There are several reasons why Ferguson may have been so concerned with flooring. Information from the United States which had embarked on numerous concerted rat-proofing campaigns in cities such as San Francisco revealed that rats could burrow into properties from underground.[48] Earth floors were thus framed as a great danger as they did nothing to prevent burrowing rats from commingling with humans inside homes. South African rat-proofing regulations, which were legally enforced on commercial premises that stored or sold food or hides and were strongly encouraged for homes, likewise stipulated that any foundations of less than 18 inches deep in hard soil or 24 inches deep in soft soil were "unsatisfactory" on account of the possibility "for rats to burrow underneath and so enter the building". Meanwhile, buildings with floors "of earth, of defective boards or of bricks laid in clay", were pathologized as "entirely unsuitable for permanent use as stores or shops in which foodstuffs, produce, or other goods are kept" and thus should be "condemned and demolished at once". Homes with earth floors, likewise, were dismissed as spaces that "can never be rodent-proof" and thus should not be permitted.[49] Updated regulations of 1930 pushed the case of concrete as a solution to these problems, insisting that all ground floors must be of concrete or "similar solid rat-proof material".[50]

Ferguson's concern with sub-floor ventilation may appear to hearken back to an earlier period in which plague was thought to be propagated by the soil.[51] However, by 1938, these concerns had been reframed in accordance with the perceived agency

---

45 Maurits Bastiaan Meerwijk, Bamboo Dwellers. Plague, Photography, and the House in Colonial Java, in: Plague Image and Imagination from Medieval to Modern Times, Cham 2021, 205–34.

46 Case No. 83. Lot 58 of ERF 48, Durban Road, Report 31 March 1938 (note 44).

47 Case No. 100. Lot 17 of ERF 11, Stemela Street, Korsten, MOH Report 11 June 1938, WCARS, 3/PEZ, 1/3/2/6/11.

48 Rupert Blue, Bubonic Plague Control in California in 1903. Origin of Ratproofing as a Control Measure, in: California and Western Medicine 40/5 (1934), 363–65.

49 All quotes since note 48 from: J.A. Mitchell, Circular No. 19 of 1928, Dept of Public Health, 28 September 1928, 4/PEZ 4/1/61. (Underlining according to the original document.)

50 J.A. Mitchell, Government Notice No. 1380 of 1930, 3/PEZ, 4/1/1/1326.

51 Lynteris, A Suitable Soil (note 14).

of rats. In a memorandum, Louis Fourie, a noted plague expert, stated that providing "light and air" in sub-floor spaces would "do much to minimise rodent infestation in this area", but failed to explain why.[52] This probably relates to perceptions of the rat as an animal frequenting dark and musty spaces, and avoiding the light.[53]

A second routine complaint of Ferguson's was the state of kitchens and other food preparation areas. Disgusted that most residents cooked in their bedrooms, he constantly flagged this as a "structural defect". Even at times where separate kitchens existed, these were typically in "scrap wood-and-iron" yard structures which were supposedly "coated with filth" and often had "earth" floors.[54] Bedroom cooking was pathologized because it risked attracting rats into the most intimate space of the home, where their fleas might hop onto sleeping humans.

These structural concerns framed Korsten houses as places that rats had inhabited, and from which they could never be evicted. The pathological architecture of Korsten had transformed human homes into rodent homes that had become "infected"[55] by rats. According to Ferguson, the construction of these wood-and-iron buildings was so defective, that it completely prevented any attempts to control rats or fleas within them.[56] The supposed inability to remove rodents from these homes placed residents in a double bind. Their homes were allegedly overrun with rats and insects, but they also could not be made rat-proof.

This was not only because the structures were supposedly filthy and dilapidated but referred to two practical problems. Firstly, according to Ferguson, the buildings were so haphazardly constructed as to render rat-proofing impossible. By 1938, South African rat-proofing regulations specified a suite of material interventions that property owners or occupiers could use to exclude rodents from their premises. Two of the most important of these were screens and barriers. Screens made of "rat-proof netting" – any sturdy netted material such as chicken-wire – were placed over ventilation shafts, gutters, and any open areas exposed to the elements. Barriers such as a layer of concrete flooring, or sturdy materials fitted to the bottoms of doors were installed to prevent

52 Plague Precautions, 10 September 1938, 3/PEZ, 4/1/1/1326.

53 Ventilation was another pertinent complaint of Ferguson's. Many of the structures he investigated had few or no windows which resulted in a "dark and gloomy appearance" allegedly favoured by rats. Case No. 79. Lots 6 and 7, ERF 82, Makuten Street, Korsten, MOH Report 19 March 1938, 3/PEZ, 1/3/2/6/10. The lack of windows in many of these houses was not only an issue from a lighting perspective, but they also caused ventilation problems. Case No. 97. Lots 8a and 9a of ERF 15, Daisy Street, Korsten, 10 June 1938, 3/PEZ, 1/3/2/6/11.

54 Case No. 100. Lot 17 of ERF 11, Stemela Street, Korsten, MOH Report 11 June 1938, 3/PEZ, 1/3/2/6/11.

55 Fourie refers to the buildings as well as the neighbourhood as "infected". Louis Fourie to Secretary of Public Health (note 2).

56 The MOH Reports on 22 July, 1938, 3/PEZ, 1/3/2/6/11.

rodents from burrowing or gnawing in or out of buildings.[57] However, these measures only worked when other entry points to a building – such as floors, ceilings, roofs, and walls – were securely constructed. According to medical officials, none of these measures could viably be installed in many Korsten homes.

Secondly, temporary measures such as fumigation were described as highly ineffective in Korsten's structures. In a letter to Ferguson, W.A. Larmuth, the manager of the South African Fumigation Company, claimed that eliminating rodents in Korsten homes was "extremely difficult" because rats could escape into "rat holes and harbourages under the floors and in foundations" and that HCN (hydrogen cyanide) gas would be "rapidly absorbed if the ground was at all damp".[58] Edward North Thornton, the Chief Health Officer of South Africa, concurred with Larmuth's assessment. Because these buildings were "jammed down on the ground as they were constructed of galvanised iron flat against the wood it naturally followed that" even after fumigation, "a number of" rat "carcases" would be left in "crevices on such premises".[59] Simultaneously, Korsten dwellings had "leaks and gaps in the walls", and although intensive fumigation might kill fleas, it would not eliminate "the eggs which were ready to hatch out".[60] This made it impossible to "say with certainty that the plague could be eradicated from these buildings."[61] In the eyes of sanitary officials, the wood-and-iron human homes of Korsten were thus fundamentally interlinked with rodent homes in the same neighbourhood. One could not be eliminated without destroying the other: to rid Korsten of rat harbourage, so too did human wood-and-iron homes need to go. This was because "contact between rats and humans in this area is intimate and encourages the spread of plague".[62]

The widespread presence of wood-and-iron buildings in Korsten transformed a problem of individual homes into one affecting an entire neighbourhood. Until "better dwellings were erected", argued Ferguson, "there could be no certainty in deratting" in Korsten.[63] Thornton, recounting a home inspection where he had witnessed a "case of plague lying on the floor in a hovel in Korsten literally alive with fleas", claimed that housing conditions were "unique" in Korsten. Such buildings, he wrote, could "not be treated in any other way but by being burnt".[64]

---

57 J.A. Mitchell, Circular No. 19 of 1928, Department of Public Health, 28 September 1928, 4/PEZ 4/1/61; J.A. Mitchell, Government Notice No. 1380 of 1930, 3/PEZ 4/1/1/1326.

58 Larmuth to Medical Officer of Health, 25 May 1938, 3/PEZ, 4/1/1/1326.

59 Notes of Meeting of Special Plague Committee, held on 16 April 1938, 3/PEZ 4/1/1/1326.

60 Notes of Proceedings, 12 April 1938 (note 5).

61 Ibid.

62 The MOH Reports on 22 July, 1938, 3/PEZ, 1/3/2/6/11.

63 Notes of Proceedings, 18 July 1938 (note 4). Fourie likewise emphasised that it was urgent to focus plague control efforts places where "housing conditions are bad and rodents are living in close contact with the occupants of dwellings". Louis Fourie to Secretary of Public Health (note 2).

64 Notes of Proceedings, 12 April 1938 (note 5).

For Thornton, it was strictly this architectural problem that had rendered Korsten a pathological space. Thornton, unlike Ferguson, was careful to pathologize *only* the material aspects of Korsten – building materials, objects, architecture – rather than its human population. Korsten's structures were its primarily issue, rather than its mixing of races, or the state of hygiene of its inhabitants. In a discussion on whether railway staff who dealt with "all classes of people" should be vaccinated, Thornton was insistent that this was unnecessary. Rather than suggesting vaccinating those exposed to "native" bodies, Thornton argued instead that vaccines be offered to people "brought into contact with the type of house in which the people of Korsten were living".[65] However, despite his insistence that the materiality of Korsten rather than its human inhabitants were the problem, Thornton's arguments nevertheless reinforced segregationist sentiments, and reveal how architecture and materiality could justify segregation on the grounds of public health. In a nod to the New Brighton scheme, Thornton claimed that it would be much easier to manage plague there, as "natives" were under greater surveillance.[66]

Ultimately, whatever their views on segregation, all scientists involved in plague-control in Korsten agreed that its wood-and-iron buildings could not be "deverminised". Human homes were thus framed as rodent harbourage in Korsten: almost every aspect of these wood and iron buildings were condemned as providing spaces in which rodents could nest, proliferate, and infect humans with plague. Perceived human, flea, and rodent intimacies within "plague infected houses", thus justified forcibly removing people from their homes and preventing them from reoccupying them.[67]

Yet despite the colonial framing of human homes in Korsten as little more than a series of rodent harbourages, the actual presence of rats in Korsten homes was rare.[68] Colonial archives themselves reveal that the wood-and-iron buildings actually had fewer infected rats than other parts of the city. One of the only properties in which Ferguson found "two plague infected rodents" in Korsten, was a brick building.[69] According to Fourie, by July, only a "dozen mummified carcases had been found" in the demolished buildings.[70] Rats were, however, readily found in other parts of the city. A white-occupied wood-and-iron house in North End, a district closer to the city centre, was found to be "infested with rodents" and subsequently flagged for demolition.[71] Cases of "plague-infested" rodents

65 Ibid.

66 Ibid.

67 The MOH Reports on 22 July 1938, 3/PEZ, 1/3/2/6/11.

68 Louis Fourie to Secretary of Public Health (note 2).

69 Case No. 95. No. 17, Dobson Street and Nos. 17, 19 and 21, Brassel Street, MOH Report 30 May 1938, 3/PEZ, 1/3/2/6/11.

70 Notes of Proceedings, 18 July 1938 (note 4).

71 Case No. 132. No. 19, Doyle Street, MOH Report 25 July, 1938, 3/PEZ 1/3/2/6/12.

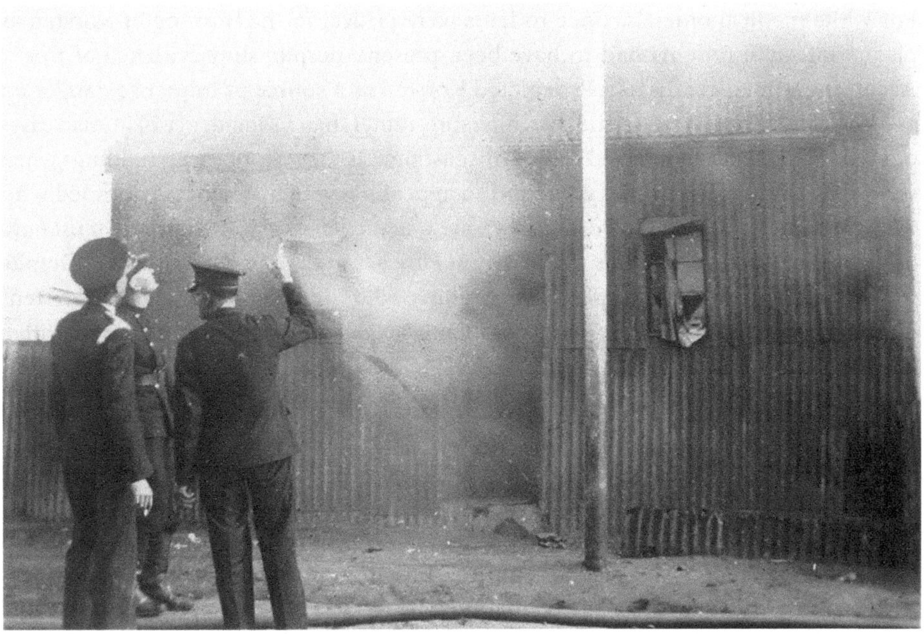

Fig. 2 "The Green House", an example of a wood-and-iron building in Korsten, Porth Elizabeth, 1938.

were also discovered in Strand Street,[72] and the Feather Market Hall, both in the centre of the city.[73] By August, only two infected rats had actually been found in Korsten itself, while six were found in other parts of the city, three of which were in North End.[74] In spite of this lack of evidence of Korsten rodent infection, Fourie insisted that he had

> no hesitation in stating that, in Korsten, the epizootic had started among the rats in the south-western corner of the township at least a year or probably more ago and it has since been smouldering and spreading slowly outwards from the primary focus of infection.[75]

72 Notes of Proceedings of Special Committee re[garding] Outbreak of Plague, meeting held on 29 April 1938, 3/PEZ 4/1/1/1326

73 Ibid.

74 The majority of rats inspected for plague were found in an area "from the South End of the City and New Brighton Location". Louis Fourie to Secretary of Public Health, Port Elizabeth, 28 August 1938, 3/PEZ 4/1/1/1326.

75 Ibid.

For white medical officials, since rodents were critical in the framing of Korsten as plague infected, rodents had to have been present, despite slim evidence of this.[76] Accordingly, medical discourse depicted Korsten as a source of immense danger on account of its allegedly rat-friendly architecture, rather than its incidence of human cases or even the presence of infected rats. So disgusting was the state of these buildings when viewed by middle class white men, and so appealing were they when examined with what these men imagined to be a rats-eye-view, that officials assumed plague *must have* originated in Korsten, and thus all cases *must have* been related to this district.[77] Despite the discovery of an infected person in Walmer who "denied having visited Korsten", Thornton emphasised that the "native evidently acquired in some way a contact with a Korsten flea".[78]

3. Reception of the Removals: Contesting the Architectural Pathology

The shaky epistemological ground upon which Korsten had been constructed as a "focus of infection" rendered the plague removals a highly controversial measure that was supported by some, and sharply condemned by others. With comparatively few rats found in the area and a small human case load, Ferguson, Thornton, and Fourie's arguments about Korsten's pathological nature hinged tightly on arguing that architecture itself was a driver of zoonosis. This enabled residents and landlords to attack them for not allowing them to put their properties in order, to make arguments that "slum" is a culturally contingent category, or to dismiss the operation as a smokescreen for segregation.

Several articles in white-owned media supported the measures and continued to reify Ferguson's framing of Korsten houses as rodent homes. A 1949 article in *The Rotarian,* is a case in point. This publication, the mouthpiece of the Rotary Club, a charitable organisation which had provided financial assistance for plague control and the construction of McNamee Village itself, described the operation as "the most important present-day social experiment in subequatorial Africa".[79] The publication, describing Korsten in zoomorphic terms, argued that Port Elizabeth's slums (including Korsten) were irredeemably infested with rodents, and infected by disease. These "festering congeries"[80],

76 This constitutes an example of what Lynteris has called the "imperative ontology" of plague. See Christos Lynteris, The Imperative Origins of COVID-19, in: L'Homme 234–235/2–3 (2020), 21–32.

77 For more on this rats-eye-view approach to architecture see Jules Skotnes-Brown, Scurrying Seafarers. Shipboard Rats, Plague, and the Land/Sea Border, in: Journal of Global History 18/1 (2023), 108–130.

78 Notes of Meeting of Special Plague Committee, Meeting held 16 April 1938, 3/PEZ 4/1/1/1326.

79 From Slums to McNamee, in: The Rotarian (1949), 26.

80 Ibid.

it claimed, were utterly unfit for humans and constituted "filthy warrens"[81] in which "Vermin swarmed".[82] By contrast, according to the article, McNamee consisted of houses "made gay with flower gardens, pocket-size lawns, and rustic adornments".[83] In 1939, the *South African Medical Journal,* likewise framed McNamee as a success story. One author argued that unlike the disease-riddled "warrens" of Korsten in which rodents putatively nested, houses in New Brighton were "built rodent-proof".[84] A reporter for *Umteteli wa Bantu,* a quadrilingual English, isiXhosa, isiZulu, and Sesotho newspaper under white oversight, but with a large nationwide Black readership, likewise praised the slum clearance project.[85] The reporter, likely a Port Elizabeth correspondent, writing under the pseudonym "Man-On-The-Spot" reiterated Ferguson, Thornton, and Fourie's pathology of architecture, declaring that the "danger spots…are the dwellings, where the human cases come from".[86]

Some individuals living in or owning property in Korsten likewise supported the removals and actively aided the government in destroying their infected properties. Property-owner S. Matheson, for example, offered his properties to the city council, "free of charge" in order to assist them in their slum clearance project.[87] Certain Coloured and Black landowners, such as Sadie Dampies, Willem van Staden, and Salomon Matebe, likewise, were happy to move out of homes in Korsten in exchange for compensation in the form of money or plots of ground in other areas.[88]

Other residents and landlords, however, sharply contested the condemnation of their properties, homes, and possessions as a series of plague-infested rodent harbourages, and a controversy over Ferguson's pathology of wood-and-iron emerged. One of the first committed challenges was articulated by the Korsten Vigilance Committee, a community group of Korsten residents and property owners. Although some of their members agreed that their homes were in a pathological state, they resented the council for "not giving them an opportunity to put their houses in order". Others contested the categorisation of Korsten houses as slums: the committee stated that their properties were "only slums from a European's point of view". Moreover, the Port Elizabeth City Council was partially responsible for turning Korsten into an infected neighbourhood. Despite

81 Ibid., 27.

82 Ibid., 26.

83 Ibid., 27.

84 New Brighton Village, in: South African Medical Journal 13 (1939), 431.

85 Natasha Erlank, Umteteli Wa Bantu and the Constitution of Social Publics in the 1920s and 1930s, Social Dynamics 45/1 (2019), 75–102.

86 Man-On-The-Spot, African Affairs at Port Elizabeth, in: Umteteli wa Bantu, 30 April 1938.

87 S. Matheson to A. Schauder, 7 May 1938, 3/PEZ, 1/3/2/6/10.

88 W.T. Jarman, Compensation of Slum Owners, Undated (likely August 1938), 3/PEZ 1/3/2/6/11.

paying rates, residents had received no electric lights, drainage, kerbing, guttering or proper access to running water.[89]

Slumlord extraordinaire Sidney Wells, who stood to lose a considerable amount of money, came out in support of these residents and, enraged, penned a series of letters to the city council. In one, he complained that his properties were not the problem. It was, in fact, the "council or public property which consists of so-called roads flooded with water and muck" that was creating a sanitary menace. Wells argued that his tenants and loan recipients had been "persecuted and taken from their homes and treated worse than animals".[90] In another, he described the condemnation of his buildings as "Hitler actions" where the "three Hitlers, the Docotr [sic] and two inspectors" were "persecuting me and others by the most vindictive actions possible". Councillors had treated Korsten residents, he fumed, like "dirt" and accordingly Wells issued a veiled threat of violence against the council.[91]

In the arc of the twentieth century, as apartheid policies came to pass, some Black residents of Korsten came to interpret the event as another in a long history of forced removals. Some of those residents interviewed by Vista University students remembered and had internalised Ferguson's pathology of wood-and-iron. One former resident, for example, stated that since he was living in a "brick building", he was "safe" and thus he was "not involved in that removal".[92] Others had correlated Korsten with rats, or forced removals with the presence of rats, despite the lack of actual evidence of rat infestations in the neighbourhood. Mrs Maleki, for example, was under the impression that only those whose houses were infested with rats were removed. According to her, the "whites would enter a house and check whether there were rats or not. If they found rats, the house would be condemned". Contrastingly, those who "had no rats in their houses stood far away from the scene".[93]

Others, however, were not convinced that plague was a genuine problem, and dismissed it as little more than an excuse to remove them from the neighbourhood. One unnamed resident of Korsten claimed that there were "always rumours that Korsten was going to be proclaimed a coloured township and that all blacks should be removed to New Brighton".[94] Fezile Teka, who was removed in 1938, likewise dismissed plague as an "invented disease", rather than a real problem.[95] Another former resident, identified as "old man", recounted that the entire process of removal was fraudulent. Plague was allegedly "sparked off by a women who was admitted to the Provincial Hospital", and

89 All quotes since note 88 from: Secretary of Korsten Vigilance Committee, 19 July 1938, 3/PEZ, 1/3/2/6/11.

90 Sidney Wells, 5 August 1938, 3/PEZ, 1/3/2/6/11.

91 Sidney Wells to Slum Committee, 22 Sep 1938, 3/PEZ, 1/3/2/6/12.

92 Quoted in Cherry, Blot (note 7), 51.

93 All quotes since note 92 from: Mrs Maleki, quoted in Cherry, Blot (note 7), 54.

94 Unnamed interlocutor, quoted in Cherry, Blot (note 7), 51.

95 Fezile Teka, quoted in Cherry, Blot (note 7), 52.

"caused by the mice in the black dwelling area". When "the people came from work", he recounted "they found that some of their houses were destroyed during the big hunt for the rats", however, it was "untrue to say that the woman admitted to hospital was suffering from rat plague". The entire affair was little more than a "scapegoat" to segregate Black from Coloured people.[96] For these residents, if plague was a hoax, then, so too was the pathologisation of many Korsten homes. One anonymous domestic worker claimed that in the 1930s, Korsten was "better at that time than the shacks you find today [1987] in the townships – it was very clean."[97] Finally, many residents who had accepted housing in New Brighton found the neighbourhood, despite the grandiose propagandistic claims of city officials, an extremely unsanitary place. These tenants complained "bitterly" about the unhygienic, and ramshackle state of their new homes, one claiming, in terms close to Ferguson's home reports, that it was "really awkward and surprising to think of it for human beings to live in this manner".[98]

4. Conclusion

This case has demonstrated that colonial suspicions about architecture, materiality, and multispecies intimacies, in addition to medicalised fears of racial mixing, were mobilised in justification of segregating Korsten residents. Although Ferguson and numerous racist others undoubtedly considered Korsten's status as a multiracial neighbourhood to be a source of disease, its alleged architectural and material "defects" ultimately were thought to have transformed it into a plague spot. The wood-and-iron buildings of the region were condemned as little more than a series of rodent harbourages that would enable rats to infect the entire city, and eventually other Indian Ocean ports. The capacity to blame architecture for plague, even in the face of few human cases and no ratfalls, represented a moment in which rat-proofing had become a dominant strategy of urban plague control in South Africa, coupled as it was with nascent strategies of "separate development". For medical officials, the perceived impossibility of excluding rodents from Korsten homes was enough to justify the destruction of much of the neighbourhood and forced removal of many its residents. Simultaneously, the mobilisation of alleged architectural "defects" and rodent "harbourages" in support of segregation also enabled to residents of Korsten to contest the condemnation of their homes, even if their appeals were ultimately ignored.

In controlling plague in Korsten, sanitary officials treated Black and Coloured homes as if they were rodent homes. To cleanse the bodies of their inhabitants for diagno-

96 All quotes from "Old man", quoted in Cherry, Blot (note 7), 53.

97 Domestic worker, quoted in Cherry, Blot (note 7), 50.

98 Reference from Native Affairs Committee, meeting held on 13 September 1938, 3/PEZ, 1/3/2/6/12.

sis and examination, both rats and humans were dipped in chemicals to kill fleas. To destroy rodent harbourages, officials believed they also needed to destroy Black and Coloured homes, furniture, and other possessions. Although residents and landlords of Korsten complained about the indignities of dipping and contested such architectural pathologies, there was little they could do against the draconian legislation that enabled officials to take almost any action to contain plague. Ultimately the plague outbreak became a point of great bitterness in the collective memory of Korsten. Former residents, recognising the shaky epistemological foundations upon which Korsten had been deemed a plague spot came to view it as yet another episode in the terrible history of South African forced removals and redevelopment.

Photo credits

Fig. 1 "Thousands of bags being deverminized at the FED" (Formidable Epidemic Diseases Hospital), Port Elizabeth, 1938. © Adolf Schauder Collection, Cory Library, Rhodes University, PIC/A 4279.

Fig. 2 "The Green House", Porth Elizabeth, 1938. © Adolf Schauder Collection, Cory Library, Rhodes University, PIC/A 4279.

Abstract:
This chapter argues that in the context of the 1938 plague outbreak in Port Elizabeth (now Gqeberha), sanitary measures imposed to control the movements of rats were extended to the attempted control of Black and Coloured people living in the suburb of Korsten. In the reports and recommendations of public health officials, numerous houses in Korsten were framed as rat habitats, which allegedly enabled the rodents to breed, nest, and disseminate disease to humans, objects, and other structures in Port Elizabeth. Humans living in this neighbourhood were forcibly removed from their homes, placed under quarantine, and encouraged to move to the model township of New Brighton, a 'hygienic', 'rat-proof', segregationists' utopia. Thus, the process of removing undesirable animals – rats and other rodent residents from Korsten – was also a process of removing Black Africans from the same area. Despite numerous protests from residents and landlords who contested the colonial pathologisation of their homes and properties as rat habitats, 3145 people were evicted. Ultimately, anti-rat measures became segregationist measures, shaping official policy, and also African memories of the removals.

Keywords:
rats | plague | segregation | South Africa | forced removals

Matheus Alves Duarte da Silva

A Global War against Wild Rodents

Sanitary Tensions, Anti-Rodent Measures, and the Spectre of Sylvatic Plague, 1927–1950s

The role played by black and brown rats as potential carriers and spreaders of the plague bacillus was central to the sanitary management of the third plague pandemic, which occurred between 1894 and 1950. Thus in the first decades of the twentieth century, rat-catching, rat-proofing, and rat-poisoning practices flourished in many cities around the world that sought to diminish rat populations in order to control or prevent local plague outbreaks.[1] Moreover, in international forums, a consensus was progressively reached on the necessity of destroying rats not only to curb disease, but also to prevent the loss of goods and food the animals caused.[2] This kind of debate was particularly important in the maritime sphere, and different countries began imposing mandatory deratization on international trade ships in the early 1900s, a measure formalized globally at the International Sanitary Conference of Paris in 1926.[3] In addition, several meetings were held to create national and international leagues against rats.[4] Across these many fronts,

1 Michael Vann, Of Rats, Rice, and Race. The Great Hanoi Rat Massacre, an Episode in French Colonial History, in: French Colonial History 4/1 (2003), 191–203; Myron J. Echenberg, Plague Ports. The Global Urban Impact of Bubonic Plague, 1894–1901, New York 2007; Matheus Alves Duarte da Silva, "O Novo Commércio Oswáldico". Circulação de Conhecimento e o Controle da Peste Bubônica no Rio de Janeiro e em São Paulo (1894–1910), in: Revista Brasileira de História das Ciências 9/2 (2016), 189–202; Lukas Engelmann/Christos Lynteris, Sulphuric Utopias. A History of Maritime Fumigation, Inside Technology, Cambridge (MA) 2019; Jules Skotnes-Brown, Scurrying Seafarers. Shipboard Rats, Plague, and the Land/Sea Border, in: Journal of Global History (2022), 1–23. – I am very grateful to the co-editors of this book for their insightful comments on preliminary versions of this chapter.
Funding ID: Research leading to this article was funded by the Wellcome Trust (Grant No. ID 217988/Z/19/Z) for the project "The Global War Against the Rat and the Epistemic Emergence of Zoonosis".

2 Conférence internationale du rat, Première Conférence Internationale du Rat (Paris–Le Havre, 16–22 Mai 1928). Documents réunis et publiés par Gabriel Petit, Paris 1931; Conférence internationale du rat, Deuxième Conférence Internationale et Congrès Colonial du Rat et de la Peste. Paris, 7–12 Octobre 1931. Documents réunis et publiés par le Professeur Gabriel Petit, Paris 1932.

3 Office International d'Hygiène Publique [OIHP], Modèle de Certificat de Dératisation (Ou d'exemption de Dératisation) Adopté par l'OIHP dans sa Session de Novembre 1927, in: Bulletin Mensuel de l'OIHP XX/2 (1928), 295.

4 Ligue Sanitaire Française Contre la Mouche et le Rat, in: Bulletin No 1, 1914; Conférence, Première Conférence (note 2); Conférence, Deuxième Conférence (note 2); Karen Sayer, The "Modern" Management of Rats. British Agricultural Science in Farm and Field during the Twentieth Century, in: BJHS Themes 2 (2017), 235–263.

a truly global war against the rat, declared in the first decade of the twentieth century,[5] unfolded over its first fifty years.

Alongside that war, however, this period also witnessed debates on the potential of wild rodents to "perpetuate" the plague bacillus and eventually spread it within national or even across international borders, which themselves prompted a varied range of anti-rodent measures. While not comparable in magnitude or in geographical range with the war against the rat, the sanitary actions against wild rodents shaped a sort of secondary global war, which could be divided into two "fronts": on the one hand, locales where a plague reservoir among wild rodents had already been constituted – namely South Africa, the USA, China, and the Soviet Union; and on the other, those places that tried to avoid the constitution of such a reservoir among wild rodents. In a previous study, I explored the emergence and transformations of the idea of sylvatic plague, a term coined to explain the persistence of plague among wild rodents around the world.[6] In this chapter, I examine the reverse side of the medal, e. g., how measures were deployed against wild rodents in the 1930s, 1940s, and 1950s to avoid the formation of sylvatic plague reservoirs. I argue that the concept of sylvatic plague became understood in several countries as a sort of prophecy of a last stage of plague that could not be eradicated. Nonetheless, anti-rodent precautions were taken in the hopes of avoiding the fulfilment of this prophecy.

After briefly highlighting the novelty afforded by the concept of sylvatic plague, coined by the Portuguese doctor Ricardo Jorge, I focus on three different contexts – Angola, the UK, and Brazil – to discuss how local actors engaged with this new idea and which sort of anti-rodent measures were applied, ranging from direct destruction to quarantine and rodent-proofing. I focus first on Angola, which in 1932 was confronted with the menace of a plague invasion connected to migratory gerbils from South Africa and South West Africa (present-day Namibia). In response, the Portuguese government created a service whose goals, among others, was the direct and indirect destruction of wild rodents. In 1932, the idea of sylvatic plague was not completely established in Angola, but by 1935, after exchanges between Jorge and Portuguese doctors based in the colony, it had become an important justification for the country's anti-rodent actions. Next, I examine the discussion on the risks of plague seeding and constituting a permanent sylvatic reservoir in the UK via wild rodents imported from the US for exhibition in zoological gardens. This point was addressed by Charles Elton in 1938–1939 after he read works on sylvatic plague written in the US by Karl Meyer, who was informed by Jorge's work. The outcome of the debate led by Elton was the imposition of a three-month quarantine over all rodents imported to the UK susceptible to catching and

5 Albert Calmette, Déclarons la Guerre aux Rats, in: La Revue du Mois 3/28 (1908), 432–444.

6 Matheus Alves Duarte da Silva, Between Deserts and Jungles. The Emergence and Circulation of Sylvatic Plague (1920–1950), in: Medical Anthropology, 2023.

dying from plague. Finally, I investigate the debates on the possible role played by wild rodents on conserving the plague bacillus in north-eastern Brazil in the late 1930s and a national anti-plague campaign starting in 1941 conducted by the Brazilian national plague service. Influenced by the works of the Chilean doctor Atilio Macchiavello, who was central in the circulation of the concept of sylvatic plague in Brazil, this campaign aimed to control plague cases related to rats and avoid the constitution of an independent reservoir among wild rodents. To achieve its goals, the Brazilian national plague service focused on the destruction of rats and wild rodents, as well as on measures to stop interaction between the two groups of animals.

By examining these three cases, I aim to contribute to the history of plague and of plague management, and to the history of the entanglements between animals and epidemics. I will show how, in the second quarter of the twentieth century, plague management, on a global scale, was no longer exclusively focused on destroying rats in big cities and ports. Indeed, alert to the idea of sylvatic plague and its risks, several countries passed legislation to deal with wild rodents, and as a result new spaces of sanitary interventions appeared, such as zoological gardens, farms, rural villages, and wild areas.

1. The Invention of Sylvatic Plague

Plague re-emerged as a global menace in 1894, when the disease broke out in the British colony of Hong Kong, an important economic hub. This outbreak led not only to the discovery of the causative bacillus of the plague, but was also considered the beginning of the third plague pandemic, which ultimately killed more than 12 million people by the 1950s, most of them in India.[7] While rats were primarily framed as epidemic villains, the relationship between wild rodents and the plague bacillus was already being studied and discussed in the earliest years of the pandemic. For instance, Chinese and Russian (and later Soviet) scholars were deeply concerned about the role played by Siberian marmots in conserving the plague bacillus, which could explain historical outbreaks of plague in Manchuria, and especially the huge and violent epidemic of pneumonic plague in 1910–1911. Consequently, not only these animals, but also their burrows and hibernation cycles were studied, scrutinized, and often blamed as primary causes for

7 Henri H. Mollaret/Jacqueline Brossollet, Alexandre Yersin, 1863–1943. Un Pasteurien en Indochine, Paris 1993; Echenberg, Plague Ports (note 1); Prashant Kidambi, "An Infection of Locality". Plague, Pythogenesis and the Poor in Bombay, c. 1896–1905, in: Urban History 31/2 (2004), 249–267; Matheus Alves Duarte da Silva, Quand la Peste Connectait le Monde. Production et Circulation de Savoirs Microbiologiques entre Brésil, Inde et France (1894–1922), Thèse de Doctorat, Paris, Ecole des Hautes Etudes en Sciences Sociales, 2020.

the persistence of plague in Manchuria.[8] In the US and South Africa, the role played by ground squirrels and gerbils, respectively, in maintaining and possibly spreading the plague bacillus to humans in California and the Orange Free State was also studied in the 1910s and 1920s. These studies gave birth to the concepts of squirrel plague in the US, and of veld plague in South Africa,[9] and were coupled with the adoption of destructive measures in the form of direct hunting, poisoning, and the creation of rodent-free zones.[10]

In international forums, however, such as the International Sanitary Conferences and the *Office International d'Hygiène Publique* (OIHP),[11] the role played by wild rodents in maintaining or spreading plague did not receive significant attention until the early 1920s. Indeed, in the 1910s these phenomena were understood as local particularities which posed no risk outside the areas where infected wild rodents were endemic. This attitude was based on the assumption that the circulation or migration of these animals was limited or negligible when compared to the sanitary risks posed by the international circulation of domestic rats.[12] An initial revision of this viewpoint, and an important milestone for the global awareness of the relationship between wild rodents and plague, was achieved only in 1924, when the OIHP, following a proposal made by Jorge, the Portuguese delegate in that agency,[13] decided to sponsor a global survey on the possible

8 Christos Lynteris, Tarbagan's Winter Lair. Framing Drivers of Plague Persistence in Inner Asia, in: id. (ed.) Framing Animals as Epidemic Villains, Cham 2019, 65–90, Susan D. Jones/Anna A. Amramina, Entangled Histories of Plague Ecology in Russia and the USSR, in: History and Philosophy of the Life Sciences 40/3 (2018) 49.

9 George W. McCoy, Some Features of the Squirrel Plague Problem, in: California State Journal of Medicine 9/3 (1911), 105–109; James Hunter Harvey Pirie, Plague on the Veld, in: id./James Alexander Mitchell/ Alexander Ingram, The Plague Problem in South Africa. Historical, Bacteriological, and Entomological Studies, Johannesburg 1927, 138–162.

10 Jules Skotnes-Brown/Christos Lynteris, blog, From Mink to the Wild. COVID-19 through the Mirror of Sylvatic Plague, in: Somatosphere, http://somatosphere.net/2021/mink-covid-sylvatic-plague.html/ (April 2021); Jules Skotnes-Brown, Preventing Plague, Bringing Balance. Wildlife Protection as Public Health in the Interwar Union of South Africa, in: Bulletin of the History of Medicine 95/4 (2021), 464–496.

11 The OIHP was created in 1907 and dismantled after WWII. On its history, see Céline Paillette, Épidémies, santé et ordre mondial. Le rôle des organisations sanitaires internationales, 1903–1923, in: Monde(s) 2/2 (2012), 235–256; Marcos Cueto/Theodore M. Brown/Elizabeth Fee, The World Health Organization. A History, Cambridge (UK) 2019, 32–36.

12 Henri Pottevin, La Dératisation. Rapport sur l'État Actuel des Méthodes Applicables à la Destruction des Rongeurs et de leurs Parasites Établi pour Être Presenté au Comitê Permanent de l'OIHP par M. Le Docteur Henri Pottevin, Secrétaire Général de l'Offfice, in: Bulletin Mensuel de l'OIHP II/4 (1910), 542.

13 On Ricardo Jorge, see Maria Antónia Pires Almeida, Fighting Disease and Epidemics. Ricardo Jorge and the Internationalization of Portuguese Science, in: Vesalius. Acta Internationales Historiae Medicinae 19/1 (2013), 19–23; Jaime Larry Benchimol, Ricardo Jorge e as Relações entre Portugal, Brasil e África. O Caso da Febre Amarela, in: Carlos Fiolhais/Décio Martins/Carlota Simões (eds.), História da Ciência Luso-Brasileira. Coimbra entre Portugal e o Brasil. Imprensa da Universidade de Coimbra, Coimbra 2013, 229–249; Rui Manuel Pinto Costa, Caminhos Batidos de um Peregrino do Saber. Ricardo Jorge

connections between domestic rats, wild rodents, their ectoparasites, and the plague bacillus. The agency invited its members, who represented more than thirty countries, to share their local observations on the role played by these animals in connection with the disease.[14]

The survey, presented by Jorge between 1926 and 1927, concluded that there were two "types" of plague, both caused by the same bacillus, but conserved and/or spread by two separate sets of animals in two sets of landscapes. The more common was the "pandemic plague", conveyed by domestic rats present in almost every port and city on the planet. The other type Jorge called the "sylvatic plague" (*peste selvatique*, in the original French), described by him as the plague infection among wild rodents living in what he referred to as "desert-like" environments.[15] According to Jorge, four hotspots (*foyers*) of sylvatic plague had been identified by 1926: the "African *foyer*", in the South African veld; the "European *foyer*", in the steppes of Astrakan; the "Asiatic *foyer*", in the steppes of Manchuria and Transbaikalia; and the "American *foyer*", in California.[16] In each of these places, a few species of rodents played a central role in maintaining the plague infection, constituting what Jorge called a "living virus reservoir": the gerbil in Africa; the sousliks in Europe; the Siberian marmot (also known as tarbagan) in Asia; and the ground squirrel in North America.[17]

As I have argued elsewhere, with his idea of sylvatic plague, Jorge invented a generic space of plague maintenance among wild rodents, which unified different landscapes – steppes, deserts, the veld.[18] As he wrote: "The sylvatic plague should not be confused with the plague of wild rodents that sometimes invade houses. The sylvatic plague occurs in the desert".[19] I have also discussed elsewhere the ambiguities of the desert as the locus of sylvatic plague, stressing how it could mean either a place with low rainfall or simply an uninhabited place.[20] Here, it is worth emphasizing the main point of Jorge's idea: to him, the sylvatic form of plague was constituted by a cycle of transmission among wild rodents living in so-called desert-like landscapes, a cycle that was maintained without the concurrence of humans and domestic rats.

---

no Contexto Científico Europeu, in Maria Manuela Tavares Ribeiro et al. (eds.), Cidadania, Política, Segurança e Cultura Científica, Coimbra 2018, 345–385.

14 OIHP, Session Extraordinaire d'Avril-Mai 1924 du Conseil Permanent de l'OIHP. Procès-Verbaux des Séances, Paris 1924, 205.

15 Ricardo Jorge, Les Faunes des Rongeurs et des Puces dans leurs Rapports avec la Peste (Deuxième Partie), in: Bulletin Mensuel de l'OIHP, XIX/9, 1927, 1257–1288.

16 Ibid., 1272–1280.

17 Ibid., 1272 and 1280; OIHP, Session Extraordinaire d'avril-mai 1927 du Conseil Permanent de l'OIHP. Procès-Verbaux des Séances. Paris, 90.

18 Silva, Between Deserts and Jungles (note 6).

19 OIHP, Session Extraordinaire d'avril-mai 1927 (note 17), 90.

20 Silva, Between Deserts and Jungles (note 6).

Jorge did not aim to propose any new sanitary policies with this categorization. He supported measures already employed in the four sylvatic plague hotspots, such as the imposition of rodent-free and rat-free zones in areas where domestic rats and wild rodents could meet, or measures already under discussion, such as the regulation of the tarbagan fur trade.[21] In that sense, the purpose of his system of categorization was above all academic, intending to provide a global standard for describing plague maintenance among wild rodents. In countries where sylvatic plague was not present in 1927, the subject passed almost unnoticed. However, from the 1930s onwards, some countries which had previously been free from this type of plague started to seriously consider the risks of sylvatic plague appearing in their territories and used the new concept, and the condition it described, to justify preventive measures.

2. Sylvatic Plague in Angola, 1932–1937

In January 1932, a plague epidemic was declared in the Ovamboland, in the north of South West Africa, a former German colony under South African mandate since the end of WWI. To study the situation, the South African government dispatched Louis Fourie, an assistant health officer of the South African Department of Public Health, and a former South West African medical officer.[22] Following fieldwork conducted between April and May 1932, Fourie affirmed that the Ovamboland epidemic was linked to a plague epizootic among gerbils, the same wild rodents responsible for several plague outbreaks in South Africa. Furthermore, Fourie concluded that the Ovamboland outbreak "was caused by the spread of an epizootic of rodent plague from the Union [of South Africa] northwards through the Kalahari [Desert]" in the wake of the gerbils' migration.[23]

In the Portuguese colony of Angola, which bordered the Ovamboland, this episode was met with apprehension. The first plague outbreak in Angola, linked to domestic rats, had occurred in 1921, when the disease reached the capital, Luanda. From that year onwards, other outbreaks emerged around the coast and its hinterland, but a plague "invasion" connected to wild rodents coming from the southern border had seemed, until then, highly unlikely.[24] Such a prospect threatened the politically fraught Baixo Cunene region, which had only been incorporated into the Portuguese Empire in the first decades of the twentieth century, and where insurrections and resistance were still

21 Jorge, Les Faunes (note 15), 1286.

22 E. N. Thornton, La Peste dans l'Union Sud-Africaine et le Territoire Sous Mandat du Sud-Ouest Africain, in: Bulletin Trimestriel de l'organisation d'hygiène II/1 (1933), 79–81.

23 Louis Fourie, Report on Plague in Ovamboland, South West Africa, Annual Report of the Department of Public Health, Year Ended 30th June, 1932, Pretoria, 1932, 79.

24 Ricardo Jorge, La Peste en Angola, Paris 1935, 1–2.

frequent.[25] The Ovamboland episode thus sparked both imperial anxieties and sanitary concerns, which led to the creation of a scientific mission financed by the Angolan colonial government. Directed by Francisco Venâncio da Silva, a medical doctor, the mission was sent to Baixo Cunene in June 1932.[26] Silva carried out studies on the local rodent fauna, catching and examining them with the help of the local population,[27] and sending some specimens to the Bocage Museum in Lisbon.[28] Furthermore, Silva gathered evidence to support the presumption that some wild rodents previously unknown to the population of Baixo Cunene were "invading" the Baixo Cunene coming from the Ovamboland, where they were linked to the plague outbreak.[29]

Based on Fourie's report and Silva's initial observations, the Portuguese colonial government concluded that a plague outbreak in Baixo Cunene was probably just a matter of time, given that the region shared the same environment and several species of wild rodents with the contaminated parts of South West Africa and South Africa. In the face of this menace, Silva's mission was promoted to a permanent plague service in November 1932.[30] In the first communications by Portuguese officials about the outbreak in the Ovamboland, they did not use the term sylvatic plague, but spoke merely of plague among wild rodents. However, in a confidential report sent to Jorge, written in 1935, Silva began to mobilize the new concept to describe the situation he was observing on the border between the Ovamboland and Baixo Cunene. Silva's use of the term could thus be due to this direct interaction with its inventor.[31]

From its beginning, Silva's plague service targeted wild rodents. Silva himself travelled throughout the Baixo Cunene region demanding that the indigenous population make their dwellings rodent-proof, chase rodents from the vicinities of their villages, and protect the rodents' natural enemies, such as snakes and birds, in an effort to break the chain of human-rodent interactions.[32] In addition, the local population was pressed to inform Silva's service of any case of plague among humans or any epizootic among wild rodents. The service would then come to the village in question, vaccinate its population, and pump cyanide gas into wild rodent holes in the fields nearby. These

25 Francisco Venâncio da Silva, Serviço Permanente de Prevenção e Combate à Peste Bubônica no Sul de Angola/Relatório 1933, Lisboa 1936, 6.

26 Ibid., 12–15.

27 Ibid., 16.

28 Ibid., 138.

29 Francisco Venâncio da Silva, Animais Bravos nas Suas Relações com os Problemas Sanitários do Sul de Angola, Luanda 1939, 25.

30 Ministério das Colônias/Gabinete do Ministro, Decreto n. 21:866, in: Diário do Governo I/270, 17 November 1932, 2231–2233.

31 Francisco Venâncio da Silva, Relatório Sobre a Peste Selvática em Angola. Elaborado a Pedido do Prof. Dr. Ricardo Jorge, 25 June 1935, Biblioteca Nacional de Portugal - Reservados. Espólio 18, caixa 18, maço 5, Biblioteca Nacional de Portugal - Reservados.

32 Jorge, La Peste en Angola (note 24), 6–7.

measures sought to kill both the rodents and their parasites, reducing the risk of plague outbreaks among humans and breaking the chain of infection among rodents.[33]

In 1933, fears of an invasion of plague in the Baixo Cunene became a reality when eleven cases of plague among humans, nine of them fatal, were observed in the locality of Namacunda, not far from the Ovamboland border.[34] In the following years, however, although important epizootics among wild rodents were registered in the Baixo Cunene, very few human cases were reported or officially diagnosed.[35] After 1937, plague cases among humans and animals ceased to be reported entirely. After that date, the "epidemic wave" was considered over and the risk of plague taking root in southern Angola was officially dismissed. Nevertheless, as Silva wrote in 1953, the disappearance of human cases did not mean that sylvatic plague had vanished from Angola; on the contrary, it likely remained a "latent problem" that could re-emerge at any time.[36]

3. The Risk of Sylvatic Plague in the UK via Imported Rodents from the US, 1938–1939

Sylvatic plague as a new concept, as well as the awareness of the risks posed by wild rodents in conserving and spreading the plague bacillus, gained global traction in the 1930s, following the publication of a new report by Jorge, this time focused exclusively on Africa and deeply connected with the situation of South West Africa and Angola.[37] In the US, a Sylvatic Plague Committee, led by Karl F. Meyer, was created in 1935 to study and address the presence of plague among wild rodents in California and other states on the West Coast.[38] As Meyer admitted, he was informed by Jorge's works and described the Portuguese doctor as an important reference for understanding the different problems posed by the plague among wild rodents when compared with the more common case of plague among domestic rats.[39] In October 1938, as part of a research trip to Canada and the US, the prominent English ecologist Charles Elton visited Meyer and his colleagues in California. Elton discussed the problem of plague in

33 Silva, Serviço Permanente (note 25), 151.

34 Silva, Relatório, (note 31), XII.

35 Ibid., XII–XIV.

36 Francisco Venâncio da Silva, Peste Selvática, Problema Sempre Latente em Angola, in: Anais do Instituto de Medicina Tropical X/3 (1953), 976.

37 Ricardo Jorge, La Peste Africaine, in: Bulletin Mensuel de l'Office International d'Hygiène Publique XXVII/9 (Supplement) (1935), 1–67.

38 W. P. Shepard, Concerning Sylvatic Plague, in: California and Western Medicine 43/5 (1935), 386–387.

39 Karl F. Meyer, The Sylvatic Plague Committee, in: American Journal of Public Health and the Nation's Health 26/10 (1936), 961.

rodents in the US with them and studied techniques to trap squirrels and collect their parasites.[40]

Elton's interest in wild rodents and the plague was not new, especially when it came to the latter's role in regulating animal populations. However, Elton's trip to North America had another effect: it consolidated his fears about the risk of sylvatic plague seeding in the UK via imported wild rodents to be exhibited in zoological gardens. In fact, a few months earlier, in March 1938, Elton had already written to his friend Julian Huxley, a biologist and secretary of the Zoological Society of London, expressing his concerns. He first explained to Huxley in general terms the problem of plague among wild rodents, affirming that he

> had been reading all the recent reports from the United States on sylvatic plague, that is, bubonic plague which has become established in the wild rodent population, much in the same way as it has in South Africa during the last twenty years, and from time immemorial in Siberia.[41]

Then, based on his reading of the recent research in the US, Elton told Huxley about the risks sylvatic plague posed to the UK:

> Although thousands of specimens of ground squirrels have been examined in different places [in the US], lesions are very seldom discovered. But when pooled quotas of fleas from a number of individuals are ground up and injected into guinea pigs, bubonic plague develops. It is that there is a real danger of introducing bubonic plague into this country [Britain] or other countries through the medium of specimens which any quarantine officer would pass as for as their individual health is concerned. The implication […] is obvious: that you [Huxley] should keep a careful watch on the situation, especially if you are going to import prairie dogs or other marmots and squirrels, especially from the West and Western regions of North America.[42]

In this letter, Elton also clarified that the primary problem was not that the imported wild rodents could spread the disease among humans, as domestic rats were feared to do, but rather that a permanent plague reservoir could be constituted among Britain's wild animals. This was not without precedent, as Elton pointed out: in 1910, a small plague outbreak among humans occurred in East Anglia,[43] which was related to plague

---

40 Charles Elton, Typescript diary of a visit to Canada and USA 29 August–17 October 1938, Bodleian Library, Oxford, UK [hereafter BoL]. Catalogued Archives MS. Eng. C. 3329, C. 24.

41 Charles Elton to Julian Huxley, 9 March 1938, Zoology Elton Archive: Correspondence about sylvatic plague 1938–1939, Bol. Catalogued Archives MS. Eng. C. 3329, C. 24. 22/1/1.

42 Ibid.

43 On that outbreak, see Karen Sayer, Vermin Landscapes. Suffolk, England, Shaped by Plague, Rat and Flea (1906–1920), in Christos Lynteris (ed), Framing Animals as Epidemic Villains, Cham 2019, 27–64.

epizootics among field rodents and rabbits.[44] Therefore, if plague could be newly imported via wild rodents, and if the infection then spread to England's native rodents and other animals, Elton worried that "there [was] practically no chance of eliminating it [sylvatic plague] by any measure at present known by us".[45]

Elton was not exactly clear, however, on how plague could pass from imported wild rodents to Britain's native animals. Therefore, we can only wonder whether Elton feared that wild rodents would escape from the zoological gardens and meet local animals, or that rats or other animals could encounter caged wild rodents on the premises of the zoos, or whether his concerns were, in fact, that wild rodents' ectoparasites infected with the plague bacillus could leave their hosts and establish themselves among local animals.

Elton's pleas were at first rejected by Huxley, who considered them quite "alarmist".[46] Elton then decided to contact the Minister of Health, Sir Arthur MacNalty.[47] MacNalty took Elton's concerns more seriously, and in November 1938 imposed a compulsory quarantine of three months on "all animals known to be commonly susceptible to epizootic plague" imported to the UK via zoological gardens. It was also decided that these rodents had to be submitted to a periodical removal of their fleas and parasites.[48] Elton considered this solution: "If this advice is consistently carried out", he wrote, "it will greatly reduce the chance of sylvatic plague getting into this country".[49] The quarantine solution was nonetheless criticized by Huxley for the problems it created for zoological gardens. In fact, since wild rodents had very short lifespans, their exposition time to the public was considerably reduced after a three-month quarantine. The issue triggered new discussions between Elton and Huxley, this time on the possibility of British zoological gardens breeding rodents instead of importing them.[50]

---

44 Charles Elton to Julian Huxley (note 41).

45 Charles Elton to Arthur MacNalty, 18 November 1938, Zoology Elton Archive: Correspondence about sylvatic plague 1938–1939, Bol. Catalogued Archives MS. Eng. C. 3329, C. 24. 22/1/1.

46 Julian Huxley to Charles Elton, 10 March 1938. Zoology Elton Archive: Correspondence about sylvatic plague 1938–1939, Bol, Catalogued Archives MS. Eng. C. 3329, C. 24. 22/1/1.

47 Charles Elton to Arthur MacNalty, 24 March 1938. Zoology Elton Archive: Correspondence about sylvatic plague 1938–1939, Bol. Catalogued Archives MS. Eng. C. 3329, C. 24. 22/1/1.

48 Arthur MacNalty to Charles Elton, 14 November 1938. Zoology Elton Archive: Correspondence about sylvatic plague 1938–1939, Bol. Catalogued Archives MS. Eng. C. 3329, C. 24. 22/1/1.

49 Charles Elton to Arthur MacNalty, 18 November 1938, Zoology Elton Archive: Correspondence about sylvatic plague 1938–1939, Bol. Catalogued Archives MS. Eng. C. 3329, C. 24. 22/1/1. I could not find any information if these quarantines practices stayed in place after 1938.

50 Julian Huxley to Charles Elton, 3 July 1939, Zoology Elton Archive: Correspondence about sylvatic plague 1938–1939, Bol, Catalogued Archives MS. Eng. C. 3329, C. 24. 22/1/1 and Charles Elton to Julian Huxley, 4 July 1939, Zoology Elton Archive: Correspondence about sylvatic plague 1938–1939, Bol, Catalogued Archives MS. Eng. C. 3329, C. 24. 22/1/1.

In short, to Elton, British zoological gardens were seen as a kind of intermediary space where a connection, albeit one neither fully described nor understood, would be achieved between the sylvatic plague *foyer* in North America and wild rodents in Britain. In that sense, what was feared was not immediate human outbreaks, as in Angola, but the plague bacillus's circulation among British wild rodents and the formation of an independent and ineradicable local sylvatic plague reservoir. The idea of sylvatic plague thus appeared in Elton's writings both as a standardized concept to describe plague among wild rodents in several parts of the world and as a justification for imposing preventive measures against wild rodents in Britain.

4. The Transformation of Plague into Sylvatic, Brazil, 1940s and 1950s

The Angolan and British cases exposed the risk of plague being carried across international borders by migratory rodents or via the circulation of wild rodents by humans, respectively. The fight against wild rodents in Brazil in the 1940s reveals some interesting correlations and particularities. In Brazil, while there was a fear that a sylvatic reservoir would be formed, the danger was seen to lie not in importations from foreign countries, but rather in the local expansion from a reservoir among domestic rats into one among wild rodents.

Plague arrived in Brazil in 1899 and caused several important outbreaks in the country's main ports, and especially in its capital, Rio de Janeiro, in the first decade of the twentieth century.[51] After a resolute campaign of deratization starting in 1903, the disease progressively decreased in Rio de Janeiro.[52] Nevertheless, in the 1920s, scattered outbreaks appeared in mid-sized cities and rural villages far from the coast.[53] This was a problem especially in the backlands (*sertões*), a region in the north-east prone to recurrent drought. A series of decisive missions to study these outbreaks was carried out in 1935 and 1936, covering the states of Pernambuco, Ceará, and Paraíba. They took place in a moment of increased centralization of public health in Brazil during

---

51 Dilene Raimundo do Nascimento/Matheus Alves Duarte da Silva, "Não é Meu Intuito Estabelecer Polêmica". A Chegada da Peste ao Brasil, Análise de uma Controvérsia, 1899, in: História, Ciências, Saúde-Manguinhos 20/1 (2013), 1271–1285.

52 Silva, Quand la Peste Connectait le Monde (note 7).

53 It does not mean, though, that plague completely disappeared from the Brazilian coast. The city of Fortaleza, the capital of Ceará state, localized in the Atlantic coast, was touched in 1934, which created a momentum for the 1935–1936 missions. See Amadeu Fialho, Estudos Sobre a Peste Bubônica no Ceará, in: Revista de Hygiene e Saúde Pública IX/6 (1935), 183.

the Vargas regime[54] and were intended "to collect data and study the local conditions aiming to elaborate a general plan to eradicate the plague".[55]

These missions initially arrived at a rather a classical conclusion, pointing out that most of the human outbreaks in the north-east could be traced to infected domestic rats, which nested in the poor houses, granaries, and cotton storage facilities abundant in rural villages.[56] These experts also noticed that some wild rodents, such as *preás*, *punarés*, and *mocós*,[57] commonly found close to rural villages and valued as bush meat by locals, seemed potentially implicated in the plague outbreaks. As hunters, farmers, and other local actors informed the plague experts in 1935 and 1936, human outbreaks in the backlands were commonly preceded by wide annual epizootic waves, which affected both wild rodents and domestic rats.[58] While no one was certain of the cause of these epizootics, some experts were thoroughly convinced that it was the plague.[59] The enquiries conducted between 1935–36 left open the question of whether wild rodents could be considered the main reservoir of plague in Brazil's north-east or whether, on the contrary, their infection was only incidental and dependent upon their contact with infected domestic rats, who would therefore be the main reservoir of the disease. Brazilian authorities, however, remained convinced that the plague would be best controlled by focusing on domestic rats, since their connection to human plague outbreaks was well established. Consequently, the main measure adopted in the late 1930s in farms and villages in the north-east was rat poisoning, coupled with anti-plague vaccination and the support, albeit feeble, of rat-proofing practices.[60]

In July 1939, the Pan-American Health Organization, in agreement with the Brazilian authorities, commissioned the Chilean doctor Atilio Macchiavello to study the plague in the north-east of Brazil.[61] At the end of his mission, in 1940, Macchiavello affirmed that domestic rats played the crucial role of spreading and conserving the plague, but conceded that local wild rodents could likewise be infected by the plague and die from it in epizootic outbreaks. However, he found no evidence "of a primary wild rodents epi-

54 Getúlio Vargas ruled Brazil from 1930–34 as a "temporary president", from 1934–1937, as elected president, and from 1937–1945 as dictator. From 1950 until his suicide in 1954, he was again Brazilian President, elected by popular vote.

55 Mario da Camara Motta, O Problema da Peste no Estado da Parahyba, in: Archivos de Hygiene VI/1 (1936), 210.

56 Decio Parreiras, Notas e Estudos Sobre a Peste no Nordeste do Brasil, Problema Nacional, 1935, 429.

57 Respectively *Cavia aperea*, *Thrichomys apereoides*, *Kerodon rupestris*. While the *preá* can be found in other South American countries, the *punaré* and *mocó* are endemic to Brazil.

58 Marcelo Silva Junior, 'Peste no Ceará', in: Archivos de Hygiene VI/1 (1936), 177.

59 Fialho, Estudos (note 53), 198.

60 João de Barros Barreto, A Peste no Brasil nos Últimos Cinco Anos, in: Archivos de Hygiene 8/2 (1938), 366–368.

61 Atilio Macchiavello, Contribuciones al Estudio de la Peste Bubonica en el Nordeste del Brasil, Guayaquil 1941, 9–10.

zootic"; quite the opposite: wild rodents were almost always killed by primary plague epizootics among rats, which suggested that the rats in fact represented the real plague reservoir in Brazil.[62] Macchiavello affirmed that what existed in the backlands was a condition he called "rural plague", characterized by its widespread distribution in an area of scattered population. To Macchiavello, rural plague was completely linked to domestic rats, which led him to conclude that sylvatic plague "possibly did not exist" in the country.[63]

Macchiavello played an important role in the circulation of ideas such as rural plague and sylvatic plague in Brazil. His reasoning influenced the creation of the Brazilian National Plague Service (*Serviço Nacional de Peste*, hereafter SNP) in 1941 and its mission.[64] The SNP aimed primarily to control rats in cities, villages, and rural areas, but also to prevent plague from becoming sylvatic in Brazil. As Almir de Castro, the director of the SNP, put it when explaining the evolution of plague in Brazil up to 1941 to the Minister of Health, Gustavo Capanema: "fortunately, we still have not yet reached [...] the sylvatic plague moment, whose eradication would be almost impossible".[65]

Following the creation of the SNP, the fight against rats was intensified, mainly in the north-east. The measures implemented by the new service included not only rat poisoning, but also direct hunting, trapping, and most importantly, the destruction of rats inside their holes by means of flamethrowers or toxic gas.[66] During this campaign, wild rodents occupied an ambiguous place. On the one hand, their infection was considered peripheric and often dependent on domestic rats. On the other hand, they represented a risk, because if the plague bacillus started to circulate freely among them in the north-east without depending on humans and domestic rats as hosts, and if this enzootic cycle came to affect wild rodents in the backlands and other regions, such as the Amazon, then plague would probably never be eradicated from Brazil.[67] Aware of this risk, the SNP often targeted wild rodents alongside domestic rats. When destroying rat-holes by flamethrowers, for example, the SNP commonly killed wild rodents as well, which nested close by and sometimes even in the same holes. When hunting rats by means of traps and sticks, the SNP also often destroyed a plethora of wild rodents.[68] Because of these direct hunting practices, in 1951, João Moojen de Oliveira, a zoologist attached to the Museu Nacional and Brazil's foremost rodent expert, proposed establishing a rodent collection, which

---

62 Ibid., 152–153.

63 Ibid., 101.

64 Simone Luna, O Serviço Nacional de Peste e o Controle da Peste Bubônica no Nordeste Brasileiro (1941–1956), Master's Thesis, Rio de Janeiro, Fundação Oswaldo Cruz/Casa de Oswaldo Cruz, 2021.

65 Almir de Castro, Atividades de Profilaxia Antipestosa do Departamento Nacional de Saúde do Ministério da Educação e Saúde 1937–1941, Rio de Janeiro, 31 October 1942, Fundação Getúlio Vargas Archives, 2, GC h 1940.03.11.

66 Almir de Castro, Serviço Nacional de Peste, in: Archivos de Hygiene 17/3–4 (1947), 316.

67 Roland Simon, Verificação da Sensibilidade dos Roedores da Região Neotrópica, Rio de Janeiro 1951.

68 Serviço Nacional de Peste. Boletins de Captura de Pequenos Mamíferos' (1944), Museu Nacional, Setor de Vertebrados.

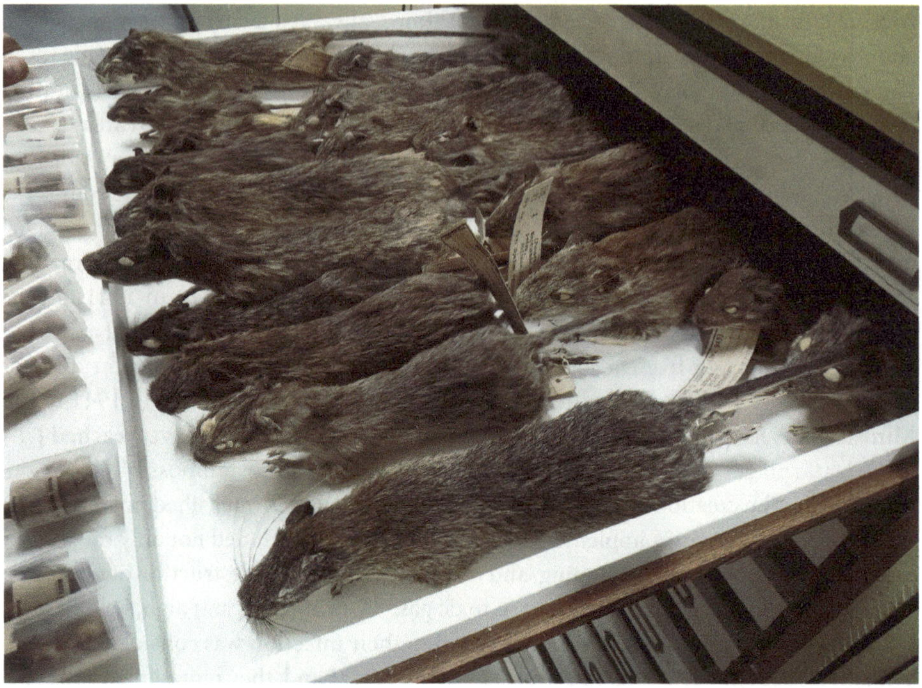

Fig. 1 Taxidermized *punarés* (Thrichomys aperoides), caught by the SNP in the Brazilian north-east from 1951–1956 (Museu Nacional, Rio de Janeiro/Brazil).

could improve knowledge of the species of rodents in the north-east, their distribution, sensibility to plague, and other related data. Moreover, the specimens collected could serve as valuable goods for exchange with other museums. One of the largest in the world, the SNP collection now contains 55,291 specimens, a testament to the SNP's capacity for catching and killing rodents (see fig. 1). In addition to direct destruction, the SNP also employed specific rodent-proofing measures, ordering the removal or increased distance of live fences (*cerca de avelós*) from the house. Frequently erected very close to rural dwellings, these live fences were seen by SNP doctors as places where wild rodents and domestic rats could meet and, therefore, where plague could spread and circulate among wild rodents.[69] In sum, although it remained dependent on anti-rat measures, the fight against wild rodents in the north-east of Brazil – informed by the menace of the possible emergence of sylvatic plague – became a central sanitary measure in the 1940s and 50s.[70]

69 Celso Arcoverde Freitas, Histórias da Peste e de Outras Endemias, Rio de Janeiro 1988, 75–76.

70 João Alves de Oliveira/Stella Maris Franco, A Coleção de Mamíferos do Serviço Nacional de Peste no Museu Nacional, Rio de Janeiro, Brasil, in: Arquivos do Museu Nacional 63/1 (2005).

In March 1956, the SNP was dismantled, partly because of the decline in plague cases in the preceding years, which rendered the service somewhat redundant. Between 1957 and 1960, some of the ideas that gave coherence and oriented SNP actions, namely the absence of sylvatic plague, started to be criticized by local and foreign plague experts working in the backlands. These new studies argued that wild rodents, instead of domestic rats, were the real reservoir of plague in Brazil, meaning that sylvatic plague had already emerged there.[71] Such an understanding became progressively more accepted after new research conducted in the city of Exú in the late 1960s and early 1970s,[72] and still remains the main paradigm for explaining the endemicity of plague in Brazil.[73]

5. Conclusion

This chapter has provided the first global history of the fight against wild rodents in the second quarter of the twentieth century. The anti-rodent sanitary measures detailed here were prompted by the fear that the plague bacillus could start circulating among wild rodents in "natural" spaces, and that plague would therefore never be eradicated from those localities. These fears are reflected in the policies adopted against wild rodents in Angola, the UK, and Brazil, three countries with different political, ecological, and geographical conditions, but nonetheless connected by their wars against wild rodents.

The anti-rodent measures in these three countries – namely, direct destruction, quarantines, and the rodent-proofing of buildings – were introduced at a time when plague did not exist among local wild rodents. In other words, these measures were implemented before a cycle of infections independent of humans and domestic rats had been established. Therefore, the purpose of framing wild rodents as potential transmitters of plague in Angola, the UK, and Brazil was to anticipate and avoid a scenario of plague maintenance in natural environments. The risk this scenario posed was a double one: the constitution of a wild reservoir would mean, firstly, that plague could never be eradicated among wild rodents, and secondly, that the disease could potentially jump from them back to rats and humans.

Independent reservoirs among wild rodents already existed in other parts of the world, a phenomenon described by Ricardo Jorge as sylvatic plague. This new concept

71 Alberto Gonçalves Neves, O Problema da Peste dos Roedores Silvestres no Nordeste Brasileiro, Rio de Janeiro 1957; José Maria de la Barrera, Relatório Sobre a Peste no Brasil, April 1960, Museu Nacional, Setor de Vertebrados.

72 Celso Tavares, Análise do Contexto, Estrutura e Processos que Caracterizaram o Plano Piloto de Peste em Exu e Sua Contribuição ao Controle da Peste no Brasil, PhD Thesis, Recife, Fundação Oswaldo Cruz/Centro de Pesquisas Aggeu Magalhães, 2007.

73 Brasil. Ministério da Saúde, Manual de vigilância e controle da peste, Brasília 2008.

had particular relevance for the three cases discussed in this chapter, where it acted not only as a descriptive notion, but also as sort of cautionary tale and prophecy. Precisely because of this prophetic aspect, anti-rodent measures seemed justified because they were intended to prevent a direr future scenario – but this scenario itself could only be imagined in Angola, the UK, and Brazil because of Jorge's new concept. Thus, while the idea of sylvatic plague justified a range of measures against wild rodents – amounting to a true global war –, these sanitary interventions served themselves to reinforce the concept, and in a way, transformed it into a new scientific paradigm for thinking about and combatting plague reservoirs.

Photo credit

Fig. 1 Taxidermized *punarés* (Thrichomys aperoides), caught by the SNP in the Brazilian northeast from 1951–1956, Museu Nacional, Rio de Janeiro/Brazil. © Photo by Matheus Alves Duarte da Silva. I am very grateful to Prof João Alves de Oliveira for letting me visit and photograph the collection.

Abstract:
The first half of the twentieth century witnessed debates on the part played by wild rodents on "conserving" the plague bacillus and eventually spreading it within national borders, and even beyond. This condition was christened by the Portuguese doctor Ricardo Jorge as sylvatic plague in 1926–1927. In the following years, sylvatic plague began to be seen as an important risk in places where an independent cycle of plague infection among wild rodents did not yet exist. This chapter examines three contexts where the spectre of sylvatic plague haunted health officers. Firstly, Angola, where the new concept framed a plague invasion by migratory gerbils coming from South Africa in 1932 and justified measures to destroy these animals. Secondly, the UK, where quarantine measures were applied in 1938–1939 against imported rodents to be exposed in zoos over the risks they could spread the sylvatic plague among local rodents. Finally, Brazil, where the menace of sylvatic plague appearing in the backlands and in the Amazon justified the creation of the Brazilian Plague National Service in 1941, and the deployment of anti-rat and anti-rodent measures in the 1940s and 1950s. Taken together, these contexts suggests that a truly global war against wild rodents unfolded in the second quarter of the twentieth century.

Keywords:
disease ecology | enzootic | global history | third plague pandemic | Charles Elton

Stephanie Zehnle

“the baboon is [...] too much like man.”

Entangled Primate History and the Beginnings of HIV in Colonial Africa

When European expeditions visited African colonies around 1900, most of them fed on any game that came in front of their rifles. Their menu even included monkey and chimpanzee meat, notwithstanding the kinship between man and ape that had been established by Darwin and his disciples. Expeditioners like the Swiss zoologist Johann Büttikofer (1850–1927) were then quite surprised to learn that, while indigenous African hunters did kill and eat monkey species, they strictly abstained from the flesh of great apes. They would kill them in defence, but never consume them. In the West African state of Liberia, Büttikofer was told via his interpreter that “the baboon” – a pidgin English term for chimpanzee – was “too much like man” to eat it.[1] The similarity of ape and human organisms does in fact increase the likelihood of trans-species infection with diseases and poses a real danger to both human and ape health. Such zoonotic infections with Simian immunodeficiency viruses (SIV) from non-human African primates to humans caused the beginning of HIV (human immunodeficiency viruses) epidemics in the 1970s. In central Africa, indigenous hunters acknowledge that chimpanzees must not be eaten because their meat would infect humans with a sort of “bloody cough.”[2] West African indigenous hunters, on the other hand, did not give health-related reasons for their taboos: The upright gait and the great ape mode of fighting with weapons were simply too similar to human behaviour to eat them.[3]

However, the Simian viruses are at least 30,000 years old, so that humans have cohabited with SIV for a long time. Why then, did HIV only emerge in the early twentieth century in colonial Africa? SIV/HIV is transmitted via bodily fluids between or within primate species. So how did inter-primate contact change in quantity and/or quality around the turn of the century, to facilitate contacts with ape and monkey blood or genital fluids? While the origins of HIV across colonial Africa have hitherto been described as the results of more general historical processes – such as destruction of ecosystems, racist tropical medicine, global mass migration, and urban prostitution – this chap-

1 Johann Büttikofer, Reisebilder aus Liberia. Resultate geographischer, naturwissenschaftlicher und ethnographischer Untersuchungen während der Jahre 1879–1882 und 1886–1887, 2 vols. Leiden 1890–1891, vol. 1, 229.

2 Robert Brisson, Mythologie des Pygmées Baka, Paris 1999, 144.

3 Büttikofer, Reisebilder (note 1), vol. 1, 230.

ter attempts to trace more local and interspecies drivers of the zoonotic viral disease HIV/AIDS. I will therefore argue that crucial alterations in human-primate interactions began well before colonialism and can thus explain the causes of HIV emergence on a more trans-local level. To follow this 'deep history' agenda, this chapter focuses on the two regions where HIV originated: the Guinean forests of West Africa, and the Central African forests of Southern Cameroon and Congo.

1. Rethinking the Global Panzootic Age

About 60% of human diseases today are caused by infections from animal vectors or animal hosts. Such animal-human infections have triggered waves of epidemics throughout the modern age, and particularly in the 'long twentieth century' – a century already being classified as the "pandemic century."[4] The history of the spread of epidemics from 1790 onwards is a global one, because "although [epidemics] are not noticeable with similar intensity everywhere in the world, they can potentially affect all inhabitants of the planet and are therefore 'global' in a maximum sense."[5] In an already globalized world, epidemics – like HIV – appear with an alleged simultaneity of break-outs.[6] As a consequence of the SARS-CoV-2 pandemic, global historians are now paying attention to "the threatening, toxic, even deadly side of 'connectivity' and global connections"[7] as well as of cultural brokerage. Stefanie Gänger and Jürgen Osterhammel, for example, have warned that if global historians did not answer historical questions about the pandemic's past and present properly, others who were less prepared would.[8] In the long run, "environmental and medical humanities – be they global or not – will drift from the peripheries of different disciplines into their centers."[9] This new expertise among global environmental historians requires methods and results from animal history, as this chapter will demonstrate.

4 See Mark Honigsbaum, The Pandemic Century. One Hundred Years of Panic, Hysteria and Hubris, London 2019.

5 Jürgen Osterhammel, China als Zentrum und Peripherie der Pandemiegeschichte, in: Geschichte und Gesellschaft 46 (2020), 507–521, 507: "Erstens machen sie sich zwar nicht überall auf der Welt mit gleichmäßiger Intensität bemerkbar, können aber potenziell alle Bewohnerinnen und Bewohner des Planeten betreffen und sind deshalb in einem maximalen Sinne ‚global'."

6 Mark Harrison, Pandemics, in: Mark Jackson (ed.), The Routledge History of Disease, London 2017, 129–146, 130.

7 Stefanie Gänger/Jürgen Osterhammel, Denkpause für Globalgeschichte, in: Merkur. Deutsche Zeitschrift für europäisches Denken 74/855 (2020), 79–86, 83: „Die bedrohliche, toxische, gar todbringende Seite von ‚Konnektivität' und weltweiten Verbindungen [...]."

8 Ibid., 86.

9 Ibid., 85: "Die *environmental* und *medical humanities*, ob global oder nicht, dürften von der Peripherie der verschiedenen Fächer zu deren Zentren hin driften."

So far, the causes given for the rise of new infections between humans and animals since the 1880s have tended to be similar regardless of region or pathogen: "The rise of industrial farming in the nineteenth century and the links fostered by global capitalism created new disease ecologies; truly global panzootics in this period."[10] Recent findings from global and colonial history therefore link pandemics with other crises of the Anthropocene, particuarly climate change and white supremacy.[11] Extreme weather conditions of the past, for instance, have led to hunger crises, animal epidemics, and finally to human epidemic diseases. Environmental racism – for example forcing enslaved people to live under unhygienic or mosquito-infested conditions – increases both the risk of animal-human infections and the mortality rate after exposure to pathogens. As a third nexus, global warming broadens the zones of (sub)tropical diseases and confronts new human generations with new diseases.[12] It is noteworthy that these three crises – epidemics, climate change, and racism – were all fuelled by colonial exploitation. While global history often gave universal answers to the question of global epidemics, the panzootic origin of the majority of diseases has not been sufficiently addressed, because the animal factor has been reduced to environmental degradation in the cases of HIV, Ebola, and SARS-CoV-2.[13] Human-animal histories are required to address the causes and risk factors of the global panzootic age adequately.

Awareness of global zoonotic dangers declined when antibiotics reduced mortality after bacterial infections and when vaccination campaigns against viruses proved successful – such as with the eradication of smallpox in 1977 and annual influenza vaccines from the 1970s onwards. Emerging zoonotic diseases were largely ignored, so that the world only learnt about the colonial origins of HI-viruses around 1990. This shock generated a new epidemiological paradigm that slowly started to integrate animal sciences. Hence, the first "Emerging Viruses"[14] conference was held in Washington, D.C. in May 1989, and afterwards, epidemiologists focused less on past animal-human infections and more on current or anticipated zoonoses in line with epidemiological futurism. And yet, the epidemiological methods of artificial intelligence and big data analysis also shed light on the past of zoonotic epidemics, as summarized by the historian of health and medicine Robert Peckham: "Technology has undermined the rigid temporal frame of the epidemic, accentuating simultaneity and making the 'beginning' and the 'end'

10 Kyle Harper, Germs, Genomes, and Global History in the Time of COVID-19, in: Journal of Global History 15/3 (2020), 1–13, 11.

11 Eleonora Rohland, Corona, Klima und weiße Suprematie – Multiple Krisen oder eine?, in: Michael Volkmer/Karin Werner (eds.), Die Corona-Gesellschaft. Analysen zur Lage und Perspektiven für die Zukunft. X-Texte zu Kultur und Gesellschaft, Bielefeld 2020, 45–53.

12 Ibid., 48.

13 Ibid., 48.

14 Stephen S. Morse (ed.), Emerging Viruses, New York/Oxford 1993.

harder to determine."[15] The simultaneous scientific observation of ancient and recent pathogens in humans and other living beings under the One Health paradigm blurs traditional temporal orders of human epidemics – starting with a visible breakout and ending when there are no longer masses of sick humans. One Health defines a new way of researching human and animal health and disease by focussing on their entanglements with each other and the environment. The paradigm was coined in 2004, when the Wildlife Conservation Society hosted a symposium and published a conference paper titled "Manhattan Principles on One World – One Health."[16] Although wildlife experts first introduced the term, the field nowadays encompasses both human and veterinary medicine.[17] However, the concept of One Health, as I would argue, also requires more historical expertise, because zoonotic "epidemics materialize a 'presence of the past,' a bodily and ecological inscription of history"[18] and are therefore essentially *historical*. Global and colonial history can fill this academic void because the "history of infectious disease inherently lends itself to global history."[19] But for this endeavour, global historians must move towards a "less anthropocentric perspective and semantic."[20] To sum up this diffuse and still rudimentary state of the art, global panzootic epidemics must be studied in trans-continental, trans-epochal, trans-disciplinary, and trans-species perspectives.

2. Rethinking SIV/HIV as Entangled Primate History

When scholars of veterinary and human medicine started to look at the African origins of HI-viruses in the 2000s, tropical medicine primarily considered its own dubious role in colonial history in a self-reflexive act of over-evaluation, and therefore blamed colonial doctors for multiple SIV-HIV zoonotic infections among humans. Critical anthropologists agreed and spread the theory that non-sterile vaccinations, infusions, and blood transfusions had caused the first infections of humans with primate SI-viruses, which then mutated into HIV variants. One dominant speculative theory explained that HIV-1 arose in humans through oral polio vaccinations in Congolese Kisangani

---

15 Robert Peckham, The Crisis of Crisis. Rethinking Epidemics from Hong Kong, in: Bulletin of the History of Medicine 94/4 (2020), 658–669, 668.

16 Brian R. Evans/Frederick A. Leighton, A History of One Health, in: Revue scientifique et technique (International Office of Epizootics) 33/2 (2014), 413–420, 417.

17 Cf. the Helmholtz Institute for One Health (HIOH) that was opened in Greifswald/Germany in April 2022.

18 Guillaume Lachenal/Thomas Gaëtan, Epidemics have lost the Plot, in: Bulletin of the History of Medicine 94/4 (2020), 670–689, 683.

19 Harper, Germs (note 10), 351.

20 Gänger/Osterhammel, Denkpause (note 7), 85: "eine weniger anthropozentrische Weltsicht und Semantik.".

(Stanleyville) between 1957 and 1960, right before the country became independent from Belgian colonial rule. Unknown monkey kidney cells were in fact used to cultivate the polio pathogens, and the medical doctors Ghislain Courtois and Hilary Koprowski had actually run an anti-polio campaign in what is now the Democratic Republic of the Congo, Burundi, and Rwanda. This theory was first mentioned in popular media, and in 1992, it was picked up by the medical journal *The Lancet*.[21] As a matter of fact, the oldest HI-viruses were found in blood extracts from African patients around Koprowski's research stations and clinics.[22] But this so-called OPV (Oral Polio Vaccination) theory slowly collapsed when genetic research in the early 2000s demonstrated that Central African HIV-1 actually predated the American OPV campaigns.[23] Yet even today, most researchers accept that the general increase of injections with contaminated needles in late colonial Africa must have multiplied human-to-human SIV infections, with the ape viruses finally mutating into HIV.[24] Belgian colonial forced labour camps and the inadequate medical "treatment" of these exhausted African workers, according to the remains of this theory, were an additional factor in the increase of infections.[25] Other studies highlighted the role of sexual liberation, prostitution, and venereal diseases in the emergence of HIV types in the first half of the twentieth century.

The second important theory about the origin of HIV has blamed the indigenous hunting and consumption of ape meat. The over-simplified variant of the Cut Hunter Theory claims that "late nineteenth century European colonizers imported huge numbers of firearms, and one African hunter, profiting from this arms influx, was cut or injured by a chimpanzee infected with SIV; he then travelled down the Sangha river to Kinshasa and became the 'patient zero' of the HIV/AIDS pandemic."[26] Although these

21 Walter S. Kyle, Simian Retroviruses, Poliovaccine, and Origin of AIDS, in: The Lancet 339/8793 (1992), 600–601.

22 Paul Sendziuk, Review of The River: A Journey Back to the Source of HIV and AIDS, by E. Hooper, in: Health and History 4/2 (2002), 127–130.

23 See B. Korber et al., Timing the Ancestor of the HIV-1 Pandemic Strains, in: Science 288/5472 (2000), 1789–1796. The coffin nail for this theory was this scientific article with an explicit title: M. Worobey et al., Contaminated Polio Vaccine Theory Refuted, in: Nature 428/820 (2004).

24 See for example Jacques Pepin et al., Iatrogenic Transmission of Human T Cell Lymphotropic Virus Type 1 and Hepatitis C Virus through Parenteral Treatment and Chemoprophylaxis of Sleeping Sickness in Colonial Equatorial Africa, in: Clinical Infectious Diseases 51 (2010), 777–784; Jacques Pepin/Annie-Claude Labbé, Noble Goals, Unforeseen Consequences. Control of Tropical Diseases in Colonial Central Africa and the Iatrogenic Transmission of Blood-Borne Viruses, in: Tropical Medicine & International Health 13 (2008), 744–753; Catherine A. Hogan et al., Epidemic History and Iatrogenic Transmission of Blood-borne Viruses in Mid-20th Century Kinshasa, in: The Journal of Infectious Diseases 214/3 (2016), 353–360.

25 Jim Moore, The Puzzling Origins of AIDS. Although no one Explanation has been universally accepted, four rival theories provide some important Lesson, in: American Scientist 92/6 (2004), 540–547.

26 Stephanie Rupp et al., Beyond the Cut Hunter. A Historical Epidemiology of HIV Beginnings in Central Africa, in: EcoHealth 13/4 (2016), 661–671, 661–662.

studies mention more complex socio-historical changes and disruptions as causes of HIV emergence, they all basically point at indigenous communities for having transformed "the hunting and consumption of wild animals as a food source, traditionally a subsistence activity, into a commercial enterprise termed the 'bushmeat' trade."[27] Such articles were therefore accompanied by pictures of the bloody slaughtering of primates by Africans in forests and at markets. Scientific papers about the Cut Hunter Theory either do not mention the term "colonial" at all, or only vaguely refer to human-centred implications such as urbanization.[28] Even the first critical voices from anthropology were convinced that "such hunting is traditional" in African communities.[29] So how did colonial hunting practices influence the hunting of monkeys and apes? Human-animal relations are not static, and neither were hunting and food practices in precolonial and colonial Africa. While this simplified version of the Cut Hunter Theory currently faces heavy critique from anthropologists, more complex Cut Hunter models acknowledge that animal-human blood-to-blood infections during hunting and slaughtering are generally realistic scenarios because SIV had been endemic among apes. However, some disagreed, primate hunting was only intensified after the Second World War and thus *after* the relevant zoonotic infections.[30] These critical voices referred to the "role of social changes and transport networks"[31] and not to changing human-animal relations. Speaking as a historian in this debate, I will not downplay or deny the role of indigenous legal and illegal hunting in the emergence of HIV. Rather, I want to remind discussants to explore human-ape contacts more extensively and beyond indigenous actors: European and American traders, colonial officials, pet keepers, zoo directors, tourists, and others also interacted with SIV-infected primates, so that the focus on indigenous hunting appears insufficient if not racist. For example, many zoo workers in America and Asia have tested positive for other ape viruses.[32]

Most of the hypotheses about the cause of the HIV epidemics collapsed when genetic research demonstrated that different HIV variants had emerged by zoonotic mutations

27 Beatrice H. Hahn et al., AIDS as Zoonosis. Scientific and Public Health Implications, in: Science 287 (2000), 607–614, 613.

28 Michael Worobey et al., Direct Evidence of Extensive Diversity of HIV-1 in Kinshasa by 1960, in: Nature 455 (2008), 661–664, 663.

29 Amit Chitnis/Diana Rawls/Jim Moore, Origin of HIV Type 1 in Colonial French Equatorial Africa? AIDS Research and Human Retroviruses 16 (2000), 5–8, 5.

30 João Dinis de Sousa et al., High GUD Incidence in the early 20th Century created a particularly permissive Time Window for the Origin and initial Spread of epidemic HIV Strains, in: PLoS One 5/4 (2010), 1–16, 3.

31 N. R. Faria et al., The early Spread and Epidemic Ignition of HIV-1 in Human Populations, in: Science 346 (2014), 56–61, 56.

32 Martine Peeters/Mirela D'Arc/Eric Delaporte, The Origin and Diversity of Human Retroviruses, in: AIDS Review 16 (2014), 23–34.

when transmitted from apes to humans as early as between ca. 1914 and 1945.[33] The history of the HI virus is researched by phylogenetic methods that look at today's virus variants and estimate periods of zoonotic transmissions by evolutionary similarities and differences in the DNA:

> First, phylogenies can reveal the ancestral hosts of microorganisms that have evolved to become pathogens of humans. Second, they can place evolutionary relationships in space and thus be integrated with the history of human migrations, contacts, and exchanges. Third, they can be situated in time, allowing evolutionary events such as disease emergence to be placed in historical context.[34]

By reading these results, historians can locate zoonotic human-ape contacts in space and time, at least indirectly, by an estimation procedure colloquially called the "molecular clock": "Molecular clocks estimate the time that it has taken for genetic differences to accumulate."[35] Combinations of phylogenetic and molecular clock methods have thus shown that the two most common HIV variants stemmed from colonial West and Central Africa and from two different primate species: HIV-1M jumped at least four times from Central African gorillas and/or chimpanzees to humans between about 1921 and 1945; the rarer West African variant (HIV-2) crossed species borders at least eight times between 1940 and 1945 from the smaller sooty mangabey monkeys.[36] Animal-human infections with SIV/HIV thus occurred repeatedly and within a similar timeframe in late colonial tropical Africa. The Oral Polio Vaccination Theory relied on the wrong time period (1957–1960), and the Cut Hunter Theory was rejected because there were obviously ten or more "patients zero" involved – not a single person.

These genetic clarifications open doors for new historical research questions and analyses: Why could human-ape interactions have multiplied in this specific colonial period? Why were new contacts established between humans and apes? Did human-ape encounters change in quality, e. g., become "bloodier" or more intimate? The non-historical disciplines involved in this debate – like various medical and public health studies as well as anthropology – very often have a clear presentist research agenda and therefore tend to project today's catalysts of zoonotic tropical infections into Africa's colonial past. Had colonial historians been involved, these questions would have been posed differently: Why is the sexual transmission factor during colonialism linked with a rise of documented consensual sex work and not with less documented rape, such as

33 HIV-1 M originated between 1915 and 1941. Cf. Korber et al., Timing (note 23).

34 Harper, Germs (note 10), 356.

35 Ibid., 357.

36 Tamara Giles-Vernick et al., Social History, Biology, and the Emergence of HIV in Colonial Africa, in: Journal of African History 54 (2013), 11–30.

committed by the colonial military? Why is the bush meat factor only linked with indigenous hunting and not with colonial hunting and pet-keeping? The following sections present some ideas and preliminary hypotheses to explain the causes of HIV emergence in colonial Africa by focussing on human-animal-environment entanglements. With a comparative approach – covering West and Central Africa, HIV-2 and HIV-1 – the next sections tackle the unresolved question of "why multiple HIVs emerged at the same historical moment in widely separated parts of sub-Saharan Africa."[37]

3. The Pre-colonial Factor: Slavery, Jihad Wars, and Wildlife

To better understand the nexus of migration and hunting practices in the parallel histories of the West and Central African HIV "hotspots," we must start with similar – though slightly earlier – pre-colonial processes: the age of jihadist expansion in Africa. Starting in the sixteenth century, Islamized scholars and cattle breeders from the Fulbe ethnic group moved from Mali across the Sahel and undertook Islamic reform movements, conquests, and state-building. In the early eighteenth century, some of these Fulbe founded the Imamate of Futa Jallon in today's Guinea and, in accordance with Islamic war laws, enslaved the alleged unbelievers living in the forest peripheries towards the Atlantic coast. These captives were then taken to the harbours of European slave vessels and on to their American plantations, or they were forced to do work across the theocratic state.[38] As a result of both the jihadist expansion and the Atlantic slave trade, then, large numbers of war refugees and enslaved people lost their villages and fled into the forests of Guinea, Sierra Leone, and Liberia in search of food and shelter. The jihadist wars soon prompted secondary waves of emigration and expulsion from savannah to forest to coast, from one population to the next. Hence, the West African HIV hotspot was a major area of forced migration into the forests in the eighteenth and nineteenth centuries.

While in the Sahel of Mali, such Islamic theocracies were less expansive and organized around walled towns, similar Fulbe expansionist jihadism transformed the Central Sahel of today's northern Nigeria and Cameroon fundamentally. This jihad started in Sokoto in 1804 and included several large Emirates by the 1820s. The military pressed southwards into the forests, and by the 1830s, many of the refugees ended up enslaved in the Bight of Benin or across the Sokoto State. Some paused or resettled in unpopulated or depopulated forest areas.[39] However, the Sokoto warfare towards and enslavement

37 William H. Schneider, Introduction, in: id. (ed.), The Histories of HIVs. The Emergence of the Multiple Viruses that Caused the AIDS Epidemics, Athens 2020, 17.

38 Roman Loimeier, Muslim Societies in Africa. A Historical Anthropology, Bloomington 2013, 115.

39 Stephanie Zehnle, A Geography of Jihad. Sokoto Jihadism and the Islamic Frontier in West Africa, Berlin 2020.

of the south generated waves of flight and expulsion into the Sangha forests, as well as new contacts between gorillas, chimpanzees, and humans.[40] Enslaved informants who were trafficked from the savannahs of the Sokoto Emirates to the Atlantic coast of Nigeria and Cameroon expressed their astonishment when they first encountered apes. They described them in Kanuri as *mala gilage* ("tail bearers") or "haired humans," and some reported that these creatures – probably chimpanzees or gorillas – were exhibited in the Emirate capitals.[41] The growing Islamic State of Sokoto exoticized apes as hybrid human-animals. Stories of the region from the mid-nineteenth century had it that apes had originally been humans who were expelled into the woods as a punishment of God, where their tails grew large. While some feared apes for hunting and eating humans, other accounts claimed that they were strict herbivores. Male ape troop leaders would regularly kill male humans, it was added, only to take their human wives as concubines and rape them in the forest. Hence, women were advised to enter forests only in large groups.[42] Traumatic encounters with both human soldiers and slave traders and aggressive male chimpanzees or gorillas might have been inserted into such spine-chilling stories from nineteenth-century Nigeria and Cameroon. Therefore, more in-depth analyses are needed to clarify how the Islamic wars and slave trade networks multiplied and intensified (sexual?) violence in human-ape encounters.

In southeast Cameroon, where the HIV-1M hotspot is currently located, the residing Baka communities remember how their ancestors in the nineteenth century fled the expansion of the Adamawa Jihadist Emirate and the subsequent military expansion of Cameroun's Grassland states into the southern forests. Two categories of new human-chimpanzee relations then emerged, according to Baka oral history: (1) Some explain how chimpanzees had saved their ancestors' lives, when the hungry emigrants followed the apes into remote forests and learnt from them which fruits and nuts to eat.[43] These historical narratives of learning and receiving help from chimpanzees are usually told in a normative fable to explain why a certain Baka community has tabooed the killing and consumption of great apes. (2) Another category of emigration myth explains the opposite dynamic, how chimpanzee residents and human newcomers started to hunt, kill, and eat each other. In one community, one ape reportedly stole a human baby, initiating an era of interspecies violence in cohabitation: "He lashed out in every direction, broke everything, climbed everywhere, cried out for no reason, jumped

40 Tamara Giles-Vernick/Stephanie Rupp, "Death does not come from the forest but from the village". People, Great Apes, and Disease in the Equatorial African Rain Forest, in: Cahiers d'anthropologie sociale 8/1 (2012), 119–136, 124.

41 Zehnle, Geography of Jihad (note 39), 293.

42 Cf. the discussion in Zehnle, Geography of Jihad (note 39), 644. See also Stephanie Zehnle, War on Wilderness. The Sokoto Jihad of Pre-Colonial West Africa and its Animal Discourse, in: Critical African Studies 8/2 (2016), 216–237.

43 Giles-Vernick/Rupp, Death (note 40), 125.

everywhere, without being aware of the dangers."[44] It is impossible to actually date these incidents based only on published interview extracts, but they certainly commemorate actual conflicts with chimpanzees, because they resemble human-ape violence of the past and present: apes attacking humans working on plantations, apes stealing babies, chimpanzees and gorillas attacking hunters when accidentally injured by their traps.[45] The long history of human-ape cohabitation in Africa is indeed a violent one.[46] In Cameroon, humans and chimpanzees competed for wild mangos and other ripe fruit, so that on multiple occasions they injured each other – even if actual ape-hunting for meat was not practiced by the Baka.

With military and cultural Islamization in Nigeria and Cameroon, food taboos became more restrictive and influential. In the Sahelian food culture, monkey meat was – like pork – considered disgusting and regarded as uncivilized. Nineteenth-century imams propagated that only unbelievers would "eat dried monkey meat."[47] So while the jihad states increased competition between humans and apes for space and vegetarian food, it never deliberately increased monkey-hunting – although slaves and refugees in the forest might have started to eat monkeys and apes in the absence of crops. Moreover, warfare and refugee migration facilitated human bodies contacting formerly unknown viruses.

4. The Colonial Factor: Hunters, Traders, Planters

Colonial warfare – usually referred to euphemistically as "military expeditions" – also led to refugee migration into uncultivated forests. Nonetheless, European colonial expansion seems to have revolutionized the environment more by contract labour, coerced labour, and labour migration. In West and in Central Africa, labour was coerced for the construction of colonial infrastructure and for plantations. Especially in the forests of French Equatorial Africa (and in the Belgian Congo, of course), people fled from their villages into the forests to avoid coerced labour, which was often exhausting and fatal due to the intensity, poor sanitation and nutrition, and corporal punishment. In these Central African rainforests, ruled by France and Belgium, HIV-1 could have emerged when the non-monetarized rural population was coerced to pay the colonial

44 Brisson, Mythologie (note 2), 144: "Il frappe partout, casse tout, grimpe partout, crie pour rien, saute n'importe où, sans se rendre compte du danger." English translation from Giles-Vernick/Rupp, Death (note 40), 125.

45 See Stephanie Zehnle, Of Leopards and Lesser Animals. Trials and Tribulations of the 'Human-Leopard Murders' in Colonial Africa, in: Susan Nance (ed.), The Historical Animal, New York 2015, 221–238.

46 Sandra Swart, Baboon. A Human History, public lecture, UCT Summer School 2017, https://www.youtube.com/watch?v=0S6zDLFAjIM (30 August 2022).

47 Zehnle, Geography of Jihad (note 39), 644.

'hut tax' in rubber: They either went into the forests to harvest the rubber, or they fled into the forests to avoid punishment and coerced labour. Either way, they turned at least into part-time hunters because of the brutal enforcement of taxation. Especially in interwar Central Africa, colonial coerced labour reached the remotest villages via military and police units. These brutal colonial initiatives were thus followed by hunger, neglected farmland, and the hunting of primates.[48]

Despite the blaming of 'traditional' hunters for allegedly consuming ape meat, it was colonialism that forced former cultivators to flee from their fields and suddenly live off hunting in the forest. One can easily imagine how untrained hunters – without culturally inherited food taboos and starving to death – developed new hunting practices. They started to kill and eat apes by chance or out of despair. Moreover, forestry workers and lumberjacks in colonial forests were not provided with food, and thus used game meat as accessible nutrition. Colonial overseers of workers were equipped with firearms that made the hunting of large-apes (like chimpanzees) possible and less dangerous.[49] These apes were mobile themselves, fleeing the forests that were used and cleared for economic exploitation and sometimes attacking people on their farms. Hence, the eating of ape meat could also have resulted from the defence against intruders to the fields with firearms.

But large apes were not the only hosts of the HIV precursors:

> Simian immunodeficiency viruses (SIVs) have been identified in no fewer than 36 different nonhuman primate species in sub-Saharan Africa; however, only two SIV strains, SIVcpz from central chimpanzees (*Pan troglodytes troglodytes*) and SIVsmm from sooty mangabeys (*Cercocebus atys atys*), are known to have crossed the species barrier, generating human immunodeficiency virus type 1 (HIV-1) and HIV-2, respectively.[50]

Sierra Leone forms a hotspot of 82% of all SIV variants of sooty mangabeys turning into HIV-2. At least two zoonotic infections must have occurred in Sierra Leone in the 1940s between mangabeys and humans, which generated HIV-2 groups E and F. Historical zoological sources from early colonial Sierra Leone and Liberia support this hypothesis, which points at non-chimpanzee primates as the hosts of SIV/HIV-2, because eating chimpanzee meat was strictly taboo among the indigenous population. Chimpanzees were considered man-like animals and therefore feared. Large apes were observed to 'dance,' 'hunt,' 'drum,' or imitate humans and were therefore described

48 Tamara Giles-Vernick, Local Primatologies in Central Africa, in: Cahiers d'anthropologie sociale 18/1 (2019), 177–186, 180.

49 Cf. Giles-Vernick, Local Primatologies (note 48).

50 See Mario L. Santiago et al., Simian Immunodeficiency Virus Infection in Free-Ranging Sooty Mangabeys (*Cercocebus atys atys*) from the Taï Forest, Côte d'Ivoire. Implications for the Origin of Epidemic Human Immunodeficiency Virus Type 2, in: Journal of Virology 79/19 (2005), 12515–12527.

as uncanny relatives. Especially their capacity to kill and partly eat other primates – including young and weak humans – was acknowledged with horror.[51] Indigenous Sierra Leoneans considered man-eating in large apes a sort of cannibalism and therefore would not react to such behaviour by hunting and eating them in return – they abstained from becoming similarly "barbarous cannibals."[52] Colonialism and its expansion of plantation systems into chimpanzees' natural habitats clearly prompted chimpanzees to go crop-raiding and to inflict injuries on human farmers and their children.[53] But this increase of chimpanzee attacks on humans – especially between the 1910s and 1930s – obviously did not lead to zoonotic infections with SIVs or the HIV-2 epidemics.

Sooty Mangabeys, on the other hand, were considered less human and were therefore hunted and eaten by West African indigenous communities from time to time. Monkey-eating was practiced before indigenous hunters acquired firearms in considerable numbers from white traders and officials. Instead, these communities had built elaborate traps into which they managed to lure ten to twenty monkeys at a time with manioc.[54] It is not clear whether the hunters primarily tried to protect their crops from raiding ape troops by trapping and thus used the meat opportunistically, or if they intentionally hunted them for consumption. Europeans in this West African rainforest, by contrast, regularly shot and ate both chimpanzee and monkey meat. The zoologist Johann Büttikofer, for example, told his Black servants to skin and prepare a lesser spot-nosed monkey for breakfast.[55] Monkeys injured by European guns regularly bit the hunters in the arms and legs.[56] Büttikofer also shot and ate monkey mothers, and would then 'adopt' the orphaned child and feed it with condensed milk and bananas – or pay a local woman to breastfeed it (see fig. 1).[57] During his expeditions to Liberia and Sierra Leone, he consequently kept several smaller monkeys and was amused by how they attacked and bit children in his neighbourhood.[58] Only in the nineteenth century did indigenous communities start to capture young monkeys alive – not for themselves, but to sell on the coast: In both Liberia and Sierra Leone, freed slaves from North America and Atlantic Africa were settled at the coasts and formed Christian urban populations with a Westernized lifestyle. These groups also kept monkeys to play

51 Paul Richards, Natural Symbols and Natural History. Chimpanzees, Elephants and Experiments in Mende Thought, in: K. Milton (ed.), Environmentalism. The View from Anthropology, New York 1993, 143–157.

52 Stephanie Zehnle, Colonial Man-Eaters. Human-Animal Murder Trials and Conspiracy-Thinking in British Sierra Leone, Habilitation thesis, University of Kiel 2021.

53 Zehnle, Colonial Man-Eaters (note 53), 358.

54 Büttikofer, Reisebilder (note 1), vol. 2, 269.

55 Ibid., vol. 1, 265. For a discussion see also Stephanie Zehnle, Animal-Skinners. A Trans-Colonial Network and the Formation of West African Zoology, in: Brett Bennett/Ulrike Kirchberger (eds.), Environments of Empire. Networks and Agents of Ecological Change, Chapel Hill 2020, 151–175.

56 Büttikofer, Reisebilder (note 1), vol. 2, 269.

57 Ibid., vol. 2, 355.

58 Ibid., vol. 1, 385.

Fig. 1 Liberian woman with Johann Büttikofer's suckling monkey and her own baby on the back. Illustration from Büttikofer's account, 1891. While this drawing from the 1880s suggests indigenous African practices of monkey-taming, Büttikofer's travel journal reveals that he engaged (or forced?) African mothers to breastfeed monkeys.

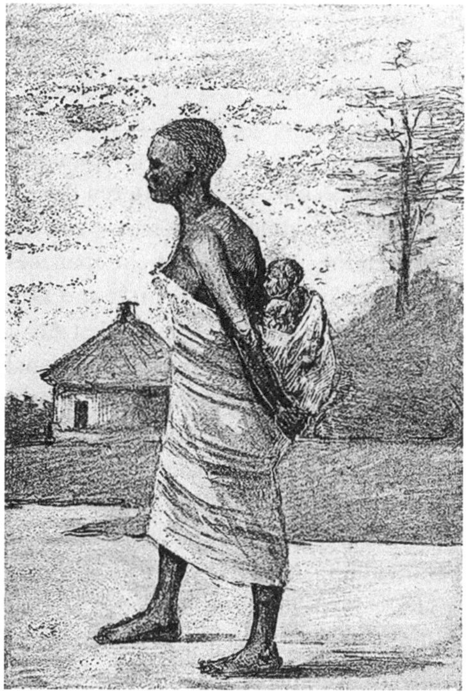

with their children, to collect firewood, or to drive birds away from the rice farms.[59] In the late nineteenth century, before the boom in the chimpanzee trade, many monkeys were shipped from Sierra Leone and Liberia to European pet-keepers and zoos, so that Büttikofer reported about "masses" of them on the steamers.[60]

The sooty mangabeys that probably transmitted SIVs to humans in the 1940s were very common in Liberia and Sierra Leone. Americo-Liberian settlers called them 'ground-monkeys' because of their lifestyle. These monkeys lived on the ground and were easily caught and tamed as pets or as export animals for European zoos.[61] Hence, from the late nineteenth century, maritime trade, Euro-colonial networks, and the colonization of the Guinean coast with freed slaves as settlers and traders increased interaction between humans and sooty mangabeys. Since European hunters only rarely managed to capture and keep juvenile monkeys alive, indigenous hunters trapped and sold them towards the coast; Black settlers then kept them in their households or sold them to Europe. Therefore, the consumption of sooty mangabey meat by indigenous hunters might not even have increased during the colonization of West Africa, whereas

59 Ibid., vol. 2, 350.

60 Ibid., vol. 2, 358.

61 Ibid., vol. 2, 359.

the colonial demand for monkey meat, pets, and zoo animals encouraged the commodification of these monkeys and thus increased contacts with animal blood – for instance, when untrained pet-keepers were bitten.

Two decades after Büttikofer's travels to Africa, another zoologist visited Sierra Leone and Liberia and reported on the commodification of monkeys tamed in Sierra Leonean villages to become pets.[62] Between the zoological expeditions of the 1880s and 1906, some African entrepreneurs had obviously turned from monkey traders to pet-keepers. However, the special role of chimpanzees was still respected, so that these primates were excluded from the menu,[63] and European chimpanzee consumption was not a relevant quantitative factor. In West Africa, hunting in general was not as important and widespread as a colonial recreational sport compared to Southern and Eastern Africa due to the thick vegetation: Most European colonial officials lacked the skill, experience, and patience to hunt in rainforest areas. They were either almost completely dependent on indigenous hunters or simply abstained from hunting. It may therefore not be surprising that the West African HIV-2 did not stem from chimpanzees, whose slaughter was taboo to the indigenous communities, whereas sooty mangabeys were both traditionally eaten by the local population and used as pets in a Western tradition from the 1880s onwards. Nevertheless, thorough studies on human-mangabey relations focusing on the 1920s to 1940s are still required.[64] To sum up, contacts between living mangabeys and colonial officials, missionaries, traders, and Black settlers intensified (see fig. 2), whereas West African food culture – at first glance – appears to have changed to a lesser extent. Based on these assumptions, we can question the unsubstantiated thesis that indigenous Africans must have been the first humans to be infected with HIV-2 from mangabeys.

In both regions of Africa, in the West and the Central rainforests, the expanding plantation economy attracted hungry (and displaced) chimpanzees, which led to a spiral of violence.[65] But in Central Africa, the dimensions of flight and migration were larger. The boundaries between human settlements and chimpanzee habitats were constantly shifting as forests were cleared, villagers found refuge in the forest, and coerced labourers were transferred into the woods. Indigenous hunting, once again, does not seem to be a major reason for the emergence of HIV in this area. The Baka of southeast Cameroon and the Congo – like Sierra Leonean and Liberian indigenous groups – "neither eat

62 Walter Volz, Reise durch das Hinterland von Liberia im Winter 1906–1907. Nach seinen Tagebüchern, Bern 1911, 33.

63 Ibid., 64.

64 A major historical ERC project on the Ivorian 'hotspot' of Ebola and HIV-2 by Gregg Mitman has just started at the Rachel-Carson-Center for Environment and Society, LMU Munich (https://www.carsoncenter.uni-muenchen.de/news/news_events/2020-news/mitman_erc/index.html, 24.08.2022).

65 Rupp et al., Beyond the Cut Hunter (note 26).

Fig. 2 British missionary Booth riding his donkey in northern Sierra Leone with his tamed monkey on his back. Illustration to W. H. Maude, More about Limbah, in: At Home and Abroad 6 (1884), 50. Keeping tamed monkeys became a trend among missionary and colonial officials well before this practice spread across the indigenous population.

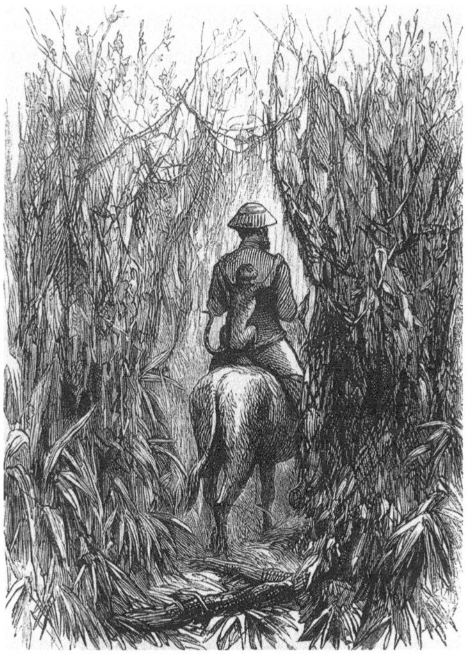

gorilla nor chimpanzee meat, nor do they hunt these animals of their own accord."[66] They would only kill great apes in defence or as a service for a paying patron. And like West African traditional hunters, the Baka have carefully observed great ape behaviour and consider them almost human, and therefore deem eating them a form of forbidden cannibalism.[67] While the Baka imagine themselves linked to chimpanzees and their shy lifestyle in the forests, they regard neighbouring farmers as equal to gorillas.[68] Future research questions must take a closer and more historically informed look at hunting and food taboos among these various groups and how they changed in the course of colonization. When and why was monkey and ape meat declared edible or taboo in West and Central Africa? Such analyses must highlight non-indigenous residents in this region: inner-African newcomers and middlemen of Western trade. Both West and Central Africa faced an increase in live primate trade: On the Congo's tributaries, for example, colonial companies from Belgium and the Netherlands bought large amounts of ivory, but also live baby apes from the Baka. From the 1920s onwards, Baka women wove new kinds of baskets or cages in which monkeys or young chimpanzees were

66 Axel Köhler, Of Apes and Men. Baka and Bantu Attitudes to Wildlife and the Making of Eco-Goodies and Baddies, in: Conservation and Society 3/2 (2005), 407–435, 416.

67 Ibid., 417.

68 Ibid., 419.

transported to Kinshasa.[69] It is therefore also possible that the decisive infections took place via Europeans as monkey traders and owners: "Although the index patient of HIV-1M may have been an African male hunter, other people – colonial soldiers, European administrators, company agents – [...] could also have been the index patient."[70]

Then again, the conspiracy theories about medical research stations generating ape-to-human infections are plausible on a less techno-scientific, and perhaps more trivial level of colonial change: Koprowski's Lindi Station for chimpanzee research close to the Belgian-Congolese town of Stanleyville must indeed have encouraged indigenous hunters and traders to reach more isolated forest habitats in search of chimpanzees: "If it became known that Americans were paying good money for young apes in Kisangani, it would be almost surprising if some hunters had not made the trip upriver."[71] Medical research stations like this one therefore increased contacts between hunters, medical staff, and remote primate groups by hunting, taming, and operating. Moreover, all of these interactions could provoke aggressive animal behaviour like biting or scratching and become a bloody business. The prohibition of African hunting as poaching and the establishment of colonial conservation areas also increased the risk of zoonotic infection for indigenous hunters in the twentieth century, since large apes now had to be slaughtered secretly and quickly in the forest, so that the meat would not be recognized by park rangers. Hurried slaughter probably resulted in more knife injuries and in incomplete cooking or smoking of primate meat. In Cameroon, the meat was now slaughtered and cooked in the forest by inexperienced men instead of in the village by experienced women.[72] In addition, because trapping required at least two secret visits to protected areas, hunters switched to hunting with firearms.

However, two important factors in the increase of bloody human-ape contact are completely missing in current studies about the emergence of HIV: (1) Since zoonotic transmission probably took place in Central Africa between 1921 and 1945, it is astonishing that the influence of German colonial rule in Cameroon (1884–1919) has not been brought into the spotlight. The German colonial empire acquired the eastern and southern districts in 1911 from France, and launched a series of 'border expeditions' in the following years. The indigenous population (including the Baka) were reported to be "hostile"[73] towards the German expeditioners who mapped the rainforest region and demanded that residents provide food. Due to these expeditions, the eight years

69 Rupp et al., Beyond the Cut Hunter (note 26), 666.

70 Ibid., 667.

71 Moore, Puzzling Origins of AIDS (note 25), 543.

72 Victor Narat et al., Using Physical Contact Heterogeneity and Frequency to Characterize Dynamics of Human Exposure to Nonhuman Primate Bodily Fluids in Central Africa, in: PLOS Neglected Tropical Diseases 12/12 (2018), e0006976, 10–11.

73 "Die Bevölkerung verhält sich sehr ablehnend, teilweise direkt feindlich". Hauptmann Johannes Abel to Reichskolonialamt, 25 February 1913, Bundesarchiv, R1001/3775, fol. 108.

of German colonial rule in what they called "Neukamerun" left behind comparatively extensive documentation of the area, which can contribute to a human-ape history of this rainforest region. (2) The Baka and some of their farming neighbours organized male initiation in secluded forests, where the camps were set up by secret societies that established supernatural and physical contact to wildlife: "The circumciser and instructor in a ritual for the initiation of young men into adulthood is significantly named after the male gorilla in both Bekwii, the Bakwele language and in Li-Baka."[74] Similar initiation practices are also known from West African forests – though with leopards as iconic animals of guidance and transformative power.[75] In both regional cases, however, the rituals involved the loss of blood during male circumcision (and sometimes during ritual scarification of face, back, and belly, too). In both areas, the borders between villages and forests, human environments and other primate habitats, were crossed by larger groups of initiates who were also often instructed to hunt. Infections – sometimes fatal – during forest initiation were regularly reported in colonial Sierra Leone, such that the risk of zoonotic transmission may have increased because of the boys' wounds and hunting activities.

5. Conclusion

This chapter has attempted to address current questions around the emergence of HIVs in the colonial period in Africa. "In engaging with these questions, we track the interconnections between disease, environmental change, and a profit-driven plantation system reliant on migrant labor."[76] But beyond such global trends, we must also focus on the specific African history of physical inter-primate encounters that were multiplied and escalated by pre-colonial warfare, slave trade, colonial taxation and coerced labour, the exotic animal trade, hunting regulations, food cultures, and medical research. Historians must resist the tendency to translate phylogenetic timeframes of zoonotic viral transmissions into research periods, and reconsider the decades before the estimated 'first' infections – the time prior to patient(s) zero. Equipped with this longue durée animal history perspective, this chapter has offered some preliminary results to enrich research in global pandemic history: Humans have lived next to SIV-infected primates for thousands of years in tropical Africa, but they kept a stable distance from these animals by taboos regarding hunting, eating, and taming. The nineteenth century, however, was marked by human migration because of inner-African wars, state expansion, the

74 Köhler, Of Apes and Men (note 66), 418.

75 Stephanie Zehnle, The Liminal Youth between Town and Bush. Humans, Leopards and Initiation in Colonial West Africa, in: Clemens Wischermann/Aline Steinbrecher/Philip Howell (eds.), Animal History in the Modern City. Exploring Liminality, London 2018, 161–180.

76 Robert Peckham, Epidemics in Modern Asia. New Approaches to Asian History, Cambridge 2016, 144.

continental and trans-continental slave trade, animal trade, and European colonization, so that human-primate encounters multiplied without following the traditional taboos. Harassed and driven from their habitats, primate troops started plundering crops and became more aggressive towards humans. These drivers of human-ape encounter and violence demonstrate that, firstly, the colonial plantation economy was not the only and maybe not even the main cause for the emergence of HIV and that, secondly, Africans were maybe not the first HIV-infected persons in history, or at least not exclusively. The colonial factor in HIV origins is more complicated, subtle, and indirect than the Cut Hunter Theory had previously assumed. Traditional ape hunting and eating was not intensified, but refugee, colonial, European, or global demands for primates – dead or alive – were increasingly met. Examples in this chapter have demonstrated that it was not African food cultures that changed around 1900, but human-primate relationships, which became more intimate, more frequent, and more violent.

Photo credits

Fig. 1 Liberian woman with Johann Büttikofer's suckling monkey and her own baby on the back. Taken from: Johann Büttikofer, Reisebilder aus Liberia. Resultate geographischer, naturwissenschaftlicher und ethnographischer Untersuchungen während der Jahre 1879–1882 und 1886–1887, 2 vols. Leiden 1890–1891, vol. 2, 299.

Fig. 2 British missionary Booth riding his donkey in northern Sierra Leone with his tamed monkey on his back. Illustration to W. H. Maude, More about Limbah, in: At Home and Abroad 6 (1884), 50.

Abstract:

The historical causes of the emergence of the human immunodeficiency viruses (HIV) in colonial Africa are typically investigated at the interface of medical sciences, genetics, and anthropology. This chapter develops a genuine historical approach towards the origins of zoonotic transmissions from monkeys and apes to humans from the 1910s to the 1940s by framing an entangled primate history of the colonial HIV 'hotspots' in West and Central Africa. To actually discover the ruptures in the history of inter-primate relationships, the author compares pre-colonial to colonial settings, Western to Central African forests, indigenous voices to migrants, and genetic research to historical archive material. This search for the causes of HIV reveals how humans have dealt with the similarities of primate behaviour, habitat, genetics, and bodies – similarities that were acknowledged across all cultures involved in these case studies. Neither Africans nor European migrants and researchers had anticipated the emergence of HIV before it became a global epidemic in the 1970s. But they were united by the fear of the thin red line between humans and other primates, which was, for example, expressed by food taboos or practices of animal 'adoption.' Based on recent phylogenetic and ethological research, this historical analysis evaluates outdated theories about the historical causes of HIV, goes beyond methods identifying general environmental destruction as the major cause, and offers prospects for human-animal historians based on new research methods.

Keywords:
primates | HIV epidemics | colonialism | Africa | hunting

Brett Mizelle

Mass Killings of Pigs and the Challenge of Multispecies Justice

Epidemics and the Entangled Lives of Humans and Animals from the 1970s to the Present

1. Introduction

As the world dealt with the Covid-19 pandemic which emerged in Wuhan, China in December 2019 another highly infectious disease was quietly sweeping the globe, one that also began in China but for which there is yet no vaccine and no treatment. African Swine Fever, a hemorrhagic illness in pigs which poses no risk to humans, was first described in East Africa in 1921, spreading between wild swine and warthogs and farmed animals. Outbreaks across the last century have been devastating for pigs, the humans who live with them, and the livestock industry. In August 2018 the first Chinese African Swine Fever outbreak was reported in Liaoning province. Within two years this virus had spread to all parts of China, throughout Southeast Asia, and into India. In China alone more than 100 million pigs were killed at a cost of hundreds of billions of dollars, creating a global deficit in pork production that helped to increase meat prices worldwide.[1]

Media coverage of the recent African Swine Fever panzootic has largely focused on the implications for global dinner plates, as opposed to the costs to pigs themselves and to those human communities whose lives are enmeshed with these animals. This is not all that surprising. After all, for most people, pigs are experienced primarily as pork, something that reflects the long-standing contradiction between our idealized view of pigs and the reality of the ways in which pigs have been transformed and killed to fulfill human desires for meat and other products made from the animals' bodies.[2] While humans have shaped the pig and pigs have shaped us, most people have paid scant attention to the global transition (albeit an uneven one depending on time and place) from subsistence foodways and community traditions of raising and killing hogs to a

1 See, e. g. "Quarter of world's pig population to die due to African swine fever", in: The Guardian, 31 October 2019, https://www.theguardian.com/world/2019/oct/31/quarter-of-worlds-pig-population-to-die-of-african-swine-fever (9 January 2023) and Mike Ives/Catherine Li, "As swine fever roils Asia, hogs are culled and dinner plans change", in: The New York Times, 14 May 2019, https://www.nytimes.com/2019/05/14/world/asia/african-swine-fever-asia-china.html (9 January 2023).

2 Brett Mizelle, Pig, London 2011.

horrifying industrial meat complex, one quite familiar to us all but amazingly difficult to dismantle.

I have been especially interested in how both living pigs and the places where they are killed for food have largely vanished from view at the same time that representations of pigs have proliferated. In the United States, for example, few people are ever likely to see a living pig, whether a domesticated animal on an increasing rare family farm or their wild-living relatives. Images of pigs are used to market pork products and barbeque joints and representations of pigs are common in children's literature and popular culture, but one is not likely to see a farrowing barn, finishing facility, or a pork processing plant. The disappearance of pigs from everyday life reflects how "distance and concealment operate as mechanisms of power in modern society," as Timothy Pachirat has succinctly put it in the introduction to his important ethnographic study of the modern industrial cattle slaughterhouse.[3] The largely unacknowledged lives and deaths of food animals, more than 8.5 billion of which are slaughtered annually in the United States, highlights how the production of meat is thus perhaps the most revealing aspect of a human-animal relationship where, as Anat Pick notes, "relations of power operate in their exemplary purity (that is, operate with the fewest moral or material obstacles."[4]

This chapter extends my concern with the ways in which our modern pork production system reflects a larger devaluation of life itself, including both the lives of pigs and those of humans, especially the marginalized workers who are exploited within industrial agriculture.[5] However, rather than look at the quotidian raising and killing of millions of pigs for food on the farm and at the slaughterhouse, I will focus on the exceptional but increasingly more common mass extermination of pigs, a subset of the larger mass killings of kinds of animals. Mass mortality events have been on the rise across the animal kingdom since the 1940s, linked to infectious diseases, biotoxicity, and human disturbance of the environment.[6] In the agricultural sector, the intensification of industrialized farming and globalization have created an increasingly "dangerous and untidy world," one where "problems that emerged in one locale could affect an

3 Timothy Pachirat, Every Twelve Seconds. Industrialized Slaughter and the Politics of Sight, New Haven/London 2011, 3.

4 Anat Pick, Creaturely Poetics. Animality and Vulnerability in Literature and Film, New York 2011, 1.

5 See, e. g. Charlie LeDuff, "In A Slaughterhouse, Some Things Never Die", in: New York Times, 16 June 2000, reprinted in Cary Wolfe (ed.), Zooontologies. The Question of the Animal, Minneapolis 2003, 183–197, and David Bacon, How U.S. Policies Fueled Mexico's Great Migration, in: The Nation, 23 January 2012, 11–18.

6 Samuel B. Fey et al., Recent shifts in the occurrence, cause, and magnitude of animal mass mortality events, in: PNAS 112/4 (2015), 1083–1088. Fey noted that "mass die-offs result from both natural and human-driven causes" and that disease was responsible for over a quarter of all mass mortality events in Amanda Schupak, "Mass animal deaths on the rise worldwide", CBS News, 16 January 2015, https://www.cbsnews.com/news/mass-animal-deaths-on-the-rise-worldwide/ (25 March 2023).

entire nation and the world."[7] While pigs are often not isolated from other agricultural species (cows, sheep, etc.) in these orchestrated cullings in response to contagions, my examples here are about scenarios where pigs were the primary, if not only, subject of these mass killings.

The most notorious recent example of this mass killing of farmed animals is the British foot-and-mouth disease (FMD) crisis in 2001 that resulted in the slaughter of over ten million animals, mainly sheep and cattle.[8] The first case of FMD was reported in Essex in February 2001, but it was quickly clear that the disease had already spread across much of Britain, connected to infected animal products imported from the far east that were used as animal feed on pig farms. Pigs acted like "virus factories" in the spread of FMD and people in Britain and around the world were transfixed by disturbing images of animal corpses being incinerated. It took more than seven months to resolve this crisis, partly due to inadequate resources, a slow response, and a long history in Britain of "stamping out" infected and contacted stock by slaughtering animals rather than vaccinating them against a curable disease that posed little threat to human health.[9]

Although more sheep were slaughtered than any other animal in the 2001 FMD epidemic, the outbreak began with pigs who were fed infected swill and hundreds of thousands of pigs were killed. Many other less-well-known mass killings of pigs have also taken place in the last twenty years: in Malaysia in 1999 (fear over the spread of mosquito-borne Japanese encephalitis linked to the primitive conditions of the country's pig production),[10] South Korea in 2002 (where 90,000 pigs were killed in the run-up to the World Cup over fears about foot-and-mouth disease),[11] Santa Cruz Island off

---

7 Alan L. Olmstead/Paul W. Rhode, Arresting Contagion. Science, Policy, and Conflicts Over Animal Disease Control, Cambridge, Mass. 2015, 320. See also Bryony A. Jones/Delia Grace/Richard Kock/Dirk Udo Pfeiffer, Zoonoses emergence linked to agricultural intensification and environmental change, in: PNAS 110/21 (2013), 8399–8404.

8 This outbreak was traced to pigs that consumed infected garbage containing remains of infected meat that had not been properly heat-sterilized. See Department for Environment, Food and Rural Affairs, "Origin of the UK Foot-and-Mouth Disease Epidemic in 2001", June 2002. PDF available at http://archive.defra.gov.uk/foodfarm/farmanimal/diseases/atoz/fmd/documents/fmdorigins1.pdf (22 March 2022). Also see Delphine Berdah's chapter in this volume.

9 Abigail Woods, A Manufactured Plague. The History of Foot-and-Mouth Disease in Britain, London, 2004 and Robin McKie, "Foot and mouth 20 years on: what an animal virus epidemic taught UK science", in: The Guardian, 21 February 2021, http://www.theguardian.com/science/2021/feb/21/foot-and-mouth-20-years-on-what-an-animal-virus-epidemic-taught-uk-science (25 March 2023).

10 "Pig Slaughter Begins in Malaysia", in: BBC News, 21 March 1999, http://news.bbc.co.uk/2/hi/asia-pacific/300053.stm (22 March 2022); Trade Environment Database Case Studies, "Outbreak of Japanese Encephalitis (Pig Virus) in Malaysia", http://www1.american.edu/ted/pigvirus.htm (22 March 2022), and Mazrura Sahani et al., Nipah virus infection among abattoir workers in Malaysia, 1998–1999, in: International Journal of Epidemiology 30 (2001), 1017–1020.

11 Jun Kwanwoo, "South Korea steps up mass pig slaughter to contain foot-and-mouth," in: Agence France Presse, 13 May 2002, http://www.organicconsumers.org/madcow/korea51302.cfm (22 March 2022).

the coast of California in 2005–2006 (where wild-living pigs were killed to save the endangered Channel Islands fox),[12] Liberia in 2009 (where wild-living pigs were killed because they contaminated of the water supply and threatened public health),[13] and Japan in 2010 (where 200,000 pigs were killed to protect other livestock from a foot-and-mouth disease outbreak in Miyazaki Prefecture, a region known for its high quality meats).[14]

In these examples we see a mix of concern about different types of pigs, both wild-living and domesticated. One of the "problems" with these pigs is that they (and, in the case of domesticated pigs, their owners as well) are unruly subjects: they were not domesticated enough, not sufficiently controlled or not raised using "standard" scientific and modern practices according to Western pork industry standards. With the notable exception of the mass killing of pigs off the California coast in the name of the environment, disease is the commonality here. Two types of diseases are of interest: *epizootic* diseases that could spread from animal to animal, threatening profits from the sale and export of living animals and meat in an era of globalized capitalism and transnational trade agreements, and *zoonotic* diseases, which can spread from animals to humans and include everything from salmonella, Lyme disease, rabies, and plague to the West Nile virus, influenza A virus subtype H1N1 ("hee-nee", popularly known as the "swine flu"), Ebola hemorrhagic fever, and, of course, SARS-CoV-2, the virus behind the Covid pandemic.[15]

---

12 "Wild Pig Hunt Aims to Save California Island Foxes", in: National Geographic News, news.nationalgeographic.com/news/2005/03/0316_050316_tvferalpigs_2.html (30 September 2009); Gregory W. Griggs, "Eradication of Santa Cruz Island pigs deemed a success", in: Los Angeles Times, August 30, 2007; "Feral pigs create ecological havoc on California's Channel Islands", in: University of California Newsroom, www.universityofcalifornia.edu/news/article/3817 (30 September 2009); Gary W. Roemer/G. W. C. /Josh Donlan/Franck Courchamp, Golden eagles, feral pigs and insular carnivores. How exotic species turn native predators into prey, in: Proceedings of the National Academy of Sciences 99/2 (22 January 2002), 791–796; Shannon Davis, "Return of the Natives," in: Backpacker, June 2008, 21–28.

13 Jefferson Massah, "Liberia: Mass Slaughter of Pigs in Bong", in: The Informer (Monrovia), 18 June 2009 http://allafrica.com/stories/200906180898.html (22 March 2022).

14 "Miyazaki faces mass cow, pig cull", in: Japan Times, 20 May 2010, http://www.japantimes.co.jp/text/nn20100520a1.html (22 March 2022).

15 Greater historical attention has been given to swine zoonoses that can spread from pigs and cause serious illness in humans, including swine influenza, which killed somewhere between 50 and 100 million people worldwide in the 1918 flu pandemic. See e. g. Gina Kolata, Flu. The Story of the Great Influenza Pandemic of 1918 and the Search for the Virus that Caused It, New York, 2001.

2. Mass Killings in Haiti, Egypt, South Korea, and the US

In the following, I will focus on four instances where pigs were the targets of mass killings of animals – cases that show the connections between speciesism, racism, imperialism, and ethnocentrism amidst the larger context of the expansion and intensification of corporate agriculture. The first of these stories takes place in Haiti and involves African Swine Fever, a disease caused by a double-stranded DNA virus that is endemic in sub-Saharan Africa among warthogs, bushpigs, and wild pigs. African Swine Fever was restricted to Africa until 1957, when it spread to Portugal after wild pigs ate food discarded by an African airline, making it a disease tied to growing postwar international trade and tourism.[16]

In the late 1970s, African Swine Fever was detected in pigs in the Dominican Republic and Haiti. Fearing the spread of the disease into its pork industry, the US government backed a multinational campaign to eradicate all the pigs in both countries.[17] In Haiti, nearly 1.3 million pigs were destroyed, with devastating effects for both the human and non-human animals interacting in this environment, in the complex entanglements of this multispecies relationship.[18] In the time before these mass killings, the people's pigs (known as *kochon kreyol*) were hearty but scrawny black pigs well adapted to local conditions. More importantly, they served as literal "piggy banks" for rural Haitians, providing them with a living savings account that could be sold or slaughtered to pay for religious ceremonies, health care, or schooling. Within months of the completion of pig eradication in 1984, school attendance dropped, malnutrition increased and religious life – both Catholic and *vodoun* – was disrupted. In the long term, this neo-imperialist pig eradication accelerated the movement of rural Haitians into cities and contributed to the deforestation crisis, as people turned to cutting down trees to make charcoal to sell to augment their incomes.

---

16 S. Costard et al., Epidemiology of African swine fever virus, in: Virus Research 173/1 (2013), 191–197. Zoonotic diseases are on the increase because of "intensive livestock farming and agriculture, international trade of exotic animals, and increased human encroachment into wildlife habitats, alongside international travel networks and urbanization." See "Zoonoses: beyond the human-animal-environment interface", in: The Lancet 396 (4 July 2020), 1.

17 The American pork industry was especially wary of ASF given the hundred-year long struggle with hog cholera. Hog cholera was a disease American farmers and policy makers had largely decided to live with until the emergence of ASF as a concern in the late 1950s and early 1960s. Because hog cholera and ASF are hard to distinguish clinically, fears of the spread of ASF led to a 1961 decision to eradicate hog cholera, an effort that was successful by 1978. For a detailed history of this effort, see Alan L. Olmstead/Paul W. Rhode, Arresting Contagion. Science, Policy, and Conflicts Over Animal Disease Control, Cambridge, Mass. 2015, 138–155.

18 For an overview of multispecies studies, see Thom Van Dooren/Eben Kirksey/Ursula Münster, Multispecies Studies: Cultivating Arts of Attentiveness, in: Environmental Humanities 8/1 (2016), 1–23. See also Donna J. Haraway, Staying with the Trouble. Making Kin in the Chthulucene, Durham 2016.

To make matters worse, the pigs sent to replace the *kochon kreyol* were much more fragile and only thrived on expensive enriched feed. The costs of preparing for and feeding one of these replacement pigs (which became known locally as *prince a quatre pieds*, or "four-footed princes") exceeded most Haitians' annual income. To even receive an American *kochon blanc*, one had to agree to construct a tin-roofed and concrete-floored shelter for the animals, a dwelling that in some cases was superior to the homes of the Haitians themselves! This operation was, in short, a disaster, one seen in racial and class terms by Haitians, who identified with the black but hearty pigs doomed for the sake of fat, white, spoiled pigs from the north. The eradication of the *kochon kreyol* is now seen as a classic example of how foreign aid undermines the aided. As one Haitian summed up his feelings: "Now they come back and make money selling us their hotdogs!"[19]

Efforts to respond to this debacle started in the late 1980s and are ongoing. French and Haitian agronomists have worked to breed a new pig that had the qualities of the original *kochon kreyol* and activist groups such as Grassroots International, which links progressive funders in the US with social movements in the Global South to improve the income and living standards of farmers by promoting sustainable local communities, have been involved in fundraising and development work in support of Haitian groups such as the National Congress of Papaye Peasant Movement. On the Grassroots International website one can download materials needed to have a "pig party" that raises awareness and funds to help provide replacement pigs to Haitians,[20] a program similar to those of Heifer International, a global nonprofit founded in 1944 by an Ohio farmer who realized while working as a relief worker during the Spanish Civil War that refugees would benefit more from the gift of a cow than from a cup of milk.

In my second example of mass extermination, Egypt began to slaughter approximately 350,000 pigs in April 2009 to stop the spread of the H1N1 influenza, even though there were no cases of swine flu reported in the country. Joseph Domenech, the chief veterinary officer at the UN Food and Agriculture Organization, immediately noted that the Egyptian order was "a real mistake. There is no reason to do that. It's not a swine influenza, it's a human influenza,"[21] although that distinction was lost on many throughout the world.

Because of Islamic restrictions on pork, Egyptian pig farmers are Christian and poor, subsisting on the collection of garbage, the sale of recycling, and the raising of pigs. The most heavily affected group were the Zabbaleen (lit: "pig-pen operators") garbage

---

19 Jennie M. Smith, When the Hands Are Many. Community Organization and Social Change in Rural Haiti, Ithaca, New York 2001, 28–30.

20 See https://grassrootsonline.org/blog/swine-flu-deja-vu/ (9 January 2023).

21 Nadim Audi, "Culling Pigs in Flu Fight, Egypt Angers Herders and Dismays UN", in: New York Times, 1 May 2009; Phillipe Naughton, "Egyptian Christians Riot After Swine Flu Cull", in: The Times (London), 29 April 2009.

collectors who depend on the pigs for their livelihood. For generations the Zabbaleen have been paid a small amount to collect, recycle and process Cairo's garbage. They raised pigs, among nature's best recyclers, on Cairo's organic waste; these pigs could then be consumed or sold, playing a crucial role in the Zabbaleen's ability to survive in one of the world's largest cities. Unsurprisingly, in response to the government culling order, the Zabbaleen blocked streets and stoned vehicles of the health ministry. They viewed the extermination of their pigs as yet another attack on their minority community, one that would inevitably lead to a waste disposal crisis. These predictions turned out to be correct: four months later the streets of Cairo were full of organic rubbish, ironically creating a greater likelihood for the spread of disease. As Moussa Ratab, a former garbage collector put it: "They killed the pigs, let them clean the city."[22]

So, what was really going on in Egypt? The mass killing of pigs here seems related to broader governmental efforts to support the interests of the private multinational waste disposal corporations that were contracted to collect the trash in Cairo in 2003. This transition has been charted in Mai Iskander's film *Garbage Dreams* (2009), which follows the lives of three teenage boys born into the trash trade and living in the world's largest garbage village.[23] Iskander shows how much less efficient these multinational corporations are at handling the waste of the largest city in the Middle East and Africa and how the Zabbaleen have seen their way of life disappear as garbage began being carted to nearby landfills.

The possible role of religious animosity in this case cannot be ignored, of course. Although Imam Samaan Ibrahim said "The bottom line is pigs are not welcome in Egypt,"[24] a foreign correspondent named Per Björklund on the scene at the time observed that "Actually, no one I spoke to brought up this issue or portrayed the decision to slaughter the pigs as an attack on Christians as a religious group."[25] In killing the Zabbaleen's pigs, the government promised a humane slaughter, butchering the pigs according to Islamic law and freezing the meat for distribution to the community, but Egyptian reporters witnessed a brutal and savage slaughter, leading to additional outcry in Egypt and around the world.[26]

Ultimately, the killing of the Zabbaleen pigs exemplifies the larger process of urban renewal, one that has historically involved driving non-human animals out of cities. For

22 Michael Slackman, "Belatedly, Egypt Spots Flaws in Wiping Out Pigs", in: New York Times, 19 September 2009, http://www.nytimes.com/2009/09/20/world/africa/20cairo.html (22 March 2022).

23 The official website for the film is http://www.garbagedreams.com/ (22 March 2022). In the United States, it was sponsored by PBS's Independent Lens: http://www.pbs.org/independentlens/garbage-dreams/ (22 March 2022).

24 Michael Slackman, "Cleaning Cairo, But Taking a Livelihood", in: New York Times, 24 May 2009.

25 Per Björklund, "Crisis Management, Egypt Style", in: Egypt and Beyond Blog, http://scandegypt.blogspot.com/2009/04/crisis-management-egypt-style.html (22 March 2022).

26 Slackman, "Cleaning Cairo" (note 23).

example, through the mid-19th century the streets of American cities and towns were full of free-roaming pigs that were simultaneously important players in urban ecologies and public nuisances. New York City tried (and failed) to deal with its urban pig problem starting in the 17th century and saw extensive debate around an 1817 law that declared that any pig found running loose could be taken to a public pound. Defenders of the city's pigs saw these reform efforts as a war on the poor, but after an 1819 trial the principle was established that pigs in the streets were a public nuisance. New York's streets were largely cleared of pigs by the late 1860s. Pig-removal was hotly contested in Manhattan, where working-class New Yorkers and members of the marginalized Irish and African American communities that depended upon their pigs unsuccessfully resisted efforts to confiscate their animals.[27] In Cairo, the extermination of the Zabbaleen pigs was linked to interest in the redevelopment of their land. As one Zabbaleen pig owner observed: "This is nothing new. Some people have been propagating against the pig farms for a long time. The reason is that there is influential people who want our land, to build expensive apartments. They take this opportunity to get rid of us once and for all."[28]

To provide some contrast with these stories of the effects of the mass extermination of animals on multispecies communities in the developing world, my third example from recent history comes from South Korea, where starting in late-2010 an outbreak of foot-and-mouth disease (FMD) led to the extermination of several million pigs. Approximately twelve percent of the domestic pig population in Korea was culled without much notice from the world's media until it was reported that many of the pigs were, contrary to international protocols, buried alive.[29] Groups including Compassion in World Farming (CIWF) and People for the Ethical Treatment of Animals (PETA) were aghast that mass killing and not vaccination was the primary response to the outbreak.[30] Images of living pigs being dumped into mass graves moved from activist sites into the mainstream media, raising additional questions about the haste of the process and concerns about the possible long-term effects on water quality from the burial of these

27 See Mizelle, Pig (note 2), 54–58, and Catherine McNeur, "The Swinish Multitude". Controversies over Hogs in Antebellum New York City, in: Journal of Urban History 37 (2011), 639–660.

28 Quoted in Per Björklund, "Crisis Management, Egypt Style", in: Egypt and Beyond Blog, http://scandegypt.blogspot.com/2009/04/crisis-management-egypt-style.html (22 March 2022). The crisis in Egypt also reveals the complicated relationship between ideologies that believe privatization and markets are the solution to all problems and the need for government regulation and policy, with policy in this instance helping to promote neoliberal forms of urban land usage.

29 Evan Ramstad and Jaeyeon Woo, "Foot-and-Mouth Disease Roils Korean Farms," in: Wall Street Journal, 11 January 2011.

30 Kat Higgins, "South Korea Buries One Million Pigs Alive", 7 January 2011, http://news.sky.com/home/world-news/article/15887024 (22 March 2022).

animals.[31] This killing threw the nation into crisis, leading many, including South Korea's political leaders, to wonder how foot-and-mouth disease could get so out of control as to result in the destruction of 140,000 cattle and an estimated 3.3 million pigs at a cost of over $1.6 billion (USD). President Lee Myung-bak promised to improve South Korea's vaccination capabilities[32] in the future, knowing full well that imports of both pigs and pork would be necessary to restore the country's pork industry.[33] As in Haiti twenty-five years earlier, United States agriculture rushed to the rescue, sending an initial shipment of 235 genetically modified pigs to South Korea to start repopulating their hog and pig industry. Three 747 airplanes full of hogs from Clayton Agri-Marketing, Inc. of Jefferson City, Missouri were shipped to Korea to help re-start their pork industry in a rare example, given concerns about the spread of epizootics, of the exporting of live hogs from American producers.[34]

As the epidemiologist Michael Ward has noted, "long-distance, transboundary spread of highly contagious and pathogenic diseases is a worse-case scenario" for agriculture, something perhaps best understood as an "analog of Covid-19."[35] Ward was writing about the threat of the 2018–2020 African Swine Fever panzootic to North American agriculture, a concern that led to an emergency appropriation of $500 million dollars to help prevent the spread of African Swine Fever into the United States after it was detected in Haiti and the Dominican Republic in July 2021.[36] These emergency funds were sent to the Dominican Republic to help respond to African Swine Fever outbreaks there as well as being used to increase inspections for illegal pork that might be brought to the US from those countries. Such increased spending and surveillance were seen as a bargain compared to the possible impact of African Swine Fever on the American pork industry, which exports 7 billion dollars of pork products to the rest of the world. While

---

31 See Yoon Du-Huk, quoted in Lorraine Murray, "South Korea's Animal Culls", in: Advocacy for Animals, http://advocacy.britannica.com/blog/advocacy/2011/05/buried-alive-south-koreas-animal-culls/ (22 March 2022).

32 Jaeyeon Woo, "Korea Foot-and-Mouth Impact Widens", in: Wall Street Journal Korea Real Time blog, 28 January 2011, http://blogs.wsj.com/korearealtime/2011/01/28/korea-foot-and-mouth-impact-widens/ (22 March 2022).

33 One result of the FMD epidemic was that beef passed pork as the most consumed meat in South Korea. See "Beef Overtakes Pork", in: The Chosunilbo, 5 December 2011, http://english.chosun.com/site/data/html_dir/2011/12/05/2011120501166.html (22 March 2022).

34 Bob Burgdorfer, "Special U.S. pigs take flight to rebuild South Korea herd", in: Reuters, 25 April 2011, http://www.reuters.com/article/2011/04/25/us-pigs-korea-interview-idUSTRE73O5A120110425 (22 March 2022).

35 Quoted in Maryn McKenna, "Another global pandemic is spreading – among pigs", in: Wired, 12 October 2021, https://www.wired.com/story/another-global-pandemic-is-spreading-among-pigs/ (9 January 2023).

36 Tom Polansek, "U.S. pledges up to $500 million to prevent African Swine Fever", in: Reuters, 29 September 2021, https://www.reuters.com/article/us-usa-swine-fever/u-s-pledges-up-to-500-million-to-prevent-african-swine-fever-idUSKBN2GP1SQ (9 January 2023).

there has been some progress towards a long-awaited African Swine Fever vaccine, the reaction to an outbreak in the United States would be the immediate "depopulation" of animals at and around the area of the incident, a "national movement standstill" that would prevent all transportation of pigs (and pig semen used in artificial insemination) for at least 72 hours, and an effort to hunt and kill any feral hogs that might be involved in disease transmission.[37] So far the United States has avoided a major African Swine Fever-related crisis, but as Raymond Robert Rowland, a pathobiologist and veterinarian at the University of Illinois reminds us, African Swine Fever, which has been found in more than fifty countries, is spread by movement at a time when the world is linked together more than ever before. He concludes:

> Name a country in the world: Eastern Europe, China, Africa. All areas that have African Swine Fever. You can easily think of a scenario where someone brings in a contaminated product, discards it into compost or garbage, and feral pigs come along and pick it up.[38]

3. Global Patterns: The Biopolitics of Killing Pigs

In all of these stories of epizootic outbreaks among swine, mass killings of pigs proved a disaster for many humans and all these pigs. In all of these instances, and in most of the other cases I have examined, hasty decisions were made without thinking through the consequences. Local farmers, residents, and others, including activists from non-governmental organizations, some scientists, and, in the case of Egypt, officials from the UN, had all predicted negative impacts before these mass killings took place but proved powerless to stop them. This lack of understanding (or, perhaps worse, a lack of interest in wanting to understand) the ways in which human and non-human animal well-being was entangled in these multispecies communities proved crucial to these disasters.

In Haiti, the whole debacle, notes University of Toronto historian Melanie Newton, "proceeded from the assumption that Haitians don't know what they're doing, don't have any understanding of agriculture and their practices are somehow a danger to the west." Similarly, in Egypt, Syada Greiss, member of Parliament and chairwoman of the Association for Protection of the Environment noted of her government: "They don't have a good understanding of what this means to the livelihood of the rubbish collectors." Government officials did not understand the intertwined lives of humans

37 See United States Department of Agriculture (USDA) APHIS Veterinary Services, Planning and Preparing for African Swine Fever (November 2021), https://www.aphis.usda.gov/animal_health/emergency_management/downloads/asf-briefing-plan-prepare.pdf (9 January 2023).

38 Quoted in McKenna, "Another global pandemic" (note 35). Ironically the human pandemic and its restrictions on travel may have enabled us to avoid a greater African Swine Fever panzootic.

and animals in Cairo's urban ecology and accordingly "did not have a full grasp of the economics or social implications" for the Zabbaleen.[39]

While the mass culling in South Korea devastated farmers, most of whom were adhering to best practices in animal husbandry and were compensated by the government for the loss of their animals, in Haiti and Egypt, the effect, if not the intention, was to drive subsistence producers off their own sources of protein and into a relationship with a globalized food production system. Recall the Haitian who complained that "now they sell us their hot dogs!". What happened in Haiti and in Cairo can thus be seen as a recapitulation of processes that had taken place earlier in other parts of the world as traditional pig farming and meat processing were replaced by "modern" systems and corporate practices that provided seemingly cheap meat to a public increasingly distant from the sources of their food.

The separation of humans and pigs here thus reflects the broader shift from subsistence production and a lived connection with animals to a relationship centered on increasing consumption of pigs as pork. The way these pigs were kept, or more precisely in the case of Haiti and Cairo, *not* kept in the style of modern intensive hog farming, with its separation of humans from animals, is critical here. In this sense, these mass killings have clear disciplining effects: in addition to their violence against animals they have been used to transform local pork production around the world, forcing local farmers already facing trauma from the loss of their animals to adapt to new conditions of animal husbandry imposed by the globalized meat industry.[40]

In the process, societies that lack clear boundaries between their human and animal populations are seen as "traditional," usually meaning backwards, antimodern, and literally diseased or sick. This was clear in Cairo, when Madgy Rady, a government spokesman, said that "If you see the conditions of the swine farms in Egypt, they are not healthy at all. They are hazards in themselves, even without the swine flu. That's why people are really getting afraid."[41] The politics of fear in the face of a possibly zoonotic disease, combined with pressures for development and religious and ethnic animosity, created socially ghettoized and materially sacrificed populations of animals, both human and non-human.

We should be concerned about the violent effects of speculation about disease, which in some cases has led to results for humans and animals far worse than the actual

39 Quoted in Slackman, "Cleaning Cairo" (note 23).

40 Dinesh Joseph Wadiwel examines the links between systemic violence towards animals in the context of our food system; cf. Dinesh J. Wadiwel, A Handshake between Anthropocentrism and Capitalism: Reflections on Animal Life within Industrial Food Systems, in: Linda Tallberg/Lindsay Hamilton (eds.), The Oxford Handbook of Animal Organization Studies, Oxford 2022 (Online Edition). See also Id., Biopolitics, in: Lori Gruen (ed.), Critical Terms for Animal Studies, Chicago 2018, 79–98.

41 "Swine flu. Egypt orders cull of all pig herds", in: The Telegraph, 30 April 2009, http://www.telegraph.co.uk/health/swine-flu/5247771/Swine-flu-Egypt-orders-cull-of-all-pig-herds.html (22 March 2022).

disease itself. Our concerns, legitimate or otherwise, about pandemic diseases serve as an important reminder of how our desire and our fear of intimate connection with non-human animals is mutually constituted. As Nicole Shukin notes in her important book *Animal Capital*:

> A fixation in pandemic discourse on zoonotic diseases–diseases capable of leaping from animal to human bodies via microbial agents such as the H5N1 avian flu virus–is symptomatic of how formerly distinct barriers separating humans and other species are imaginatively, and physically, disintegrating under current conditions of globalization.[42]

As Alex Blanchette has recently noted, the collapsing barriers between humans and animals are prompting a redefinition of what it means to be human for those who work amidst concentrations of animal life. In 2013 many cases of Porcine Epidemic Diarrhea virus (PEDv) emerged in the Great Plains and spread throughout North American hog herds. Within a year, more than seven million animals, approximately ten percent of all the pigs in the United States, had been killed. To help contain the spread of PEDv new biosecurity regimes of corporate governance emerged that redefined human workers and their families as potential carriers of disease that threatened breeding stock. As Blanchette notes, "workers are reimagined as a threat to the vitality of industrial hogs in ways that subtly alter the value of human livelihood and autonomy in this region," marking yet another step in the long transformation of the human-pig relationship that has remade both partners to fit the needs of industrial capitalist animality.[43]

4. Conclusion: Defining the Way Forward

So, what might all this mean for efforts to create a livable sustainable planet, one that might honor multispecies relationships in all their complexity? In my concluding remarks, I would like to end with a few challenges, aware that I am raising more problems than solutions.

For starters, how do we respond to the authority of science, especially the medical discourse about pandemics? Epizootics and zoonoses frequently create a sense of panic in which the priority is containing the outbreak, which usually means promptly killing

---

42 Nicole Shukin, Animal Capital. Rendering Life in Biopolitical Times, Minneapolis 2009, 46. She adds elsewhere, "Indeed, novel diseases erupting out of the closed loop of animal capital – mad cow disease, avian influenza – are one material sign of how the immanent terrain of market life becomes susceptible, paradoxically, to the pandemic potential of 'nature' that early modern discourses of biopower originally sought to circumscribe […]." (16)

43 Alex Blanchette, Herding Species. Biosecurity, Posthuman Labor, and the American Industrial Pig, in: Cultural Anthropology 30/4, 640–669.

animals rather than vaccinating them.[44] Amidst these panics this constructed sense of urgency drives immediate action when the spread of the disease and its actual effects on humans and animals are not yet certain. The result is a substantial overkill, especially of animals that may not actually be sick. For example, in the 2001 British foot-and-mouth disease epidemic it was estimated that 80% of the animals killed did not have the disease. In the confusion and panic, one sees surprisingly little concern about the health of the animals, which often can live with these diseases, which are painful but not necessarily fatal. The message that foot-and-mouth disease is usually nonfatal for adult animals and that the culling of animals takes place primarily to stop the spread of the disease and to prevent trade bans from being imposed on affected countries has, unfortunately, failed to generate much purchase.[45]

Given the ways in which distance and concealment operate in the way power works on animals, perhaps we can find some hope in the work of activist groups that have used the internet and social media to get the word out about these mass exterminations. For example, much of what we learned about the killing of more than three million animals, mainly pigs, in South Korea came from activists and from government workers and officials horrified by the haste and cruelty of this killing. Groups like Korea Animal Rights Advocates (KARA) put the story before Koreans and helped spread it via the global animal rights community, although they were concerned about the pigs being buried alive, not the farmers or workers in Korean agriculture, a reminder of the difficulties involved in thinking about what might be best or most sustainable for multispecies communities.

Given the relative invisibility of both the human and non-human animals involved, it comes as little surprise that these mass killings often take place without much public awareness or comment. As in Haiti and Egypt, the affected humans are themselves often always already marginal in these societies. Pigs also have a long history of being viewed negatively, making it inevitable that industry-driven economic imperatives and national concerns about imports and exports dominate over any concerns about the animals and the (often marginal) people who share their lives and space.

One further question emerges for those of us engaged in animal studies as both an academic inquiry and an activist pursuit: Can we imagine ourselves supporting or working to restore a multispecies relationship that will still involve the commodification and killing of pigs by these subaltern communities? Given the critical stance we take toward the nostalgic human-pig relationship currently fetishized in the slow food movement, heritage farming, and popular writings about food and agriculture (all of which raise important questions about race, class, and privilege), even if a return to

---

44 See the chapter by Delphine Berdah in this volume.

45 The disease is quite painful to animals, as it leads to blisters on the feet and mouth, but only has a mortality rate of two to five percent.

traditional animal husbandry were an effective way to improve the lives of all members in in multispecies communities, how would we address global poverty and hunger on such a massive scale? After all, it is almost certainly not possible to use traditional agriculture to feed the almost seven billion people on the planet.[46]

There have been some efforts to think about how to integrate modern agriculture with the contemporary city, seen most notably in a 2001 proposal in which living pigs would be returned by the thousands to urban spaces to live in high-rise farms. The Dutch architectural firm MVRDV has proposed a "pig city" as a way to raise pigs organically in the crowded Netherlands landscape. These pigs would be kept comfortable in "apartments" with balconies and trees. Each 80-meter tower would contain a central slaughterhouse, a rooftop fish farm to supply some of the needed food, and a waste-processing station that would produce energy for the building through biogas. They argue, "If pigs are efficiently kept in stacked "apartments" in such a way that they enjoy better conditions, the meat acquires a better taste, livestock transport becomes unnecessary, diseases are eliminated, and the Netherlands acquires more space."[47]

This provocative effort to rethink urban ecology and the human-pig relationship was primarily intended as a critique of contemporary industrial agriculture. It has finally been put into practice, however, in Ezhou, a city in Hubei province in China. There a 26-story pig farm and slaughterhouse went into operation in October 2022 when the first 3700 sows were admitted to the farm. The building has a capacity for 650,000 animals and, it is hoped, will provide a more efficient, bio-secure, and environmentally friendly model of meat production in a country that consumes half of the world's pork. While this high-rise farm should minimize the interactions between these farmed pigs and wild animals and their diseases (a vector of transmission seen as the key to the origins of the Covid-19 pandemic), experts worry about the effects of this higher density of animals on the spread, amplification, and possible mutation of infectious pathogens.[48]

Combatting the ongoing transformation of the human-pig relationship and the environment in the Anthropocene with even more Anthropocene-thinking, this project highlights our failure to see ecologically and to see non-human animals as part of human environments as co-creators of our world. All of which begs my final two questions: Given the intimate entanglements of human and animal lives, how do we get beyond the

46 Kendra Coulter has argued that stopping the trade in exotic animals, embracing a OneHealth framework that sees human, animal, and environmental health as inextricably connected, and dismantling industrial agriculture are all essential to the future of the planet. See Kendra Coulter, "Coronavirus shows we must get serious about the well-being of animals", in: The Conversation, 24 May 2020: https://theconversation.com/coronavirus-shows-we-must-get-serious-about-the-well-being-of-animals-138872 (9 January 2023).

47 See http://www.mvrdv.nl/#/projects/181pigcity (22 March 2022).

48 "China's 26-storey pig skyscraper ready to slaughter 1 million pigs a year", in: The Guardian, 25 November 2022, https://www.theguardian.com/environment/2022/nov/25/chinas-26-storey-pig-skyscraper-ready-to-produce-1-million-pigs-a-year (9 January 2023).

productivist and reductionist emphasis of intensive agriculture to focus on relationships between animals (human and non-human), communities, and the earth? Or, to put it differently, how will a complex, enlightened and sustainable green society involve actual animals?

Abstract:
This chapter examines epizootic episodes across global pig populations and the typical response to them: the mass killings of pigs and other livestock in the name of disease prevention and eradication. Tracing the impact of these eradication programs on humans and other animals in multispecies communities, I show how the mass slaughter of pigs to prevent the spread of infectious diseases has emerged in conjunction with the growth of concentrated animal breeding and feeding operations and the consolidation of a globalized corporate meat-production industry. Examining recent mass killings of pigs in Haiti, Egypt, Korea, China, and elsewhere, I suggest that modernization in the global south has partly taken the form of mass killings of pigs in the name of disease prevention without much, if any, consideration of the intertwined lives of people and animals. By looking at the history of pigs and epidemics, the resulting mass killings of pigs, and responses to the destruction and re-orientation of human-pig relationships (which include efforts to restore native pig breeds and recuperate these multispecies relationships), this paper highlights the need for multispecies justice in efforts to both combat epizootic disease events and improve the entangled lives of human and non-human animals.

Keywords:
epizootic diseases | pigs | multispecies communities | industrial agriculture | killing animals

The *Longue Durée*

Timothy P. Newfield

Premodern European Animal Plagues

Common but Enigmatic?

The history of non-human animal plagues in premodernity very much remains in its infancy.[1] While our understanding of premodern animal disease has advanced considerably in recent years, specifically in regards to the fourteenth- and eighteenth-century European bovine panzootics, much remains unknown about the disease outbreaks domesticated and undomesticated animals suffered centuries and millennia ago across all world regions. This article seeks to survey the state of our knowledge about animal plagues in western Eurasia, focusing on the Middle Ages. It employs case studies of animal plagues observed in the sixth, early-ninth, late-tenth and early-fourteenth centuries to probe the limits of what we can glean about premodern animal plagues from written sources alone, to tease out the relevance of recent and ongoing work in the paleo- and phylo-genetic sciences, and to advance a framework for studying animal disease outbreaks in the distant past. There is much work to do and no one discipline or scholar can do it alone. To contextual recent histories of epizootic and zoonotic disease, to begin to establish trends in outbreaks over time and space, and to start to identify triggers of, and risk factors for, historical animal disease outbreaks, we must advance a new agenda, one that seeks to interdisciplinarily interrogate the diverse evidence we have for past animal disease and to establish what data we might look to produce. This article is a step in that direction.

1 The Social Sciences and Humanities Research Council of Canada supported the researching and writing of this article, which has a long history and has benefited from the comments of Bruce M.S. Campbell, Louisa Gidney, Richard Hoffmann, William Chester Jordan, Dan P. McCarthy, Scott McGill, Alexander Murray, Philip Slavin, Paolo Squatriti, Richard Thomas and Faith Wallis. Note that translations of passages from the Anglo-Saxon Chronicle, Chronicon ex Chronicis, Gregory of Tours' Libri Historiarum X and De Virtutibus Sancti Martini Episcopi, and Agnellus of Ravenna's Liber Pontificalis Ecclesiae Ravennatis are based on the translations cited, but have been altered in some respects following consultation of the editions of these texts also cited. Also note that "plague" is used here as a generic term for a disease outbreak. It is not treated interchangeably with the disease plague, caused by *Yersinia pestis*. Similarly, "cattle plague" does not refer here to the rinderpest virus, unless specified, but simply an outbreak of disease in cattle.

1. Introduction

The history of premodern European epizootic disease remains in its infancy. Ancient, medieval and early modern written evidence for non-human animal health and illness has been overlooked or dealt with uncritically for generations, and few livestock plagues before the great cattle panzootics of the eighteenth century have attracted the attention of modern historians.[2] Several "catalogues" of premodern outbreaks of disease in domesticated animals, assembled by veterinarians, antiquarians and their kin in the eighteenth through twentieth centuries, exist, but, as is emphasized throughout this article, these present rather ahistorical accounts of ancient, medieval and early modern epizootics and should be avoided or, if consulted, examined most carefully. These catalogues – the most influential of which have been Paulet's *Recherches historiques et physiques sur les maladiés epizootiques* (1775), Fleming's *Animal Plagues* (1871) and Dieckerhoff's *Geschichte der Rinderpest und ihrer Literatur* (1890)[3] – rarely pay heed to the date or place of the composition, or textuality, of the sources for premodern animal plagues they consult. They make and perpetuate numerous unsupported claims regarding the diagnoses, consequences, and temporal and spatial parameters of plagues, contain errors in dating, rely heavily on non-contemporary sources and secondary scholarship, regularly cite one another, and often employ now outdated editions and

2 On eighteenth-century plagues see, for example, Clive A. Spinage, Cattle Plague. A History, New York 2003, 103–150, 241–262; Dominik Hünniger, Die Viehseuche von 1744–52. Deutungen und Herrschaftspraxis in Krisenzeiten, Neumünster 2011; id., Policing Epizootics. Legislation and Administration during Outbreaks of Cattle Plague in Eighteenth-Century Northern Germany as Continuous Crisis Management, in: Karen Brown/Daniel Gilfoyle (eds.), Healing the Herds. Disease, Livestock Economies and the Globalization of Veterinary Medicine, Athens, OH, 2010, 76–91; Karl Appuhn, Ecologies of Beef. Eighteenth-Century Epizootics and the Environmental History of Early Modern Europe, in: Environmental History 15 (2010), 268–287; Carsten Stühring, Der Seuche begegnen. Deutung und Bewältigung von Rinderseuchen im Kurfürstentum Bayern des 18. Jahrhunderts, Frankfurt 2011; id., Managing Epizootic Disease in Eighteenth-Century Bavaria, in: Simonetta Cavaciocchi (ed.), Le interazioni fra economia e ambiente biologico nell'Europa preindustriale, secc. XIII–XVIII. Proceedings of the 41st Study Week of the Fondazione Istituto Internazionale di Storia Economica "F. Datini", Florence 2010, 473–480.

3 Jean-Jacques Paulet, Recherches historiques et physiques sur les maladiés epizootiques avec les moyen d'y remédier dans tous les cas, Paris 1775; George Fleming, Animal Plagues. History, Nature and Prevention, London 1871; Wilhelm Dieckerhoff, Geschichte der Rinderpest und ihrer Literatur. Beitrag zur Geschichte der vergleichenden Pathologie, Berlin 1890. Also Thomas Short, A General Chronological History of the Air, Weather, Seasons and Meteors, etc., 2 vols., London 1749; J. C. Wirth, Lehrbuch der Seuchen und ansteckenden Krankheiten der Haustiere, Zurich 1838; Georges Curasson, La Peste Bovine, Paris 1932, and more recently Spinage, Cattle Plague (note 2), 81–101.

translations of primary texts.[4] Moreover, no catalogue is exhaustive in its coverage and most fail to distinguish between major and minor crises.[5]

The history of premodern epizootic disease must begin afresh. There is much work to do: the temporal and spatial contours, as well as the triggers, of many animal plagues have yet to be identified, the frequency with which epizootics occurred in different periods and regions remains to be (even roughly) established, the impact of livestock mortalities on different economies and populations, and in different regions and periods, begs for further assessment, as do the distinctive consequences for human populations of mortalities of different domesticated species. The diagnoses of most animal plagues also have yet to be addressed and those that have may require re-evaluation. Was it rinderpest (RPV), foot-and-mouth disease (FMD) or contagious bovine pleuropneumonia (CBPP)? And, importantly, why do diagnoses matter? What do we gain and what do we lose when we diagnose? The very impetus to affix modern scientific labels to premodern epizootics, not to mention the methods by which we attempt to align the premodern animal disease experience with the modern, should perhaps themselves be reconsidered, as medical historians, like Jon Arrizabalaga, Nadine Metzger and Claudia Stein, have come to reappraise the retrospective diagnosing of human epidemics.[6]

4 Support for these statements is found in the following pages. It is worth emphasizing here, however, how infrequently some catalogues draw from sources contemporary to the plagues they address. Take Fleming, Animal Plagues (note 3) for example. In his well-known work, Fleming regularly, though not universally, draws upon non-contemporary historical sources, earlier catalogues of premodern livestock disease, and secondary scholarship for evidence: of non-contemporary sources Fleming employs John Hardyng's fifteenth-century chronicle for a late-seventh-century epizootic (ibid., 42), Vaclav Hajek of Libočany's sixteenth-century annals for eighth-, ninth- and eleventh-century epizootics (ibid., 44–45, 59), Raphael Holinshed's sixteenth-century Chronicles for eleventh-, twelfth- and fourteenth-century epizootics (ibid., 64, 66, 78, 92–93), John Stow's sixteenth-century Annales or General Chronicle of England for eleventh, thirteenth and fourteenth century epizootics (ibid., 66, 79, 93), and François de Belleforest's seventeenth-century text for an early ninth-century epizootic (ibid., 48); of earlier catalogues, Fleming draws upon Short's mid-eighteenth-century accounts of tenth- through fourteenth-century livestock plagues (ibid., 40, 65, 68–73, 78–9, 90, 92–4) and Wirth's early nineteenth-century accounts of several early medieval outbreaks (ibid., 41, 47, 50); of secondary scholarship, Fleming relies heavily on James Edwin Thorold Rogers' A History of Agriculture when discussing late-twelfth- and early-thirteenth-century livestock disease (ibid., 87–9, 93). Fleming's assessments of epizootics are often based on summaries of summaries of extant evidence and are often three or four steps removed from the actual sources.

5 For instance, the early fourteenth-century panzootic addressed below either appears equal in extent and impact to epizootics far more circumscribed and less mortal, or is altogether lost in a collection of references indiscriminately plucked from medieval sources and organized in no particular way other than chronologically.

6 Jon Arrizabalaga, Problematizing Retrospective Diagnosis in the History of Disease, in: Asclepio 54 (2002), 51–70; Claudia Stein, "Getting" the Pox. Reflections by a Historian on How to Write the History of Early Modern Disease, in: Nordic Journal of Science and Technology Studies 2 (2014), 53–60; Nadine Metzger, Kynanthropy. Canine Madness in Byzantine Late Antiquity, in: History of Psychiatry 26 (2015), 318–331.

All of these issues represent important scholarly pursuits. Premodern European human economy and health was to a large extent dependent on the wellbeing of domesticated animals and recent scholarship indicates that dramatic and sudden mortalities of livestock could have devastating effects for premodern human populations.[7] Livestock not only supplied dairy and meat, as well as bone, fibers, hides, horn, sinew and tallow, but they were the trucks and tractors of premodern agriculture. They were also very highly valued for their production of manure. For most of Europe, throughout the preindustrial period, with the exception of some Mediterranean regions, cattle, which seem to have been struck more regularly by epizootic disease than other domesticates, were the principal source of the traction and fertilizer necessary for arable farming.[8] Commerce, communication and warfare were as well heavily dependent on the health of livestock, equines and bovines especially. At the same time, concepts of animal health were interwoven with those of human health and coming to terms with the ways in which animal disease was reported, understood and dealt with will have ramifications for our understanding of the ways premoderns conceived of health, good and bad.

This article intends to (re-)set the stage for the diachronic study of premodern European livestock epizootics. Via an assessment of the written evidence for six plagues of cattle (*Bos taurus*) – those of 591 and 809–810, better-known in the veterinary sciences than the humanities, the lesser-known cattle plagues of 569–570, 583–584 and 986–988, and the cattle panzootic of 1314–1325, which has been the subject of much study in

7 Ian Kershaw, The Great Famine and Agrarian Crisis in England 1315–1322, in: Past and Present 59 (1973), 14, 20–32, 34, 43, 45, 48; Carroll Gillmor, The 791 Equine Pestilence and its Impact on Charlemagne's Army, in: Journal of Medieval Military History 3 (2005), 23–45; Philip Slavin, The Fifth Rider of the Apocalypse. The Great Cattle Plague in England and Wales and its Economic Consequences, 1319–1350, in: Cavaciocchi (ed.), Le interazioni (note 2), 165–179; Philip Slavin, The Great Bovine Pestilence and its Economic and Environmental Consequences in England and Wales, 1318–50, in: Economic History Review 65 (2012), 1239–1266; Bruce M. S. Campbell, Nature as Historical Protagonist. Environment and Society in Pre-Industrial England, in: Economic History Review 63 (2010), 288–291; id., Physical Shocks, Biological Hazards, and Human Impacts. The Crisis of the Fourteenth Century Revisited, in: Cavaciocchi (ed.), Le interazioni (note 2), 24–27; Bruce M. S. Campbell, Panzootics, Pandemics and Climate Anomalies in the Fourteenth Century, in: Bernd Herrmann (ed.), Beiträge zum Göttinger Umwelthistorischen Kolloquium 2010–2011, Göttingen 2011, 194–196.

8 It was suggested that the horse came to dominate traction in agriculture across much of northern Europe in the early and high Middle Ages, but it is now known that this transition was limited to eastern and southeastern England, northern France and the Low Countries and that it began, depending on the region, between the twelfth and fourteenth centuries, See, for example, John Langdon, Horses, Oxen and Technological Innovation. the Use of Draught Animals in English Farming from 1066 to 1500, Cambridge 1986; Adriaan Verhulst, The "Agricultural Revolution" of the Middle Ages Reconsidered, in: Bernard S. Bachrach/David Nicholas (eds.), Law, Custom and the Social Fabric in Medieval Europe. Essays in Honour of Bryce Lyon, Kalamazoo 1990, 18–19, 22; John Langdon, Was England a Technological Backwater in the Middle Ages?, in: Grenville Astill/John Langdon (eds.), Medieval Farming and Technology. The Impact of Agricultural Change in Northwest Europe, Leiden 1997, 282–283; Bruce M. S. Campbell, English Seigniorial Agriculture, 1250–1450, Cambridge 2000, 123–127.

recent years – the article demonstrates the changing quantity and character of the evidence available for livestock epizootics before the great outbreaks of the eighteenth century, and the possibilities and problems that this evidence presents for an assessment of the contours, diagnoses and effects of premodern animal plagues. In studying these particular outbreaks, the article also surveys most of the existing scholarship on premodern epizootics, tests prevailing notions, rooted in the aforementioned catalogues, about the scale, consequences and pathogenic identities of the outbreaks of 591 and 809–810, and reappraises claims that written evidence for these plagues provides proof of the antiquity of rinderpest.

These six plagues are addressed individually. The article starts with the most thoroughly documented, the 1314–1325 panzootic, and works backward to the sixth century. This reverse chronology brings out in sharp resolution the ambiguous and fragmentary nature of the earlier evidence for epizootics and the difficulties encountered when using it to establish extents, impacts and diagnoses. Working backwards also demonstrates from the outset the limitations imposed by the written evidence – even when it is good. Directions for future research are highlighted in conclusion, but throughout the article stress is put on the need for inter- or multi-disciplinary efforts. Collaboration between interested scholars of multiple disciplines concerned with past animal health will be essential for a deep understanding of premodern European epizootic disease. Without rigorous collaborative efforts, such animal plagues, as common as they were, will remain enigmatic.

2. A Great "Slaughter of the Cattle" from Poland to Ireland, 1314–1325

Between 1298 and 1325, over forty contemporary or near-contemporary annals, chronicles and histories from modern-day Austria, Czechia, Denmark, England, France, Germany, Ireland, the Netherlands, Poland, Scotland, Sweden and Wales document mortalities of domestic bovines. These accounts range from short, matter-of-fact statements, such as "pestilence of cattle" encountered in the *Annales Essenbecenses* (Randers, Denmark) in 1308 and the "a pestilence killed horses, sheep and both oxen and all the cattle of field" found in the *Chronicon Regiae Aulae* (Zbraslav, Czech Republic) in 1316,[9] to longer and more descriptive reports, like that of the Tintern (Wales) version of the *Flores Historiarum*. In 1319 that text reads,

> there was the greatest mortality of animals, that is oxen, cows and other animals, on account of which people had hardly, or no, oxen to cultivate their lands. And therefore there was as

9 Annales Essenbecenses, ed. Ellen Jørgensen (Annales Danici Medii Aevi), Copenhagen 1920, 148; Chronicon Regiae Aulae ed. Johann Loserth, (Fontes rerum Austriacarum Scriptores 8) Vienna 1875, 379.

> great as possible dearth of horses, with the aforementioned pestilence beginning in Scotland, afterwards in England, and finally in the Welsh Marshes around the Feast of All Saints.[10]

The majority of the textual accounts of the plague provide only vague and indirect indications of its temporal and spatial parameters, while lengthier reports comment on the scale of the mortality, the immediate impact it had on human health and economy, and some measures contemporaries adopted to absorb losses. Although the plague has yet to register in catalogues of livestock disease or in the veterinary, virological or policy studies,[11] historians Lucas, Kershaw and Jordan drew attention to several early fourteenth-century narrative accounts of animal mortalities in their respective studies of the Great European Famine (GEF),[12] and a more exhaustive collection and assessment of the textual evidence pertaining strictly to domestic bovines appeared more recently.[13] With this evidence, it is possible to discern a pan-European outbreak of disease in cattle, irrupting c.1314/1316 in modern-day Poland and Czechia, spreading westward to modern-day Germany, the Netherlands, France, Denmark, Sweden c.1316/1318, England c.1319, Scotland c.1319/1320, Wales c.1320 and Ireland c.1321 where the disease appears to have persisted until 1325.[14] The *Chronicon* of Louth Park claims that all Christendom was affected, and Johannis de Trokelowe, a contemporary chronicler at St. Albans, reports that all of France suffered, but evidence for the outbreak in southern France, Spain or Italy is unknown.[15] Reports of cattle mortalities leading up to the famine, between 1298 and 1313, are largely restricted to central and northern Europe

10 Flores Historiarum, ed. Henry Richards Luard, London 1890, 343.

11 Short, General Chronological History (note 3), vol. I, 160, 162, only draws attention to animal mortalities in England in 1314 and 1318/21, which he attributes to poisoned grass, disease and drought. Paulet, Recherches historiques (note 3), 85–86, addresses the plague in England alone and, drawing upon the Histoire d'Angleterre of André Duchesne (1584–1640), ties the mortalities to poor weather and ruined pastures. Fleming, Animal Plagues (note 3), 91–94, employs a wider range of sources, most non-contemporary, and, like the others, does not discern a pan-European outbreak. Dieckerhoff, Geschichte der Rinderpest (note 3), 28, contains few fourteenth-century references. He notes evidence for epizootics in that century is slight. Although he is unaware of the 1314–1325 panzootic, he remarks of bovine mortalities in Germany, Belgium and England in 1315. He does not identify rinderpest as the cause. Spinage, Cattle Plague (note 2), 92–94, draws upon the studies of Lucas, Kershaw and Jordan but perhaps does not attribute the outbreak the significance it deserves.

12 Henry S. Lucas, The Great European Famine, in: Speculum 5 (1930), 343–377, 355, 358, 362; Kershaw, Great Famine (note 7), 14, 26, 30; William Chester Jordan, The Great Famine. Northern Europe in the Early Fourteenth Century, Princeton 1996, 35, 38–39.

13 Timothy P. Newfield, A Cattle Panzootic in Early Fourteenth-Century Europe, in: Agricultural History Review 57 (2009), 155–190, 159–171.

14 Newfield, Cattle Panzootic (note 13), 171–174; for Sweden see Janken Myrdal, Farming and Feudalism, 1000–1700, in: Janken Myrdal/Mats Morell (eds.), The Agrarian History of Sweden. From 4000 BCE to AD 2000, Lund, 2011, 79, 273, n.12.

15 Newfield, Cattle Panzootic (note 13), 163–164.

and may be interpreted as circumscribed outbreaks of the disease, which only in the context of the GEF managed to disseminate across a large area of Europe.[16] That said, these early mortalities could have been unrelated to the spread of disease in the context of the GEF. References to subsequent cattle mortalities in the mid-1320s in England, and in the mid-1330s in England, Ireland, Wales and Iceland, may tell of spatially restricted reoccurrences of the panzootic, though extreme weather could be to blame for some of these deaths.[17]

In addition to reports of the plague found in annals, chronicles and histories, the die-off crops up in correspondence, petitions and manorial accounts from England and Wales. These records corroborate the more qualitative narrative texts and expand our knowledge of the plague's dissemination, duration, extent, identity, impact and mortality. The Letter-Books of Christ Church Canterbury produce three references to the outbreak, one of which laments the deaths of over a thousand head of cattle and another which details the deaths of 257 oxen and 511 cows on forty manors belonging to the religious house. The abbot of Ramsey, the archbishop of Bolton Priory, and a letter from Westminster's St. James' Hospital, also tell of cattle mortalities in their respective locales. Like these letters, the four known Welsh petitions – requests for relief of dues filed by English subjects to Edward II – emphasize the magnitude of the mortality as well as provide additional indications of where cattle died. Some also remark on a subsequent "impoverishment." Petitions alone demonstrate the panzootic's presence in the counties of Anglesey, Caernarvonshire and Glamorgenshire.[18]

Of the non-narrative evidence, the manorial accounts are unquestionably the most informative. For over a century, agrarian historians of England have drawn upon select accounts to demonstrate the severity of this mortality on specific English demesnes.[19] It was not until Kershaw's seminal article on the GEF, however, that the value of these records for the study of the panzootic really became apparent.[20] Kershaw drew upon the manorial accounts of the estates belonging to Bolton Priory and Westminster,

16 Disease is reported in Poland in 1298, in Germany in 1299 and 1300, 1300, in Denmark in 1308 and 1310, in Gotland in 1300, in mainland Sweden c.1310, and possibly in Austria in 1310. See Newfield, Cattle Panzootic (note 13), 160, 175–76, 180; I owe the Swedish references to Janken Myrdal and Bruce M. S. Campbell, pers. corresp. 18 March 2010. A plague reported in 1298 in Alsace may have been associated to that documented then in Poland and Germany, though the cattle mortality reported in the Annals of Connacht (Annála Connacht. The Annals of Connacht, [A.D. 1224–1544], ed. A. Martin Freeman, Dublin, 1994, 217) and Annals of Loch Cé (Annals of Loch Cé I, ed. William M. Hennessy, London 1871, 545) of Ireland in 1308 are, considering the dearth of evidence for epizootic disease then in England, France and the Low Countries, unlikely to be related to outbreaks around that time in northern and eastern continental Europe.

17 Campbell, Physical Shocks (note 7), 27; Newfield, Cattle Panzootic (note 13), 171, 177–79.

18 Newfield, Cattle Panzootic (note 13), 155, 167–169.

19 Ibid., 157, n.10.

20 Kershaw, Great Famine (note 7), 24–26, 28.

in addition to roughly fifteen other seigniorial farms. More recently Campbell and Slavin have presented more systematic and exhaustive assessments of this evidence.[21] In successive articles, Slavin has consulted the records of 145 and 165 manors. These fiscal records of the agrarian economy of lordly farms, which document manorial yields over the agricultural year, survive from several regions of England and parts of Wales, and in great quantity between 1275 and 1425. They allow us to calculate with precision the plague's mortality on individual demesnes and to map the distribution of the disease with greater accuracy in England and Wales. The hard data acquired from these accounts may also be employed cautiously to illuminate the panzootic's continental history.

Initial scholarly estimates of the scale of the mortality ranged widely. It had been suggested that manorial losses in England varied between 20 and 70 per cent, that English herds were often reduced by 90 per cent, and that the plague killed half of all the oxen in Europe.[22] Medieval texts from central, northern and northwestern Europe do stress a large mortality: many annals, chronicles and histories write of a "great"and "large" "slaughter of cattle", of a plague of an "unheard of" scale, and of the "greatest" outbreak then known. Contemporary Robert of Reading, in the Westminster *Flores Historiarum*, remarks that "an infinite multitude" of animals were laid low and that the plague left "few [animals] in different parts" while the archbishop at Bolton Priory observes that the mortality appeared to be "universal" and the author of the *Poem on the Evil Times of Edward II*, composed in the early- or mid-1320s, that "the cattle all died quickly".[23] In his fifteenth-century *Chronicon*, based on earlier sources, Edmond of Dynter claims that the mortality was so great "that from ten [cows] hardly one survived".[24] While few of these statements are without precedent and many medieval descriptions of the scale and severity of animal plagues have much in common, that there are so many contemporary and independent reports of a large mortality signals many animals did in fact die between 1314 and 1325. On the basis of the narrative sources, however, roughly how many is wholly uncertain.

Manorial accounts confirm this reading and allow for a more exact idea of the mortality. Data relevant to the panzootic published prior to 2009 revealed a death

21 Campbell, Nature (note 7), 288–291; id., Physical Shocks (note 7), 24–27; Slavin, Fifth Rider (note 7); Slavin, Great Bovine Pestilence (note 7).

22 John Aberth, From the Brink of the Apocalypse. Confronting Famine, War, Plague, and Death in the Later Middle Ages, New York 2000, 22; H. F. Diaz et al, Climate and Human Health Linkages on Multiple Timescales, in: P. D. Jones et al. (eds.), History and Climate. Memories of the Future?, Dordrecht 2001, 275.

23 Flores Historiarum (note 10), 186–187; A Letter from Archbishop Melton to the Prior and Convent of Worksop, in: Historical Studies and Letters from the Northern Registers, ed. James Raine, London 1873, 306–307; Poem on the Evil Times of Edward II, in: The Political Songs of England VI. From the Reign of John to that of Edward II, ed. Thomas Wright, London 1839, 342–344.

24 Edmund Dynter, Chronicon, in: Chronica Nobilissimorum Ducum Lotharingiae et Brabantiae ac Regum Francorum II, ed. P. F. X. de Ram, Brussels 1856, 497.

rate on affected English manors of around 60 per cent,[25] while, in 2010, Campbell, drawing upon his database of English manorial accounts, established a mortality on seigniorial farms representing roughly 50 per cent of the combined value of bovine animals,[26] and, in 2011, a demesne cattle mortality exceeding 65 per cent.[27] Slavin, in the most exhaustive work to date, has calculated an average mortality on seigniorial farms of 62 or 63 per cent.[28] Naturally, herd mortality varied regionally and locally. Some farms escaped the disaster outright, others saw mortalities of 80 to 90 per cent, and others yet lost all their cattle. For example, Beauworth in Hampshire lost 56 of its 68 demesne bovines, Poundisford Park in Somerset 102 of 126, Knoyle in Wiltshire 120 of 123, and Pontelond in Northumberland five of five, while Belasis in Durham lost only 9 of 40, Llangwm in Monmouthshire 10 of 33, and Sedgeford in Norfolk none of 48.[29] This variation upsets the blanket claims of the narrative sources and may be attributed to a number of factors, such as the proximity of herds to markets, well-worn roads and other susceptible animals, the extent of animal malnutrition experienced during the GEF, as well as differences in regional and local cattle population density and distribution. Variation in the underlying disease burden and malnutrition may have mattered too, as sick and underfed animals may have been more likely to die. In any case, over 1,000,000 bovines likely succumbed to disease in England alone in a stretch of 12 to 18 months when the panzootic passed through the country.[30]

Manorial accounts, like correspondence, petitions, and several annals, chronicles and histories, reveal that of domesticated species cattle alone were affected and that cattle, as most of the textual reports of the disaster observe, died of disease. Indeed, while some insular and continental textual accounts of the GEF speak vaguely of crop failures, extreme weather and animal mortalities, and some English texts conflate the sheep mortalities that took place during the exceptionally wet early years of the subsistence crisis with the cattle deaths that took place in England at the tail end of the shortage,[31] the manorial data illustrate that cattle and sheep deaths were not concurrent in England. The manorial evidence also confirms, as the textual evidence implies, that deaths of cattle did not occur simultaneously across England or Europe: the disease spread geographically. The manorial accounts, as such, help us make sense of reports of animal mortalities like

25 Newfield, Cattle Panzootic (note 13), 185.

26 Campbell, Nature (note 7), 89; id., Physical Shocks (note 7), 26.

27 Campbell, Panzootics (note 7), 182, 195.

28 Slavin, Fifth Rider (note 7), 170; id., Great Bovine Pestilence (note 7), 1239, 1242.

29 Slavin, Great Bovine Pestilence (note 7), 1265–1266 (Appendix I).

30 Slavin (pers. corresp. 15 October 2011) estimates that there were 2.4 million domestic bovines in England c.1320. Campbell, Panzootics (note 6), 195, notes that in excess of 500,000 working oxen died in England alone.

31 Kershaw, Great Famine (note 7), 20–24.

that found in the *Chronicon Regiae Aulae*, which bundle together GEF-era deaths of multiple species.

In England, the panzootic first appears in manorial accounts in the southeast, in the agricultural year of 1318/1319. Trokelowe observes that the panzootic irrupted in the county of Essex around Easter 1319. Although his account should not be taken verbatim, as discussed below, it is possible that the disease did arrive first in England in the spring of 1319 in Essex from which it spread north, south and west. Welsh cattle do not appear to have been hit until mid-September 1320 (manorial data place the plague in southeastern Wales and petitions in the northwest), but the plague had arrived at the Scottish border by August 1319.[32] The manorial accounts, thus, serve to correct the path of dissemination suggested in the Tintern *Flores*. While the majority of the manorial accounts Slavin consults stem from southern and eastern counties (manorialism was not everywhere strong or present, and far from all manors are endowed with accounts for years of the outbreak), these records, when employed alongside textual evidence, correspondence and petitions, do demonstrate a nearly nation-wide spread of disease, but again that mortality, and presumably disease prevalence, varied widely.[33] For instance, a chronicle compiled in southwestern England, where manorial accounts dating to the GEF appear to be non-extant, provides the best-known direct indication that the panzootic hit Devon, though manorial accounts alone illuminate the plague in neighbouring Somerset. The accounts also illustrate that the disease persisted in England for 12 or 18 months. This corrects references to the panzootic's duration in the *Stoneleigh Ledger Book* and the *Chronicon Lanercost*, which report respectively that the plague persisted for a long time and that it lasted two years in southern England before moving north.[34]

The spatial and temporal contours, speed of dissemination, duration and mortality of the panzootic are relatively clear in England and Wales. In what is now Czechia, Denmark, France, Germany, Ireland, the Netherlands, Poland, Scotland and Sweden, on the other hand, we have only rough indications of when and where the plague was present. The sole known evidence for the panzootic in Poland, the brief "a pestilence of humans and heavy animals" found in the *Annales Bohemiae Brevissimi*,[35] the only known German reference to the plague, the "there was a great famine and a large pestilence of oxen and cattle" found in the *Anonymi Chronicon Wirceburgense*,[36] the two reports of the disaster in France (in addition to Trokelowe's note), the "great mortality of people and

32 Newfield, Cattle Panzootic (note 13), 163, 168, 172–173; Slavin, Fifth Rider (note 7), 168.

33 Newfield, Cattle Panzootic (note 13), 184 (figure 1); Slavin, Fifth Rider (note 7), 168 (figure 1).

34 Stoneleigh Abbey Leger Book, ed. Rodney H. Hilton, Stratford-upon-Avon 1960, 75; Chronicon Lanercost, 1272–1346, trans. Herbert Maxwell, Glasgow 1913, 228.

35 Annales Bohemiae Brevissimi, ed. Georg Heinrich Pertz (Monumenta Germaniae Historica [MGH], Scriptores 17), Hanover 1861, 720.

36 Anonymi Chronicon Wirceburgense, in: Commentarii de Rebus Franciae Orientalis et Episcopatus Wirceburgensis I, ed. J.G. von Eckhart, Würzburg 1729, 821.

cattle" found in a fragmented and anonymous text and the "lack of animals" and "general plague of animals" noted by contemporary Jacques de Thérines,[37] and the best evidence from Scotland, John of Fordun's "nearly all the animals were extinguished",[38] reveal very little. But close consideration of the more abundant English and Welsh material, however, can cautiously inform us of the plague's potential extent and mortality in these regions. Importantly, the textual reports of the disaster in England, together with manorial accounts, indicate that the disease did not originate in England or Wales and that in these countries it struck a "virgin" population (or a population without immunity assuming previous exposure granted it). The mortality rate in individual animals may have been close to 100 per cent, as there is no evidence for the recovery of infected cows, several sources remark that cattle died suddenly, and the wide breadth of the plague indicates it was not opportunistic.[39]

The outbreak's spread in England, Scotland, Wales and Ireland signifies a continental origin. Considering that continental cattle herds were hardly isolated prior to the take off of major European cattle trades post 1350,[40] it is unlikely that a virulent and communicable disease could have been unknown to English and Welsh cattle but well-known to animals elsewhere in northwestern, northern and central Europe. On the continent, it may be suspected, if the disease was not hosted in other animals or reliant on vectors, that the disease claimed a similar proportion of herds, persisted for an equal number of months, spread at a comparable rate, and was roughly as ubiquitous as it did or was in England and Wales. That there is more evidence in England and Wales need not mean that the disease took a greater toll or was more widespread there, though that remains a real possibility. At the same time, the disease may have achieved a wider prevalence on the continent than in England and Wales and, as such, claimed more animals, as it spread across continental Europe in the worst years of the GEF when movements of people and animals would have been most exaggerated.[41] Continental bovines may have also been more liable to succumb to disease when the plague hit their regions, considering that the crop failures and exceptionally wet weather, flooding and severe winters of 1315–1317 would have seen drastic declines in fodder allowances

37 Martin Bouquet, Fragment d'une chronique anonyme, in: Recueil des Historiens des Gaules et de la France 21 (1869), 151, n. 19; N. Valois, Un plaidoyer du XIVe siècle en faveur des Cisterciens, in: Bibliothèque de l'École des Chartes 69 (1908), 366.

38 Johannis de Fordun, Chronica gentis Scotorum, in: The Historians of Scotland I, ed. W. F. Skene, Edinburgh 1871, 349.

39 Newfield, Cattle Panzootic (note 13), 173; Slavin, Fifth Rider (note 7), 171, 172, 180; Campbell, Physical Shocks (note 7), 25–26.

40 Newfield, Cattle Panzootic (note 13), 174, n. 82; Slavin, Fifth Rider (note 7), 169.

41 Lucas, Great European Famine (note 12), 356, 359, 363, 375; Kershaw, Great Famine (note 7), 9, 11, 12; Jordan, Great Famine (note 12), 97, 111–112, 100, 134, 143–144.

and in the quantity and quality of available pasture.[42] In other words, cattle may have been severely malnourished and immunologically weaker than they were in England later. This is supported by Slavin's most recent study of the English manorial evidence,[43] which finds a correlation between crop failure and cattle mortality on affected demesnes: mortality in herds was generally greater c.1320 on the manors that suffered the worst harvests in 1315, 1316 and 1317. Slavin also finds that mature female cattle appear to have been somewhat more susceptible to contract and die of the disease than bulls, oxen or immatures,[44] possibly on account of the nutrient taxing conditions of pregnancy and lactation. Still, the pathogen clearly did not prey on animals with poor nutritional standing and compromised immune function. Cattle of all sorts suffered acute disease. The pathogen appears to have claimed most of the animals it infected, young and mature, female and male, and it was virulent in England, Wales and Ireland after the hardest years of the GEF, that is, when many famine-afflicted cattle may have been slaughtered, replaced or recovered.

There is also little reason to doubt that large mortalities occurred outside of England, as contemporary reports of the disease from Ireland to Poland stress, considering that manorial accounts verify fundamentally similar qualitative reports of widespread cattle mortalities in England and Wales. At the same time, poor data and generalizations must be identified as such, and without a firm grasp of the disease's transmission mechanics broad stroke claims must be avoided. Although the disease may have persisted for 12 or 18 months in most regions, in areas densely populated with cattle, such as southwestern Jutland in Denmark, Schleswig-Holstein in northern Germany, Frisia and Holland in the Netherlands, and highland Scotland, it may have lasted for upwards of four years, as contemporary sources indicate it did in cattle-rich Ireland.[45]

The available evidence suggests, though does not confirm, that the disease was not enzootic to central, northern or northwestern Europe, before or after the plague. The origins of the outbreaks may lay east of Poland, where it is first surely attested. It is not impossible that cattle mortalities in early fourteenth-century Europe are tied to mortalities described in contemporary texts in Asia. West Asian authors describe a mass mortality of cattle during the reign of Tohtu Khan (1291–1312), Russian chronicles record cattle epizootics in 1298 and 1309, and, at the opposite end of Eurasia, a Chinese text documents multiple cattle mortalities in Mongolia between 1288 and 1331.[46] The

42 Lucas, Great European Famine (note 12), 350–351, 354, 359, 361, 365, 374, 376–377; Kershaw, Great Famine (note 7), 6–10, 13, 15–6, 19–20; Jordan, Great Famine (note 12), 17–9; 37, 119, 207; Campbell, Nature (note 7), 287–89, 291, 293, 299–301; id., Physical Shocks (note 7), 15–24, 26; id.., Panzootics (note 7), 184–192; Slavin, Great Bovine Pestilence (note 7), 1263.

43 Slavin, Great Bovine Pestilence (note 7), 1245–1247.

44 Ibid., 1247 (table 3).

45 Newfield, Cattle Panzootic (note 13), 175.

46 Addressed in Slavin, Fifth Rider (note 7), 167–168; Newfield, Cattle Panzootic (note 13), 160.

possibility remains, however, that these mortalities are entirely distinct from those of Europe and themselves unrelated. It likewise remains a possibility that the plague emerged not far from where it was first reported and represents, for instance, a European emergence of a novel pathogenic disease. Once in European cattle, the disease plausibly spread via the transfers of cattle between farms, local and regional sales of cattle at markets, transhumance and warfare.[47]

Why the panzootic broke out in central Europe from the east, and spread as widely as it did, when it did, is up for debate. That it appears to have generally adhered, spatially and temporally, to famine-afflicted Europe has fostered two interrelated theories as to the timing of its European irruption: one which holds that the socio-economic and political dislocation generated or accelerated by the extreme shortage conditions of 1315, 1316 and 1317 facilitated the dissemination of disease into and through central, northern and northwestern Europe;[48] and another which holds that the plague's spread was more directly associated to the severe weather at the root of the failed crops that initiated the GEF.[49] As much palaeoclimatic evidence amassed by Campbell demonstrates, the panzootic took place in a period characterized by profound climatic change and climate variability.[50] Although the plague irrupted and spread across Europe in the midst of a late thirteenth- and fourteenth-century climatic anomaly, cattle are not known to have succumbed to disease in all regions affected by the anomaly (around the Aegean or in northern Fennoscandia for example) and the panzootic does not temporally correspond with much precision to any particular European climatic or weather phenomenon within the anomaly.[51] There is no indication, however, that the pathogen was conditioned by particular environmental conditions or that its mortality was seasonal. The disease flourished across a large breadth of Europe, seemingly in all seasons, and in spanning the duration of the GEF, it appears to have done well in years characterized by heavy rains and a difficult winter (1314–1317), drought (1320–1321), and "normal" conditions (1318, 1319 and, at least in Ireland, 1322–1325).

The dramatic scale of the climatic anomaly in general, and the extreme weather of 1314–1317 in particular, may account in part for the wide breadth of the plague's spread, in that they fostered one of the longest sequences of disastrous harvests in recorded European history. Manorial accounts demonstrate that the mean net grain yield per

47 Newfield, Cattle Panzootic (note 13), 175–176; Slavin, Fifth Rider (note 7), 169; Campbell, Physical Shocks (note 7), 26.

48 Newfield, Cattle Panzootic (note 13), 176–177.

49 Campbell, Nature (note 7), 293; id., Physical Shocks (note 7), 13–14, 19–23; id., Panzootics (note 7), 192–194.

50 Campbell, Physical Shocks (note 7), 15–24, 31–32; id., Nature (note 7), 293–294, 299–300, 306; id., Panzootics (note 7) 184–192.

51 But it does fit neatly within a growth inversion detectable between "New" and "Old" World trees. Campbell, Physical Shocks (note 7), 22–23; id., Panzootics (note 7), 193–194.

seed in England was 39 per cent below average in 1315, 63 per cent below average in 1316, and 10 per cent below average in 1317.[52] A change in climate, however, might not itself be thought to account for the plague's European irruption or dissemination. The disease irrupted and spread in Europe only after crops failed. Prior to these failures, and despite the then already ongoing period of climatic change, the European occurrence of the plague appears to have been limited. It is possible that the notable climatic events in Asia in the late 1200s, highlighted by Campbell,[53] may have spurred the initial diffusion of the disease there, if the disease responsible for mortalities in Europe was ever present in Asia. Conflict in famine-afflicted Europe – in the early years of the GEF between Austria and Bavaria, and the French and the Flemings, until 1319 in Scandinavia, and throughout the GEF along the Celtic fringe – may have also contributed to the outbreak's wide geographical spread, though only one contemporary text is known to link war (on the Scottish border) to the panzootic.[54] In any case, conflict, like climatic anomalies and extreme weather, is not a proven catalyst for the spread of infectious diseases in livestock.[55] As stressed below, and as modern historians of eighteenth- through twenty-first century epizootics underscore,[56] as well as modern veterinary manuals for plagues such as CBPP, FMDV and RPV,[57] direct contact between sick and susceptible animals and trade in live animals, has proven to be the most common ingredient for the outbreak of communicable diseases in cattle.

A wide variety of sources speak to the impact of the panzootic, in England especially. Reports of barren fields in the immediate aftermath of the mortality encountered in some correspondence and petitions, and several chronicles such as the Tintern *Flores*, *Chronicon de Lanercost* and Henry Knighton's *Leycestrensis Chronicon*, signify a contraction of arable and an inability to till.[58] The *Chronicon de Lanercost* documents the employment of equines in traction and the Tintern *Flores* suggests that the supply

52 Campbell, Nature (note 7), 288, 300–301; Slavin, Great Bovine Pestilence (note 7), 1239.

53 Campbell, Panzootics (note 7), 196–197.

54 Newfield, Cattle Panzootic (note 13), 164.

55 See Roger Cooter, Of War and Epidemics. Unnatural Couplings, Problematic Conceptions, in: Social History of Medicine 16 (2003), 283–302.

56 Hünniger, Policing Epizootics (note 2), 85–86; Peter A. Koolmees, Epizootic Diseases in the Netherlands, 1713–2002. Veterinary Science, Agricultural Policy, and Public Response, in: Brown/Gilfoyle (eds.), Healing the Herds (note 2), 19–24, 26, 30–31; Martine Barwegen, For Better or Worse? The Impact of the Veterinary Service on the Development of the Agricultural Society in Java (Indonesia) in the Nineteenth Century, in: Brown/Gilfoyle (eds.), Healing the Herds (note 2), 99, 102–103.

57 J. Anderson et al., Manual on the Diagnosis of Rinderpest (Food and Agricultural Organization), Rome 1967; T. U. Obi et al., Manual on the Preparation of Rinderpest Contingency Plans, Rome 1999, 5–6; Food and Agricultural Organization, Recognizing Contagious Bovine Pleuropneumonia, Rome 2002, 4; William A. Geering/William Amanfu, Preparation of Contagious Bovine Pleuropneumonia Plans, Rome 2002, 6; William A. Geering/Juan Lubroth, Preparation of Foot-and-Mouth Disease Contingency Plans, Rome 2002, 1, 7, 25, 27–28, 34–35.

58 Henry Knighton, Leycestrensis chronicon II, ed. Jospeh R. Lumby, London 1965, 412.

of stots was incapable of repairing the draught vacuum. Robert of Reading remarks that rich and poor alike were affected, while the *Chronicon* of Louth Park Abbey reports that the outbreak "ruined the substance" of that religious house and the *Chronicon Monasterii de Melsa* notes that on account of the GEF and panzootic "many villages of England were ruined."[59] The *Gesta Edwardi de Carnarvon* observes that by 1321 "many farmers" throughout England who were once wealthy in livestock "are now forced to beg through the lands," and the *Poem on the Evil Times of Edward II* implies that the mortality resulted in a grain shortage, as does Ireland's *Annals of Innisfallen*.[60] The Prior and Chapter of Canterbury also remarked that his lands were unusually barren and that the aggregate quantity of grain produced on his estates diminished, the bishop at Bangor writes of general impoverishment in the wake of the plague, and the letter from St. James's Hospital speaks of a poverty of resources at Westminster.[61]

Manorial accounts support these observations.[62] As Slavin and Campbell demonstrate, these records reveal that the ability to replenish cattle stocks was significantly curbed, that arable cultivation generally contracted with the loss of the primary draught animal, and that the supply of manure, like the output of milk and the availability of dairy products, declined sharply. Unsurprisingly, the focus in restocking was on draught animals, which many wealthy estates acquired relatively quickly, unlike lesser estates and, presumably, peasants. By and large, restocking was a long process. Manors relied on inter-manorial transfers, the market, natural reproduction, and tenant dues to replace their animals. The accounts show that though some manorial herds, the draught cohorts in particular, were restocked in five years, most were not: the "national" herd did not retain its pre-panzootic level for over thirty years. By 1331, the "national" seigniorial ox herd was 84 per cent of its pre-panzootic level, and by 1341, dairy stocks had only reached 90 per cent of their pre-panzootic level.[63] A mere 9 per cent of manors belonging to wealthier ecclesiastical landlords were able to restock their herds within five years. The lesser cattle mortalities of the mid-1320s, 1330s and 1340s undoubtedly slowed the recovery. Manorial accounts also shine light on the decline in arable. The combined arable acreage of the Winchester estates, for example, was nearly 18,000 acres in 1319 but only 9,000 in 1321.[64] While similar declines are witnessed on manors in other regions of the country, and the aggregate quantity of grain produced did contract,

---

59 Chronicon abbatie de Parco Lude, ed. Edmund Venables, Horncastle 1891, 24, 27; Chronica Monasterii de Melsa, ed. Edward A. Bond, London 1867, 333.

60 Gesta Edwardi de Carnarvon auctore Canonico Bridlingtoniensi, in: Chronicles of the Reigns of Edward I and Edward II, ed. William Stubbs, London 1883, 48.

61 Newfield, Cattle Panzootic (note 13), 161–171.

62 Slavin, Fifth Rider (note 7), 171–181; id., Great Bovine Pestilence (note 7); Campbell, Nature (note 7), 288–90; id., Physical Shocks (note 7), 24–27; id., Panzootics (note 7), 195–196.

63 Slavin, Fifth Rider (note 7), 179.

64 Ibid., 169, 177.

many manors belonging to large ecclesiastical landlords in southern and eastern England were clearly able to maintain their arable acreage on account of the expansion of their horse cohorts.[65] The aggregate quantity of milk produced and the yield of milk from cows remaining in the wake of the plague also fell dramatically. Winchester cows produced over 130 gallons of milk a year in the 1310s and a mere 39 gallons in 1320. Not surprisingly, the price of butter, from 1320, and cheese, from 1321, climbed and remained high until 1323. A general scarcity of milk resources ran into the 1330s.[66]

Recent scholarship has emphasized that medieval farmers and estate managers could effectively manage their operations to absorb natural crises,[67] and the manorial accounts do illustrate a multifaceted attempt to limit losses during and after the plague. In the midst of the mortality, for instance, some manors sold large portions of their herds to minimize losses. Of course, these "panic sales" may have furthered the spread of the disease and could possibly help explain the aforementioned variation in herd mortality. Campbell suggests that a flooding of the market with cattle, together with a fear of buying sick stock, explains the panzootic's apparent failure to generate a significant increase in the price of bovine animals. Indeed, in 1320 available data indicate the price of oxen fell from 14 to 4.5 shillings, and cows from 12 to 6 shillings, and between 1317/1318 and 1321/1322, the price of oxen and cows rose by only 8 and 20 per cent. Thereafter, however, prices climbed dramatically and remained high into the mid-1320s. A small number of manors preemptively culled their bovine stocks, and others yet slaughtered sick animals, again likely to limit financial losses. As some texts observe, and manorial accounts demonstrate, those who owned or could afford horses employed them in traction. While the wealthy ecclesiastical landlords of the south and east were able to expand their working-horse stocks by roughly 40 per cent,[68] others were likely less fortunate. Prices of equines climbed steeply after the outbreak from 13 shillings in 1318/1319 to 16 shillings in 1319/1320 and 17.5 in 1320/1321. Some estates that managed to replenish oxen or purchase horses actually expanded their arable acreage in order to make use of unused pasture. Other manors concentrated on expanding comparatively cheap ovine and swine cohorts.

The panzootic's indirect effects on human health – via dramatic declines in available milk, dairy and grain – need to be assessed in greater detail yet. In the short-term, the crop failures of the GEF, to which the cattle plague undoubtedly contributed, together with declines in milk and dairy, may have lent themselves to heightened excess human

65 Slavin, Great Bovine Pestilence (note 7), 1250, 1255–1257.

66 Slavin, Great Bovine Pestilence (note 7), 1258–1259; Sharon DeWitte/Philip Slavin, Between Famine and Death. Physiological Stress and Dairy Deficiency in England on the Eve of the Black Death (1315–50). New Evidence from Paleoepidemiological and Manorial Accounts, in: Journal of Interdisciplinary History 44 (2013), 51–54.

67 David Stone, Decision Making in Medieval Agriculture, Oxford 2005.

68 Slavin, Great Bovine Pestilence (note 7), 1256.

mortality throughout the famine. The plague may have also had long-term consequences via the extended shortage of dairy. DeWitte and Slavin combined the English manorial evidence for the impact of the 1314–1325 plague on milk production and an assessment of stress markers in 491 human skeletons from north London's East Smithfield Black Death cemetery, and concluded that a generation of the English population, on account of the panzootic, sustained a long-term shortage of calcium, protein and B12, which may have influenced Black Death death rates.[69]

Interestingly, meat, which made up an insignificant part of the diet for the majority of people, would have been available in large quantity in the immediate wake of the panzootic. Several texts imply, or outwardly state, that people, the poor especially, consumed plague cattle. For instance, in 1316 the aforementioned *Anonymi Chronicon Wirceburgense* of the region of modern-day Bavaria observes both "a large pestilence of oxen and cattle" and that "the poor, because of penury and famine, were eagerly consuming the flesh of dead cattle".[70] In 1319, the *Chronicon de Lanercost* of northern England also reports "a pestilence and death of cattle" and that "people ate cattle dying in the aforesaid manner".[71] Trokelowe remarks that birds and dogs that scavenged on cattle carcasses contracted the disease and died, though he borrows this detail verbatim from Matthew of Paris, an earlier chronicler working at St. Albans. Contrary to other texts, but like Dynter, Trokelowe notes that contemporaries avoided cattle that died in the plague. Yet, a wider survey of heterogeneous medieval evidence indicates that people likely did consume diseased stock in the wake of epizootics.[72]

The available evidence permits a speculative diagnosis. While revisionists among modern medical historians are right to point out that a disease is at once a biological and socio-cultural entity, that the manifestation and perception of disease are unstable, and that the language and foundations of pre-laboratory medicine and laboratory medicine are incommensurable,[73] we need not abandon all attempts to affix modern labels to ancient, medieval and early modern disease.[74] Diagnoses are not without purpose, even if appropriately identified as speculative, and some disease occurrences are more suitable for diagnosis than others. Well-documented animal plagues for which we have

---

69 Sharon DeWitte/Philip Slavin, Between Famine and Death. England on the Eve of the Black Death – Evidence from Paleoepidemiology and Manorial Accounts, in: Journal of Interdisciplinary History 44/1 (2013), 37–60, 49, 51, 56–57.

70 Anonymi Chronicon Wirceburgense (note 36), 821.

71 Chronicon de Lanercost, 240.

72 Timothy P. Newfield, Epizootics and the Consumption of Diseased Meat in the Middle Ages, in: Francesco Ammannati (ed.), Religione e istituzioni religiose nell'economia Europea, 1000–1800. Proceedings of the 43rd Study Week of the Fondazione Istituto Internazionale di Storia Economica "F. Datini", Florence 2012, 619–639.

73 Arrizabalaga, Retrospective Diagnosis (note 6).

74 Piers D. Mitchell, Retrospective Diagnosis and the Use of Historical Texts for Investigating Disease in the Past, in: International Journal of Paleopathology 1 (2011), 81–88.

knowledge of both symptoms and epizootiology, and are able to deduce properties of the latter indirectly from the sources (and thus independently from the language of the texts), generally furnish a good opportunity for a tentative diagnosis. Although descriptions of the symptoms of medieval epizootics are often few and the most persuasive diagnoses are founded upon consideration of symptoms and epizootiology,[75] a predominant focus on epizootiology is not necessarily a bad thing. It forces one to circumvent some of the problems opponents of retrospective diagnosing have identified concerning the textuality and perception of disease. Naturally, paleogenomic support of a diagnosis would be most welcome. To date, however, we have no paleogenomes for known plague-causing pathogens that afflict livestock, like RPV, FMD and CBPP.

Very little is known about the symptoms of the 1314–1325 panzootic. There is only one indication in a text from southwestern England that cattle may have experienced some intestinal or bowel related stress.[76] Much more is known about the plague's epizootiology and an assessment of the known epizootiological properties points to RPV or CBPP. The early fourteenth-century plague afflicted, of domesticated species, cattle alone, it was not at least as far as we can tell zoonotic,[77] it exhibited a mortality rate in individual animals of upwards of 100 per cent, it killed quickly, was not purely or very opportunistic, and it was, considering its rapid spread across a large span of Europe and that it claimed, on average, 63 per cent of affected herds, quite communicable and capable of achieving high morbidity. The wide breadth of the die-off, the ease with which the disease spread among herds, and the pathogen's lack of any strong seasonality and seeming indifference to severe and abrupt changes in environmental and weather conditions, emphasizes that the disease was transmitted between like species and indicates strongly that it was neither primarily soil- nor arthropod-borne.[78] Of course, the pathogen may have been disseminated on the backs of other domesticates and in wild animal populations as well, and possibly via trade in goods, not to mention human traffic.

These characteristics imply strongly that the disease could not have been anthrax, bluetongue, bovine viral diarrhea, bovine tuberculosis, brucellosis, east coast fever,

---

75 Samuel K. Cohn Jr., The Black Death Transformed. Disease and Culture in Early Renaissance Europe, London 2002, 3, 58.

76 Newfield, Cattle Panzootic (note 13), 165, 181.

77 In 1319, the abbot at Ramsey wrote that a human epidemic was expected on account of the stench of cattle carcasses infecting the air, but there is no indication that the disease was zoonotic. See J. Ambrose Raftis, Estates of Ramsey Abbey. A Study in Economic Growth and Organization, Toronto 1957, 319 (appendix G). Belief in miasma may account for the abbot's reasoning, so too the remarks of Paris, Trokelowe and Dynter. Human deaths reported in tandem with cattle deaths in some continental sources, such as the *Annales Bohemiae Brevissimi*, can be easily understood as the result of the famine or famine epidemics.

78 Timothy P. Newfield, Early Medieval Epizootics and Landscapes of Disease. The Origins and Triggers of European Livestock Pestilences, 400–1000 CE, in: Sunhild Kleingärtner et al. (eds.), Landscapes and Societies in Medieval Europe East of the Elbe. Interactions between Environmental Settings and Cultural Transformations, Toronto 2013, 91–92.

foot-and-mouth disease, haemorrhagic septicaemia, or malignant catarrhal fever, as they are known to modern science.[79] That RPV is more virulent and communicable than CBPP[80] signifies that, of the two, it irrupted in central Europe c.1314.[81]

Kershaw first imposed a rinderpest diagnosis on the c.1319–1320 English mortalities,[82] drawing upon Trow-Smith's discussion of eighteenth- and nineteenth-century panzootics to do so.[83] While Kershaw's knowledge of the fourteenth-century panzootic and the virus was somewhat rudimentary and Trow-Smith wrongly thought RPV ancient, long unchanged, and "endemic" in Britain "from very early times until its eradication in 1877," rinderpest was then and still is the best bet for the 1314–1325 plague. Yet, a RPV diagnosis of this plague, of course, is far from definite. To identify the panzootic as rinderpest, on the basis of a comparison between the epizootiology of the fourteenth-century plague with modern scientific knowledge of RPV, is to suggest that a strain of a highly mutable morbillivirus has remained more-or-less unchanged for several centuries and that the virus existed and behaved in domestic European bovines in the early 1300s as it is known to have in the nineteenth and twentieth centuries. It is also to assume that the panzootic was caused by a pathogen, or strain of, that is known to modern science. While multiple epizootiological similarities can be drawn between the fourteenth-century panzootic and eighteenth-century panzootics, this does not in itself confirm a rinderpest diagnosis, as the RPV diagnoses of eighteenth-century cattle plagues, though regularly encountered in the historical and scientific literature, are themselves not definite.[84] Palaeogenomic support for the common RPV diagnosis of all of these plagues is wanting, and until eighteenth- and fourteenth-century cattle panzootics are shown definitely to have had a common cause, the later should not be employed to help explain the earlier. Yet, even if paleogenomic diagnoses are established for these panzootics, one might question how much knowledge we should draw from the panzootics of the 1700s for our histories of the panzootic of the 1300s. Certainly, 400-years' worth of changes in animal population density, distribution, health and husbandry, not to mention landscape and trade, would have ensured the outbreaks differed. This parallels the argument that one should not heavily draw upon the Black

79 For these and other diseases discussed below see the Organisation Mondiale de la Santé Animale's Technical Disease Cards: http://www.oie.int/en/animal-health-in-the-world/technical-disease-cards/ (last visited in February 2023).

80 Obi et al., Manual (note 57), 5; Food and Agricultural Organization, Recognizing Contagious (note 57), 3, 6; Geering/Amanfu, Preparation (note 57), 6; Koolmees, Epizootic Diseases (note 56), 22, 27.

81 Newfield, Cattle Panzootic (note 13), 158–159, 188–189.

82 Kershaw, Great Famine (note 7), 24.

83 Robert Trow-Smith, A History of British Livestock Husbandry to 1700, London 1957, 240, n. 6; id., A History of British Livestock Husbandry 1700–1900, London 1959, 34–35.

84 Hünniger, Policing Epizootics (note 2), 76–77.

Death to articulate the history of the Justinianic Plague, even though both have been proven, on paleogenomic grounds, to have been *Yersinia pestis*.

As noted, there is yet no paleogenomic evidence for the rinderpest virus. Following the push to eradicate RPV stocks, there are now comparatively many modern genomes from twentieth-century samples, but being a highly fragile RNA virus, it is unlikely any paleogenomes will be reconstructed soon from archaeological remains. Several independent molecular clock studies are, however, in hand. These have to some degree illuminated the evolutionary history of rinderpest and known closely related morbilliviruses, notably measles, canine distemper and peste des petits ruminants. As molecular clocks convert genetic distance between (time-stamped modern) samples to establish rates of genetic substitution or mutation, they can thereby identify, albeit only very roughly, when lineages of these viruses and the viruses themselves diverged.

Most multiple clock studies available directly relevant to RPV's evolutionary history have focused not specifically on rinderpest, but on measles (molecular clock analyses have yet to be directed at the relative flood of recent RPV sequence data). While the estimated emergence date of rinderpest has differed between these studies, all agree on a few points. Importantly, the most robust of the analyses agree that rinderpest, as we would recognize it, had emerged by the time of the fourteenth-century panzootic. Yet, not one molecular clock study supports the common twentieth-century speculation that RPV emerged in domestic cattle multiple millennia before the Common Era. Two papers now more than a decade old, position rinderpest's emergence as early as 800–1100 CE. A more recent paper, utilizing more sequence data, notably a measles paleogenome (not a very old one – it is early twentieth century in date), has, however, argued that RPV and measles may have gone their respective ways as many as 1,700 years earlier. This analysis, the firmest to date, now suggests RPV could have emerged as early as (but possibly long after) the sixth century BCE. While this date will not hold (molecular clock dates never do, as more data is drawn upon, techniques for estimating divergence dates improve, and, particularly, as paleogenomes [even modern ones] are introduced; there is also the issue that morbillivirus diversity centuries and millennia ago remains undescribed, complicating efforts to establish definitively RPV's evolution), there is good reason to believe that rinderpest, as it is known to modern science, had come to exist sometime before the 1300s CE.

The geography of rinderpest's emergence is less certain, though for centuries interested commentators, mostly Europeans, have speculated rinderpest established enzootic foci initially around the Caspian Basin, in southern Russia and on the Steppes. This thinking, it should be stressed, however, is heavily influenced by the perceptible trajectory of the infamous eighteenth-century European panzootics, putatively rinderpest, which seem to have broken out repeatedly from a region east of Europe. That the alleged ancestral origins of the virus are thought to lie east of Europe corresponds well with the suggested origins of the fourteenth-century panzootic, but that is hardly proof of the association. Where and when the pathogen spread, and in what species it established reservoirs historically, are enigmatic.[85]

Naturally, without a definite diagnosis, what is known of the fourteenth-century panzootic, or of other supposed medieval RPV outbreaks, should not be incorporated into our modern scientific understanding of RPV. As odd as this may seem, it is crucial to recognize that many premodern cattle plagues, from late antiquity forward, have been integrated into the modern sciences of RPV, used as framing in diverse genetic, veterinary, virological and policy studies, and drawn upon to support claims that the virus is ancient, that it originated on the Steppes of Central Asia, long irrupted into Europe from enzootic regions lying east of Europe, and was for many centuries before eradication highly communicable and virulent. The fourteenth-century panzootic could be employed to support all these positions, but putting it to use for that purpose now is not recommended.[86]

Speculative diagnoses may be of limited use, but they are not completely without purpose. Economic, political and social historians of premodern Europe have long treated retrospective diagnosing as a straightforward, simple task meant only to enhance our total understanding of the past (consider Kershaw's RPV diagnosis of the fourteenth-century cattle plague and reference to liver fluke in the context of the ovine mortalities of the GEF[87]), while medical historians have increasingly in recent years demonstrated the complexity of diagnosing on the basis of written evidence alone with some arguing strongly against its practice. A middle ground seems reasonable. A tentative (rather than firm) identification of a premodern plague, made with close consideration of the symptoms and epidemiology/epizootiology of both the historical disease evident in extant sources and diseases known to modern science, can be instructive. Such speculation can provide direction for those working in the palaeogenomic and, if the disease produces skeletal stigmata, palaeopathological sciences. At the same time, one must acknowledge that such "linear" disease histories cannot reveal the whole story.

Palaeoscientific identifications of the disease, in turn, could go a long way towards establishing a definite diagnosis. With the early fourteenth-century panzootic identified in time and space, and its impact examined as far as the extant evidence permits, a firmer diagnosis could, potentially, corroborate aspects of the plague and its impact known from the historical sources as well as highlight unknowns. If the 1314–1325 panzootic was RPV, one could speak with greater confidence about the plague's modes of transmission, morbidity and mortality, plausible duration, ability to establish enzootic foci in Europe, relation to the extreme weather of 1315–1317, the climatic anomaly of the early fourteenth century and the nutritional standing of cattle, and whether the

85 Spinage, Cattle Plague (note 2), 43–55.

86 For instance, Gordon R. Scott/Alain Provost, Global Eradication of Rinderpest, Rome 1992, 1, 33; Thomas Barrett, Vaccination Spells the End for A Devastating Plague, in: Microbiology Today 34 (2007), 20.

87 Kershaw, Great Famine (note 7), 20, 24.

disease conferred immunity to survivors, affected other domesticated or wild species (and thus cut into other sources of food). One could also speak to the state of cattle post mortem, how severely, for instance, hides and flesh would have been damaged, and whether the pathogen may have been spread via trade in animal byproducts.

Yet, as stressed, with only written sources, diagnoses are exceptionally difficult to establish, as the decades of pre-paleogenomic debate over the identity of the Black Death lays bare.[88] It appears that multiple palaeoscientific assessments of cattle remains dating to the period of the panzootic from across the affected area are needed and, in lieu of paleogenomic detection, that the results of these assessments must be independently verified. Of course, identifying remains of animals that died in the panzootic may itself be a difficult task: faunal remains can often only be dated to within 50 to 100 years, and while many animals may have been buried en mass in pits,[89] which may be unearthed and cautiously dated with a higher resolution following the consultation of the written record for epizootics, many others may have been burned or abandoned in fields for scavenging wildlife,[90] and others yet slaughtered for their hides, meat, sinew, etc. Despite their diseased state, and religious restrictions on the consumption of carrion, the flesh and hides of thousands upon thousands of bovines may have been harvested. Consider that after the 1314–1325 panzootic hit England's southwest, the Earl of Cornwall's havener's accounts document the export of 280 dickers in 1322/1323, by a considerable margin the most exported any year between 1289/1290 and 1350/1351.[91] That the outward flow of hides also increased noticeably c. 1286, when disease plagued cattle in England's southwest as well,[92] strengthens the possible connection between high dicker exports and abnormal cattle deaths c. 1320. Back to the skeletal evidence, linking documented epizootics to animal remains via radiocarbon dating may prove quite complicated or even impossible as often multiple animal plagues occurred within spans of 50 and 100 years in the Middle Ages.[93]

Attention in the palaeopathological sciences to the nutritional and pathological condition of cattle in the early fourteenth century in general, and those affected in the panzootic in particular, might, however, inform us of the disease's relation to underlying health and illness. Although not opportunistic, the infection may have exacted a heavier

88 Graham Twigg, The Black Death and DNA, in: Lancet Infectious Diseases 3 (2003), 11; Vivian Nutton (ed.), Pestilential Complexities. Understanding Medieval Plague, London 2008; Lester K. Little, Plague Historians in Lab Coats, in: Past and Present 213 (2011), 267–290.

89 Newfield, Cattle Panzootic (note 13), 166.

90 Jordan, Great Famine (note 12), 37; Newfield, Epizootics (note 78), 623, 627.

91 The Havener's Accounts of the Earldom and Duchy of Cornwall, 1287–1356, ed. Maryanne Kowaleski, Exeter 2001, 36, 69. No data survives for 1318/19–1321/22.

92 Kaoru Ugawa, The Economic Development of Some Devon Manors in the Thirteenth Century, in: Transactions of the Devonshire Association 94 (1962), 647, 675; Kershaw, Great Famine (note 7), 28; Slavin, Great Bovine Pestilence (note 7), 1249.

93 Newfield, Epizootics (note 78), 629–633; Kershaw, Great Famine (note 7), 28.

toll in the particularly malnourished and chronically ill. Skeletal evidence from London for an early fourteenth-century increase in mean cattle size has been tentatively tied to a possible higher rate of survival for larger, healthier bovines during the famine and plague.[94] Of course, evidence of diseased but butchered bones would be enlightening, and there may be physical evidence for a later average age of slaughter (the noted growth of London bovines might also reflect the delayed slaughtering of breeding animals post panzootic), not to mention skeletal indications of the unusually heavy exploitation of remaining cattle in traction post panzootic (bulls, cows, immatures and oxen). When there were fewer bovines, more animals were plausibly reared into adulthood, and a higher percentage of existing animals would have been employed in draught. The early fourteenth-century mortality might have something to do with the slight increase in the slaughter age and the dramatic increase in the pathological frequency in the lower limbs of cattle from the early and mid-fourteenth-century West Midlands identified by Thomas.[95]

Several historians have commented upon the unusual and unprecedented scale of the spread of cattle disease between 1314 and 1325.[96] This panzootic was not the only great animal plague of the Middle Ages, however. More evidence exists for it than for any other ancient or medieval epizootic, but it was not necessarily unparalleled in extent or mortality.

3. England, Wales, Ireland and the *Scitta*, 986–988

Disease appears to have devastated English, Irish and Welsh cattle in the mid-980s. Appears is the key word, though, as the significance of this plague is rather obscure. Our knowledge of its spatial and temporal extent, origins and impact pales in comparison to that of the plagues of 1314–1325 and (even) 809–810 as there are at best only seven independent and contemporary, or near contemporary, references to the mortality, all but one of which are brief. In 986, the *Anglo-Saxon Chronicle* (*ASC*), reports that "the great cattle plague [*yrfcwealm*] first came to England",[97] and in 986 or 987 the three principal versions of the Welsh *Brut y Tywysogion* observe an animal mortality, each with minor differences: the Peniarth MS 20 records that "a mortality took place upon

94 Richard Thomas et al, "So bigge as bigge may be." Tracking Size and Shape in Domestic Livestock in London (AD 1220–1900), in: Journal of Archaeological Science 40 (2013), 3309–3325, 3309, 3319.

95 Richard Thomas, Diachronic Trends in Lower Limb Pathologies in Late Medieval and Post-Medieval Cattle from Britain, in: Documenta Archaeobiologiae 6 (2008), 187–201, 187, 190, 193, 196–99.

96 In England see Kershaw, Great Famine (note 7), 28–29; Richard Britnell, Britain and Ireland, 1050–1530. Economy and Society, Oxford 2004, 492; across Europe see Jordan, Great Famine (note 12), 39.

97 The Anglo-Saxon Chronicle (C), Annals 978–1017, in: English and Norse Documents Relating to the Reign of Ethelred the Unready, trans. Margaret Ashdown, Cambridge 1930, 40-41.

the cattle in all the island of Britain," the Red Book of Hergest that there was "a mortality upon the animals in all the island of Britain," and the *Brenhinedd y Saesson* that there was "a mortality upon the animals in all Wales."[98] The most thorough account of the plague is found in the English *Chronicon ex Chronicis* (*CC*). In 987, it documents that

> two plagues unknown to English people in past generations, namely a fever of humans and a plague of animals, which in English is called "shit" (*scitta*) but in Latin can be called the "flux of the bowels," have thoroughly afflicted all England, and raged indescribably in all parts of England, affecting men with a great destruction and widely consuming the animals.[99]

The *Annals of Tigernach* (*AT*), *Annals of Ulster* (*AU*) and *Chronicon Scotorum* (*CS*) of Ireland record the presence of an animal plague there in 987. Following notice of a human mortality caused by "a colic", the first observes "the beginning of a great murrain, to wit, the unknown *máelgarb*, came for the first time" and the third, clearly related to the first, reports "a sickness (…) in the east of Ireland which caused death among the people" and "the beginning of the cattle-plague, the *máelgarb*, such as had not occurred before," while the second observes "a sudden great mortality which caused a slaughter of people and cattle in England, Wales and Ireland."[100]

The Irish poem *Saltair na Rann* documents the plague as well. The poet, or an interpolator, uses the cattle deaths to identify his time of writing as 988: "from Adam of the bright signing orders" to "the great slaughter of cattle" and "from the birth of Christ (…)" until "the hundred-fold destruction of the cattle".[101] The *Saltair* also includes a list of insular and continental rulers reigning during the plague. As far as we can tell, only the Irish, Welsh and Scottish of these kings were in power when the plague possibly transversed their realms (the list includes Lothar of France, who died in March 986, and the Holy Roman Emperor Otto II, who passed in December 983). That Scotland's Cináed mac Maíl Choluim is at the head of the *Saltair's* regal list suggests bovines in his realm may have been affected. As another cattle epizootic is not encountered in

98 Brut y Tywysogyon, or Chronicle of Princes. Peniarth MS. 20 Version, ed. Thomas Jones, Cardiff 1952, 10; Brut y Tywysogyon, Red Book of Hergest Version, trans. Thomas Jones, Cardiff 1955, 17; Brenhinedd y Saesson or, The King of the Saxons. BM Cotton MS Cleopatra B v., trans. Thomas Jones, Cardiff 1971, 45.

99 Chronicon ex Chronicis, trans. Jennifer Bray/P. McGurk, Chronicle of John of Worcester II, Oxford 1995, 436–437.

100 These texts were consulted on The Corpus of Electronic Texts (CELT): http://celt.ucc.ie/publishd.html (accessed 14 and 15 March 2018). The paper version of the CS (ed. William M. Hennessy, London 1866, 231) dates the plague to 985, a date corrected to 986 on CELT. The AU passage presented here is from Hennessy's translation (Annala Uladh, Annals of Ulster I, trans. William M. Hennessy, Dublin 1887, 497), which is preferable to Mac Airt's translation found on CELT, though Hennessy dates the passage one year in arrear. Dan McCarthy assures me that the date of 987 is correct (pers. corresp. 22 July 2011).

101 Saltair na Rann, ed. Whitley Stokes, Oxford 1883, I.XII, 2337–2372.

English or Welsh sources until the 1040s,[102] it is also possible Wulfstan II, archbishop of York and bishop of Worcester, refers to this late tenth-century cattle plague in homilies penned c.1014 when writing vaguely of a recent "plague and mortality, cattle plague and disease" and of a "cattle plague or human plague through sudden diseases".[103]

This plague of the 980s crops up in catalogues of livestock disease,[104] but it has been overlooked in the humanities and modern sciences.[105] Not surprisingly, considering the known body of evidence, few aspects of the plague's history are certain. It is quite likely that these texts do refer to one and the same mortality and, considering the lack of evidence for extreme weather or a subsistence crisis, that the mortality was the result of disease, as the *ASC*, *AT*, *AU*, *CC*, *CS* and *SR* specify. It also seems, given the dating of the animal mortalities in the sources, that the disease appeared first, in northwestern insular Europe, in England in 986, and then spread westward to Wales in 986 or 987,[106] and Ireland in 987. The marking of the disease in the *ASC* as having "come to England" also suggests, as does the plague's apparent westward trajectory in England, Wales and Ireland, and alleged, or implied, wide prevalence and high mortality, that the disease was not enzootic in northwestern insular Europe but brought to England from the continent, as was the 1314–1325 panzootic. Reference in the *AT*, *CS* and *SR* to the great scale of the losses in Ireland, the dating of the plague in Irish texts to 987 and 988, and

102 The Anglo-Saxon Chronicle, trans. G. N. Garmonsway, London 1975, 163, 167.

103 Wulfstan II, Sermo Lupi ad Anglos, ed. Dorothy Whitelock, London 1952, 39–40; Wulfstan II, Be mistlican gelimpan, in: Wulfstan, Sammlung der ihm zugeschriebenen Homilien nebst Untersuchungen über ihre Echtheit, ed. Arthur Napier, Berlin 1883, XXXV, 170.

104 Short, General Chronological History (note 3), vol. I, 91; vol. II, 208; Fleming, Animal Plagues (note 3), 54, 57–58; Dieckerhoff, Geschichte der Rinderpest (note 3), 27; Spinage, Cattle Plague (note 2), 90. Short dates the plague to 987. Fleming's chronology of it is partially incorrect and he treats the 986 and 987 mortalities as separate events. Believing that the plague was zoonotic, Spinage proposes that the disease was anthrax. Spinage also implies that the CC account was initially written by Florence of Worcester and mistakenly assumes, consequently, that it is non-contemporary. Relying on a seventeenth-century summary of the CC passage, he also assigns the "flux of the bowls" reported in the CC to both humans and cattle. Dieckerhoff dates the plague to 987 and 988, limits its spread to England (but stresses that all of that country was afflicted), and separates the mortalities of humans from those of cattle. Focusing primarily on France, Paulet, Recherches historiques (note 3), 73–82, neglects this plague in his list of early medieval epizootiques.

105 There is passing mention in Fergus Kelly, Early Irish Farming. A Study Based Mainly on the Law-Texts of the 7th and 8th Centuries AD, Dublin 1997, 195–96; Benjamin T. Hudson, Vikings Pirates and Christian Princes. Dynasty, Religion, and Empire in the North Atlantic, Oxford 2005, 62, 69. Brief treatment is found in Timothy P. Newfield, Human-Bovine Plagues in the Early Middle Ages, in: Journal of Interdisciplinary History 46 (2015), 10–14.

106 The plague is dated in the "Peniarth MS. 20" to 986 (no dates are given in the Red Book or Brenhinedd y Saesson versions) but the editor of these texts proposes, based on a comparison of some passages in Peniarth, the AU and CS, that the dates given in the Peniarth from 974 to 1003 are a year in arrear. That the ASC reports an animal mortality in 986 may force us to reconsider the bumping of the plague in Wales from 986 to 987.

the implication in the *AU* that the disease appeared in England and Wales before Ireland, denote the disease did not originate in Ireland. The labeling of the disease as unknown in the *ASC*, *CC*, *AT* and *CS* also signals that it was not enzootic to northwestern insular Europe, but a continental import, though many plagues were tagged as "new" in the Middle Ages and these remarks may be tropes.

No continental evidence for an outbreak of livestock disease is known in the late tenth century prior to 986. The last significant plague occurred in the late 930s and early 940s.[107] The only known late tenth-century continental observations of epizootics are found in 989, 990, 993, 994 and 996 in the German *Annales Quedlinburgenses* (*AQ*), a text compiled at Quedlinburg Abbey in the early eleventh century from earlier sources, and the *Annales Hildesheimenses* (*AH*), drafted at Hildesheim in the eleventh century, also from earlier sources. In 989, the *AQ* reports "a great pestilence in humans and draught animals, especially oxen",[108] and in 994 a continuation of that text documents "a great pestilence of humans, pigs, oxen and sheep",[109] and in 996 "a common loss of pigs and oxen in pestilence distresses all Germany".[110] In 990, the *AH* records "no small mortality of humans and draught animals"[111] and in 993 "a great plague and mortality equally of humans and draught animals".[112] Whether these mortalities were connected to those recorded earlier in England, Wales and Ireland is unknown. An *argumentum ex silentio* is to be avoided, but if the disease were foreign to northwestern insular Europe it would have affected parts of northern continental Europe before spreading to England.[113] Continental sources are renownedly thin following the Carolingian period (esp. 950–1000 CE). Yet had a large continental die-off occurred in the early 980s it might be suspected that the deaths would have been reported in the *AQ* or *AH*. The evidence is too slight to assert that a large pan-European outbreak of cattle disease took place in the late tenth century, as in the early fourteenth, but further consideration of what the insular references tell us about the epizootiology of the epizootic does lend itself to the idea that a large number of animals fell on the continent in the 980s.

The *ASC* entry is encountered in the Abingdon II, Worcester and Laud/Peterborough *ASC* manuscripts. The latter two are likely derived from the former, the Abingdon II, which appears to provide a contemporary witness. Almost certainly based on the Abingdon I manuscript, the Abingdon II was likely composed at Abingdon in the 1040s. The Abingdon I ends in 977, at which point the Abingdon II seems to include matter

107 Timothy P. Newfield, Domesticates, Disease and Climate in Early Post-Classical Europe. The Cattle Plague of c. 940 and its Environmental Context, in: Post-Classical Archaeologies 5 (2015), 108–117.

108 Annales Quedlinburgenses, ed. Georg Heinrich Pertz (MGH, Scriptores 3), Hanover 1839, 68.

109 Ibid., 72.

110 Ibid., 73.

111 Ibid., 68.

112 Ibid., 70.

113 Newfield, Early Medieval Epizootics, 90–91, 94–97.

from non-extant local Abingdon-area annals. Compiled in part by John of Worcester, and possibly Florence of Worcester, in the late eleventh and first half of the twelfth centuries, the pre twelfth-century portions of the *CC* are largely based on the *Chronicon* of Marianus Scotus, an Irish monk who lived and wrote in Germany in the third quarter of the eleventh century, in addition to a variety of English annals, histories and *vitae*. Although the root sources for many of the English passages in the *CC* are identifiable, the origins of the 987 passage is unknown and the original source seemingly lost. Marianus Scottus says nothing of a late tenth-century animal mortality in his *Chronicon*.[114] The *CC* entry may have come from a set of annals local to Worcester, where the text was likely compiled. It is clearly distinct from the *ASC* entry and its 987 dating may indicate, assuming that it and the *ASC* entry are dated correctly, that the *CC* passage was not composed as animals were dying, but shortly thereafter, or that the plague persisted in England into 987. That the exiling from England of Aelfric of Mercia is reported in 985 in the *ASC* and 986 in the *CC*, however, suggests that the *CC*'s 987 entry is a year in arrear.

The three principal versions of the *Brut* are independent Welsh translations of a non-extant Latin text commonly referred to as the *Cronica/Historia Principium Britanniae/Wallie*, which appears to have been compiled in the late thirteenth century (no earlier than 1286) at Strata Florida and is a conflation of multiple sets of local Welsh annals, notably the lost *Annals of Strata Florida*, which until c.1100 seems to have relied primarily on a text from St. David's. Of the three versions of the *Brut*, the "Peniarth MS 20" is thought to provide the more complete, reliable and literal translation of the *Cronica*. The entries in the *AT* and *CS* plainly derive from a common source, what is often referred to as the *Annals of Clonmacnoise* or the Clonmacnoise-group text, likely composed in Clonard or Clonmancoise. It is also plausible that the *AU* entry is related to that of the *AT* and *CS*, as the *AU* shares many items with the Clonmacnoise text in the tenth and eleventh centuries. That said, the obvious differences between the *AT/CS* and *AU* entries suggests that the latter entry may not be shared and, consequently, that the *AU* represents an independent source for the plague composed in the north of Ireland, possibly at Armagh. Still, Evans warns that annalists having received "written notices of events would often partially or wholly transform the accounts into their own annalistic style, which can obscure the origins of the item,"[115] and McCarthy suggests, following an analysis of the textual elements and vocabulary of the *AU*, *AT* and *CS* entries, that the *AU* may here be a reinterpretation of the separate accounts of cattle and human disease found in the Clonmacnoise text by Ruaidhrí Ua Caiside, the principal interpolator of

114 Marianus Scottus, Chronicon, ed. G. Waitz (MGH, Scriptores 5), Hanover 1844, 554–555.

115 Nicholas Evans, The Present and the Past in Medieval Irish Chronicles, Woodbridge 2010, 91–114, 244–45.

the *AU*, in the early 1500s.[116] All or part of the relevant passage in the *SR* was possibly written at Rosscarbery in southwestern Ireland.[117]

Several of the insular references to the plague were clearly composed some distance apart. From this we may make the important inference, presuming that animals died not far from where the texts were composed or that the manuscripts did not circulate widely in the plague years, that the outbreak was indeed rather general in northwestern insular Europe, as the *AU*, *Brut* and *CC* assert, and the *ASC*, *AT*, *CS* and *SR* suggest. Wulfstan's very inclusion of a cattle plague in his homilies suggests that the plague he refers to, possibly that of 986–988, was not a trifling matter. Of course, that possibly seven independent and contemporary, or near contemporary, texts emphasize the great scale of the 986–988 mortality at the very least signals that many animals did die across much of England, Ireland and Wales. The manorial evidence for the fourteenth-century panzootic indicates that reports of large animal mortalities encountered in medieval annals, chronicles and histories should not be hastily discounted as exaggerated or as simply conforming to literary conventions. Yet establishing some idea of the breadth of the outbreak within Britain, independently from the contents of the known references, lends support to contemporary claims about a spatially vast mortality. Attention to the place of composition of the known references also indicates that the disease spread relatively quickly, lending support to the *AU's* qualifying of it as "sudden". It is possible that cattle herds in south-central England, the West Midlands, southwestern Wales, and central and northeastern Ireland were afflicted in about a year. Such a rapid dissemination of disease across a fairly large span of northwestern insular Europe strongly suggests that the pathogen was not principally arthropod- or soil-borne, but transmissible between susceptible species. With this in mind, and the likelihood that the disease was virulent and foreign to northwestern insular Europe, it may be suspected that a significant number of animals did die on the continent in the early- or mid-980s. Why the plague initially irrupted in England or on the continent is unclear and will require further consideration of the economic, environmental and political context in which the plague occurred. Although not impossible, there is no evidence to support the proposal that Danes brought the disease to England, as Spinage suggested.[118] The outbreak does not appear to correspond spatially or temporally to a subsistence crisis, climatic anomaly or a major conflict. Equally uncertain is the outbreak's duration. The dating of the *CC* passage, if correct, suggests that the plague persisted for a year or more in some regions, though the report of a cattle mortality in the *AU* in 993 may indicate that the disease persisted for several years in Ireland as did the 1314–1325 panzootic.[119]

116 McCarthy personal correspondence 18 July 2011.

117 Gearóid Mac Eoin, The Date and Authorship of Saltair na Rann, in: Zeitschrift für celtische Philologie 28 (1960/61), 51–67.

118 Spinage, Cattle Plague (note 2), 90.

119 Annals of Ulster, trans. Hennessey (note 100), 501.

However, that humans and bees are also said to have died in 993 in the *AU* suggests that the deaths of bovines then may have been the result of extreme weather and a subsistence crisis, perhaps the same crisis reported in the *Brut* in 993/994.[120]

We can press further. It seems, despite the ambiguity of some of the texts, that the disease, like that of the early fourteenth century, primarily afflicted cattle, of domesticates, as the *ASC*, *AU*, *CS*, the most reliable version of the *Brut*, and possibly Wulfstan suggest. The *yrfcwealm* and *orfcwealm* encountered respectively in the *Anglo-Saxon Chronicle* and Wulfstan II's homilies should be read as "cattle plague".[121] However, without records like the aforementioned manorial accounts, it is impossible to be certain that other animals were not also affected. Sudden and dramatic deaths of cattle may have been more noteworthy than mortalities of other domesticates, let alone wild animals on account of their important role as suppliers of traction, fertilizer, food and other consumables. It is perhaps on account of their significance for human economy and health that most species-specific references to livestock plagues encountered in medieval annals, chronicles and histories concern cattle. For example, roughly 90 per cent of the animal mortalities reported in Irish annals between 750 and 1350, most of which were clearly the result of disease, are said to have affected cattle.[122] This in itself, however, is neither an indication that plagues of other domesticates occurred less regularly or were less spatially and temporally extensive, nor that multiple species were not affected in what appear in the annals as cattle plagues. Yet references to deaths of multiple species in the *AQ* need not affect our analysis of the insular accounts of cattle mortalities in 986–988, as the association of the mortalities reported in the *AQ* with those reported in England, Wales and Ireland is imprecise. Moreover, the *AQ* annalist may have connected unrelated deaths of different animals to a single cause and very few infectious diseases, at least of those known to modern science, cause high mortality in multiple domesticated species. Anthrax may affect multiple species, but outbreaks of it are generally quite localized, as the soil-borne pathogen does not spread geographically like the 986–988 plague seems to have.[123] Further, the mortalities of humans, pigs and sheep observed in the *AQ* may have been tied to the extreme weather and subsistence crises documented in a number of continental texts in the late 980s (post 986) and 990s.[124]

120 Peniarth MS. 20, ed. Jones (note 98), 10; Red Book, ed. Jones (note 98), 19.

121 Jane Roberts et al, A Thesaurus of Old English, vol. I: Introduction and Thesaurus, Amsterdam 2000, 217; Thomas A. Bredehoft, History and Memory in the Anglo-Saxon Chronicle, in: David Johnson/Elaine Treharne (eds.), Readings in Medieval Texts. Interpreting Old and Middle English Literature, Oxford 2005, 114.

122 Newfield, Epizootics (note 72), 630–631.

123 See Spinage, Cattle Plague (note 2), 85.

124 Annales Quedlinburgenses, ed. Pertz (note 108), 67–68, 72; Annales Hildesheimenses, ed. Pertz (note 111), 67–68; Lamberti Annales, ed. Georg Heinrich Pertz (MGH, Scriptores 3), Hanover 1839, 67–68; Annales Augustani, ed. Georg Heinrich Pertz (MGH, Scriptores 3), Hanover 1839, 124; Thietmar

It is possible that this *scitta* was zoonotic. The *ASC*, *Brut* and *SR* refer not to human deaths, but the *CC*, *AT*, *CS*, *AU* and Wulfstan do. The omission of epidemic mortalities in some accounts of the plague may be interpreted as an indication that the pathogen was less prevalent or less lethal in human populations. It is possible that unrelated human and bovine deaths were conflated, but that the spread of disease among people is reported as contemporary to, and in association with, the spread of disease among cows in multiple independent sources suggests otherwise. Moreover, in this case the human deaths, unlike those reported in a small portion of the passages concerning the 1314–1325 panzootic, cannot be ascribed to famine. It is also not impossible that the best candidate for the *scitta* was zoonotic in the tenth century, as discussed below.

Nothing concrete can be said about the impact of this late tenth-century plague. The only known reference to the outbreak's repercussions is found in another version of the *Brut*, likely not derived from the lost *Cronica* and quite possibly non-contemporary. The text observes "a great mortality among the cattle in all Wales; from which ensued a great price upon articles made from milk".[125] Regardless of this passage's provenance, we can assume that the availability of dairy products would have declined and the value of butter, cheese and milk inflated, as in the early fourteenth century. It is also possible to suppose, considering the place of cattle in tenth-century agriculture and the known aftermath of the 1314–1325 panzootic, that the quantity of land brought under the plow contracted, at least slightly, and the aggregate quantity of grain reaped fell, perhaps dramatically, in the short term. Still, it is far from certain that the mortality had something to do with the food shortages reported in the *Brut* in 988/989 and 993/994,[126] particularly considering that there is no evidence for shortage in other regions affected by the cattle plague – though not every region would have been equally vulnerable. If restocking was a major burden, as it was in the early 1300s, the plague may have made contemporaries more susceptible to subsistence crisis, even several years post-plague in the mid-990s, in that it diminished their capacity to produce grain, cut into supplies of dairy and meat, and reduced purchasing power. At the same time, consumption rates of meat may have climbed radically during and immediately following the plague if diseased animals were consumed. Whether contemporaries attempted to preemptively sell stock or boost cohorts of other domestics is unknown, though some evidence for the 809–810 panzootic discussed below, indicates that the culling of sick animals, presumably to preserve the value of flesh and hides, was practiced in the early Middle Ages. Naturally,

---

of Merseburg, Chronicon, ed. C. CL. IOH. M. Lappenberg (MGH, Scriptores 3), Hanover 1839, 773; Fritz Curschmann, Hungersnöte im Mittelalter. Ein Beitrag zur Deutschen Wirtschaftsgeschichte des 8. bis 13. Jahrhunderts, Leipzig 1900, 107–108.

125 Brut y Tywysogion, trans. Cambrian Archaeological Association (Archaeologia Cambrensis X Third Series), London 1864, 36–37.

126 Peniarth MS. 20, ed. Jones (note 98), 10; Red Book, ed. Jones (note 98), 17, 19; Annales Cambriae, ed. John Williams ab Ithel, London 1860, 21.

if other domesticates were also afflicted, the impact would have been more varied and complicated.

Had people died simultaneously on a plague scale, as it seems they did, the impact of cattle loses may have been amplified in some regions and lessened in others. Concurrent mortalities in bovines and humans would have exaggerated the aggregate demographic and economic setback that the plague dealt. Large losses of people and their cows may have caused significant short-term agrarian and settlement contraction, more so than a plague of cattle or people alone. Of course, mortality may have been disproportionate. Had more cattle died than people the plague's impact would have been less severe than had both species been hit evenly. In this scenario, demand for draught, meat, milk and hides would have declined as did supply, though to a lesser overall extent. Without a better understanding of events, it is hard to make sense of the effects of this coupling of human-bovine mortalities.

A definite diagnosis would tentatively help us untangle the history of the plague, and establish with greater confidence its virulence in individual animals and the severity of the mortality in northwestern insular Europe, not to mention the disease's modes of transmission and thereby a better idea of its probable extent, and whether a significant die-off should be expected for the continent in the early 990s. Although such a diagnosis may be some ways away, a speculative diagnosis based on symptoms and epizootiology may provide direction for those in the palaeosciences.

If the disease primarily afflicted cattle, was communicable between like species and neither arthropod- nor soil-borne, likely foreign to northwestern insular Europe, and exhibited high morbidity and mortality, RPV and CBPP, of pathogens known to modern science, would again seem to be the best match. The *CC*'s identification of what was likely the plague's most noteworthy and distinct symptom – diarrhea – lends more support to a tentative RPV identification, as diarrhea is a classic sign of acute reactions to the virus and is not typical of other known highly communicable and virulent plagues of domestic bovines.[127] The labeling of the plague as "máelgarb" – "bald-rough" – in the *AT* and *CS* may speak to the effect of the disease on the coats of cattle. The focus in the Irish texts on this and not diarrhea might suggest that the latter was not universally understood as the primary sign of the disease. On the other hand, this Irish annalist may have been concerned principally with the financial repercussions of ruined hides. Like *fluxus intraneorum*, a rough coat is typical of RPV, but it is not as classic or distinguishing a symptom of the disease. Notably, the *CC*'s specific reference to *fluxus intraneorum* in the context of an animal plague appears to be unprecedented, though in different terms diarrhea is identified in a mid-sixth-century continental bovine epizootic discussed below. Despite the claim of the Irish annalist, this is not the first "máelgarb" to appear in relation to an animal plague in the Irish annals, nor the last. In 770 and 1129, "máelgarb"

127 Anderson et al., Manual (note 57), 9–10, 114–115; Obi et al., Manual (note 57), 7–10.

also spread and killed cattle, though we might doubt the term was used systematically across centuries.[128] In the latter year, pigs as well died. Naturally, it is uncertain whether the pathogens behind these three plagues were one and the same, regardless of their shared label.

That humans appear to have succumbed to the plague alongside bovines does not necessarily problematize a morbillivirus diagnosis. The most robust of the molecular clock studies (discussed above) has measles and rinderpest diverging as early as 600 BCE. That need not mean they diverged then or soon after, but that they could have, on the basis of that study, have diverged that early. Crucially, as an earlier genomic study on measles' evolution proposed, as had earlier pre-genome-era treatments of morbillivirus evolution, an ancestral morbillivirus may have been zoonotic pre-divergence, a pathogen hosted in cattle that intermittently jumped to humans (or vice versa – though that route is rarely envisioned).[129] The 986–988 *scitta* may attest to the dissemination in Europe of the ancestral zoonotic morbillivirus. Should the divergence time be pushed back, this plague may alternatively evidence the co-existence of the RPV forebearer with distinct measles and rinderpest viruses. One might hesitate before making a sport out of such speculation, however. Without more definitive answers we stand to gain only little via these very tentative diagnoses.

4. Charlemagne's Panzootic, 809–810

Towards the end of the first decade of the ninth century, a disease of cattle broke out on a large scale in Europe. Multiple contemporary and independent texts refer to the mortality. This panzootic, which appears to have afflicted bovine herds as far apart as northeastern Germany and southwestern Spain, and central Italy and Wales, has long attracted attention in catalogues of animal disease, modern veterinary manuals and virological and policy studies on the rinderpest virus.[130] The plague has been

128 Kelly, Early Irish Farming (note 105), 195–196.

129 Yuki Furuse/Akira Suzuki/Hitoshi Oshitani, Origin of Masles Virus: Divergence from Rinderpest Virus between the 11th and 12th Centuries, in Virology Journal 7 (2010), 1.

130 Early catalogues touch on this panzootic briefly. See Short, General Chronological History (note 3), vol. I, 84, and Paulet, Recherches historiques (note 3), 76–77, 80–81, both draw upon a single non-contemporary text. The former writes only that 810 was "remarkable for a great dearth of cattle," while the latter suggests that the mortality was limited to France. Paulet also wrongly associates Agobard's remarks on the mortality with the poorly documented 801 epizootic (Annales Lobienses, ed. Wilhelm Wattenbach (MGH, Scriptores 13), Hanover 1881, 230). Fleming, Animal Plagues (note 3), 45–47, consults multiple contemporary and non-contemporary sources, asserts that there is little doubt that the disease was rinderpest, speculates that the plague reached Europe from the eastern shores of the Black Sea, proposes that wars might account for its appearance and spread in Europe, and, like Paulet, improperly assigns Agobard's remarks to 801. Dieckerhoff, Geschichte der Rinderpest (note 3), 26, quotes from the Annales

described as highly mortal, pan-European, and as either cutting short or facilitating the conquests of the Carolingian emperor Charlemagne. For some time, commonly perceived knowledge of the outbreak's extent, impact and supposed RPV identity, have been mutually reinforcing, though each lacked much foundation. While treatments of the plague in these works leaves much to be desired, a recent assessment of the extant written evidence and the panzootic's diagnosis argues, as several catalogues of livestock disease and modern studies of RPV stress, that the plague was a major event and could have had, as the early fourteenth-century panzootic did, serious consequences for contemporary human economy and health.[131]

At least ten accounts of the die-off survive, eight are continental and six appear to be contemporary and independent. While we are better informed of the continental history of this ninth-century epizootic than that of the early 1300s, let alone the 980s, our overall knowledge of its spatial and temporal extent, origins, mortality and impact is far less clear than that of 1314–1325. Textual references give only vague and indirect indications of the disease's presence in what is now Austria, Belgium, England, France, Germany, Italy, Luxembourg, the Netherlands, Spain, Switzerland and Wales. Most accounts speak generally of a vast mortality, and, as in the 980s, no evidence survives that allows us to quantify the plague's toll. That multiple independent and contemporary texts stress that the disease was virulent and the plague spatially vast, does, however, suggest that many thousands of bovines died across a wide breadth of Europe. Attention to the composition of the known references as well points to an extensive mortality.

The *Chronicon Moissiancense* (*CM*) and *Annales de Gestis Caroli Magni Imperatoris* document cattle deaths in 809. Composed in the tenth century at Ripoll from earlier sources, the *CM* briefly observes a "great mortality of animals" spreading westward across Europe from the "east."[132] Here "oriens" may refer to lands east of the Elbe, as it does elsewhere in the text.[133] The *Annales* was penned c. 890 at Corvey by the

---

Fuldenses, a text then dependent on the Annales Regni Francorum. He firmly identifies the outbreak as one of rinderpest and remarks that it spread westward from the Orient and that it affected England. Spinage, Cattle Plague (note 2), 89–90, likewise mixes contemporary and non-contemporary sources, wrongly dates both Agobard's remarks on the 809–810 plague and the RFA 809–810 plague passage to 801, claims that Agobard wrote in Leyden (not Lyons), and suggests that Charlemagne having crossed the Rhine to combat the Huns (which he did not do in 809/810) introduced the disease to Europe, which, according to Spinage, following Fleming, spread westward from the eastern shores of the Black Sea and eventually to London from the Netherlands. For Spinage, the sources provide clear indications of rinderpest.

131 Timothy P. Newfield, A Great Carolingian Panzootic. The Probable Extent, Diagnosis and Impact of an Early Ninth-Century Cattle Pestilence, in: Argos. Bulletin van het Veterinair Historisch Genootschap 46 (2012), 200–210. For a Brief earlier treatment see, for example, Jean-Pierre Devroey, Économie rurale et société dans l'Europe franque (Vie–IXe siècles), Paris 2003, 66.

132 Chronicon Moissiacense, ed. Georg Heinrich Pertz (MGH, Scriptores 1), Hanover 1826, 309.

133 Ibid., 313. See also Annales Regni Francorum, ed. Friedrich Kurze (MGH, Scriptores rerum Germanicarum 6), Hanover 1895, 149–150.

so-called Saxon Poet, who, in composing his biography of Charlemagne, is known to have relied heavily on several earlier texts. Yet his account of the outbreak has little in common with other known sources and may be based on earlier poetic descriptions of livestock plagues,[134] like that encountered in Virgil's *Georgics*. Like the Augustan poet, the Saxon writes of a great mortality in Noricum (modern-day eastern Austria, southern Germany and northern Slovenia), the stench of dead cattle strewn across fields, and farmers using knifes to kill the sick. Unlike Virgil, he writes of disease in cattle alone, significant mortality beyond Noricum, indeed across Europe, and farmers cleaning stalls. Of course, the Carolingian writer may have drawn also on non-extant sources for the 809–810 plague in the eastern portions of Charlemagne's empire as well as personal knowledge of animal plagues or responses to smaller-scale episodes of animal disease in his own liftetime.

In 810, animal mortalities are encountered in a range of texts, most notably the *Annales Regni Francorum* (*ARF*), which documents a cattle plague alongside Danish attacks on Frisia and Charlemagne's campaign into the northeastern reaches of his empire.[135] The annalist, who quite possibly wrote at Aachen c. 810 and was a member of the court and well-informed about matters from across the empire, claims that the mortality was enormous, that nearly all the cattle on Charlemagne's campaign died, and that cattle were affected throughout each of the provinces of the empire – from the Mediterranean to the North Sea and English Channel, and Catalonia and the Atlantic Ocean to the Elbe and Saale rivers. In the same year, the *Annales Laurissenses Minores* (*ALM*), penned at Lorsch in the early ninth century, documents "the greatest mortality of oxen across almost all Europe and of many people",[136] while the *Annales Sancti Emmerammi Ratisponensis* (*ASER*), possibly composed at Regensburg (Bavaria), records "a great mortality of animals"[137] and the *Annales Xantenses* (*AX*) "a great mortality of oxen and other animals".[138] The *ALM* and *ASER* seem to provide contemporary and independent accounts of the plague, but the *AX* entry, perhaps compiled at Lorsch in the early 830s, is quite plausibly derived from the *ARF*.

Another contemporary and independent account of the plague is encountered in Agobard of Lyons's *De Grandine et Tonitruis*, penned in the mid-810s in his diocese of Lyons. Agobard writes of a "mortality of oxen" over a vast territory, spanning "fields and mountains, meadows and springs". Countryfolk in Agobard's area believed, according to Agobard, that the mortality was caused by a dust that a Duke Grimoald, Charlemagne's

---

134 Saxon Poet, Annales de Gestis Caroli Magni Imperatoris, ed. Georg Heinrich Pertz (MGH, Scriptores 1), Hanover 1826, 263–264.

135 Annales Regni Francorum, ed. Kurze (note 133), 132.

136 Annales Laurissenses Minores, ed. Georg Heinrich Pertz (MGH, Scriptores 1), Hanover 1826, 121.

137 Annales Sancti Emmerammi Maiores, ed. Harry Bresslau (MGH, Scriptores 30.2), Leipzig 1934, 739.

138 Annales Xantenses, ed. Bernhard von Simson (MGH, Scriptores rerum Germanicarum 12), Hanover 1909, 4.

Beneventan adversary, had spread about.[139] Adobard does not assign the mortality a date, but notes that it took place a few years ago, signaling these deaths were part of the 809–810 panzootic. A sermon attributed to Arno of Salzburg, dated to 806–811, and given at a synod in Bavaria, may also refer to bovine deaths c. 810. It speaks vaguely of an "animal mortality" and "pestilence".[140] Lastly, for the Carolingian sources, the epizootic is encountered in the *Gesta Karoli Magni Imperatoris* of Notker Balbulus. Notker briefly describes the plague wreaking havoc on Charlemagne's cattle while on campaign, killing 100 oxen in a single night.[141] Notker's late ninth-century *Gesta*, however, is not considered a reliable or independent source for Charlemagne's reign. It is likely that he based his account of the plague on that of the *ARF*. Still, it is not out of the question that Notker drew upon non-extant sources at St. Gall, where he wrote, or, as he suggests, that he used the reports of earlier monks at St. Gall.

Animal mortalities are also documented across the English Channel. In 810, the *Annales Cambriae* (*AC*), composed at St. David's, records "a mortality of cattle across Britain",[142] and the three principal versions of the *Brut* report animal deaths as well: the Peniarth MS. 20 documents "a mortality upon the animals in all the island of Britain,"[143] the Red Book "a mortality of animals throughout the island of Britain,"[144] and the *Brenhinedd y Saesson* "a mortality of animals throughout all Wales."[145] It is probable, considering the similarities between these passages, that the lost *Cronica* on which the *Brut* depends, was reliant, in its reference to the plague, on the earlier *AC*, and that only one contemporary and independent Welsh reference to the plague survives. The entry in the *AC*, though not found in the earliest extant MS of the text, was possibly composed in or shortly after 810 and is independent of the Carolingian sources. The later *CC* also reports, ultimately following the *ALM*, that in 810 "the greatest mortality of oxen devastated nearly all Europe".[146]

Together, these texts demonstrate that the disease spread across a wide area of continental Europe in addition to Wales. If animals died not far from where the texts were composed, we may identify the plague more precisely in the vicinity of Aachen, Lorsch, Lyons, Regensburg, Ripoll, St. David's, Salzburg and, possibly, Corvey. In observing animal mortalities on Charlemagne's campaign, the *ARF* reveals that northeastern

139 Agobard of Lyons, De Grandine et Tonitruis, ed. L. Van Acker (Agobardi Lugdunensis Opera Omnia), Turnhout 1981, 14–15.

140 Rudolf Pokorny, Ein unbekannter Synodalsermo Arns von Salzburg, in: Deutsches Archiv für Erforschung des Mittelalters 39 (1983), 379–394, 381, 393.

141 Notker Balbulus, Gesta Karoli Magni Imperatoris, ed. Hans F. Haefele (MGH, Scriptores rerum Germanicarum, Nova Series 12), Berlin 1959, 75–76.

142 Annales Cambriae, ed. Williams ab Ithel (note 126), 11.

143 Peniarth MS. 20, ed. Jones (note 98), 3.

144 Red Book, ed. Jones (note 98), 7.

145 Brenhinedd y Saesson, ed. Jones (note 98), 13.

146 Chronicon ex Chronicis, trans. Bray/McGurk (note 99), 234–235.

Carolingian Europe was affected too, in the regions of Wesel and Verden, and/or further east around Höhbeck.

As in the 980s and early 1300s, it is quite likely that these texts refer to a single outbreak given that each emphasizes the vastness of the plague and the unlikelihood that multiple virulent diseases affecting cattle would irrupt simultaneously in Europe on a large scale. It is also certain that the losses were the result of disease, as the *ARF*, Notker and Saxon Poet specify, and not extreme weather or food shortage, and there is little doubt that the disease primarily afflicted cattle: not only do the *AC*, *ARF*, *AX*, Notker and Saxon Poet specify domestic bovines as the susceptible species, but Agobard explicitly states that only cattle were affected. The "other animals" referred to in the *AX* may have been non-draught cattle or even young cattle, as for instance in the Domesday Book.[147] It is not impossible that the plague was zoonotic, as the *ALM* suggests, though no other source documents a mortality of humans c. 810. That the disease managed to affect cattle in southwestern Wales, northwestern Spain, central France and north-central Germany, and quite plausibly other regions of Charlemagne's empire, in about a year, strongly implies that it, like the disease of the 980s and early 1300s, was neither arthropod- nor soil-borne but transmitted (efficiently) between cattle.

Why the plague irrupted in Europe when it did and what drove its spread is unclear, as is the case with later plagues. That Charlemagne's campaign of 810 introduced the disease to Europe or played a major role in its dissemination, as has been suggested, is unlikely, considering that the 810 campaign was a comparatively limited affair geographically, that Charlemagne left Aachen with herds intact and returned empty handed, and that the plague had already, according to the *CM* and Saxon Poet, disseminated widely in Europe in 809. Departing Aachen in late spring or early summer, Charlemagne crossed the Rhine at Lippeham, pressed forward to the meeting of the Aller and Weser rivers, and then into Saxony, presumably to Höhbeck, before returning to Aachen in October.[148] Danish advances on the Obodrites, who occupied parts of northeastern Germany (Schleswig-Holstein and Mecklenburg-Vorpommern) and Carolingian attacks on the Linones and Smeldingi (other Slavic groups located between the Elbe and Oder rivers), in 808, could have aided the introduction and spread of the disease, as may have Obodrite and Saxon attacks on the Veleti, who claimed a region to the south of the Obodrites, in 809, the movement of Carolingian forces (possibly including cattle) from across the empire (*Gallia atque Germania*) to Frisia in the same year, and Danish attacks on Frisia in 810.[149] While these conflicts may have played some role in the pathogen's initial diffusion, they cannot account for its wide prevalence across Europe. Neither a food shortage nor climatic anomaly/extreme weather appear to have played a significant

147 Langdon, Horses (note 8), 294.

148 Annales Regni Francorum, ed. Kurze (note 133), 131–132.

149 Ibid., 125–131.

role in the disease's irruption or spread in Europe. The *ARF* reports an "exceptionally mild" winter in 808,[150] and in 809 the Saxon Poet observes the failure of grape vines to produce fruit in several regions,[151] while the *Annales Sancti Amandi* documents a "great flood of water,"[152] and the *Capitulare Missorum Aquisgranense Primum* speaks vaguely of a subsistence crisis.[153] But written and palaeoscientific evidence considered, the 809–810 plague did not take place in the context of a general environmental crisis.

The *ARF* and Notker report that the die-off severely impeded Charlemagne's 810 campaign, as do indications in the *ARF* (in 811 and 812) that Charlemagne's attempts to restore order in Saxony and on the Elbe in 810 were ineffective.[154] The sources say nothing else possibly relating to the plague's impact, though it is again safe to presume that arable acreage and, consequently, the aggregate quantity of grain reaped, would have contracted, possibly in many regions, and that meat and dairy supplies would have dwindled and their prices inflated. That the outbreak itself gave birth to a food shortage is unlikely, though it may have made contemporaries more susceptible to crises (possibly contributing to the dearth of 813 reported in the *Concilium Arelatense* or worsening the existing, but seemingly minor, shortage of 809[155]), particularly where restocking was difficult. Whether contemporaries attempted panic sales or preemptive culls, or augmented the cohorts of other stock, is unknown. The Saxon Poet writes of the slaughtering of sick animals, presumably in an attempt to preserve their value, though this detail may have been borrowed from Virgil and not be indicative of any general attempt to curb losses. Of course, a definitive diagnosis would, in corroborating several aspects of the 809–810 plague's epizootiology, help us establish a fuller picture of the plague's devastation, as would further consideration of the agrarian economy of early ninth-century Europe. Of pathogens known to modern science, RPV and CBPP are the best fit once more, considering that the disease targeted cattle, was very likely spread between like species and highly communicable, virulent and foreign to Europe. Of course, were the 809–810 panzootic RPV, there would be room to doubt that the 986–988 plague was a pre-divergence morbillivirus, an ancestor of measles and rinderpest, unless rinderpest's ancestor co-existed for a time with a distinct RPV, or RPV was initially less host specific. Much about the virus pre-divergence remains unknown, however, and speculation piled on speculation should be treated with great care.

150 Ibid., 125.

151 Saxon Poet, Annales, ed. Pertz (note 134), 264.

152 Annales Sancti Amandi, ed. Georg Heinrich Pertz (MGH, Scriptores 1), Hanover 1826, 14.

153 Capitulare Missorum Aquisgranense Primum, ed. Alfred Boret (MGH, Capitularia Regum Francorum 1), Hanover 1883, 151.

154 Annales Regni Francorum, ed. Kurze (note 133), 134–35, 137.

155 Concilium Arelatense, ed. Albert Werminghoff (MGH, Concilia 2.1.), Hanover 1906, 252.

5. Plagues of Cattle in Italy and France, 591, 583–584 and 569–570

Two centuries earlier the sources for livestock mortalities are fewer and farther between. Near the end of his *Libri Historiarum X* (*LHX*), in his account of the events of 591, Gregory of Tours reports that

> There was an immense drought, which destroyed all the grass pasture; thus, a severe disease began to grow strong in cattle and draught animals [oxen], and left few animals for breeding purposes, just as the prophet Habakkuk foretold: "The sheep shall be cut off from the fold, and there shall be no oxen in the stalls" [Habakkuk 3:17]. This plague not only attacked domesticates but also various kinds of wild animals. For throughout the forest glades a multitude of deer, actually of all animals, were found lying dead in impassible places.[156]

Earlier in the *LHX*, Gregory observes other animal mortalities: in 583 he writes that "a disease of cattle" followed conflict between Merovingian kings "so that hardly a head of cattle survived and it was quite a rare thing to see a bullock or set eyes on a heifer",[157] and in 584 that "a disease of cattle prevailed again so that hardly any remained".[158] In an undated passage, in Gregory's *De Virtutibus Sancti Martini Episcopi*, we also read that

> Once a devastating plague was ravaging cattle so severely that someone might think that no means was left for restoring the species. One of my [servants] went to the holy church and poured into a container oil from the lamps that were hanging from the ceiling and some water. He brought the container home, dipped his finger into the liquid, and made the sign of the Lord's cross on the foreheads and backs of the cattle that this disease had not yet infected. Since he was confident in his faith, this man also sprinkled this ointment in the mouths of the cattle that had collapsed and were lying on the ground. Soon, more swiftly than words can say, this mysterious plague was eliminated, and the herds were saved.[159]

Another sixth-century author, Marius of Avenches, documents an animal pestilence around the same time. In his *Chronica* he reports that "a virulent disease greatly afflicted

---

156 Gregory of Tours, Libri Historiarum X, ed. Bruno Krusch (MGH, Scriptores rerum Merovingicarum 1), Hanover 1937, 525; id., Libri Historiarum X/The History of the Franks, trans. Lewis Thorpe, London 1974, 592–593.

157 Id., Libri Historiarum X, ed. Krusch (note 156), 301; The History of the Franks, trans. Thorpe (note 156), 361.

158 Id., Libri Historiarum X, ed. Krusch (note 156), 317; The History of the Franks, trans. Thorpe (note 156), 377.

159 Gregory of Tours, De Virtutibus Sancti Martini Episcopi, ed. Bruno Krusch (MGH, Scriptores rerum Merovingicarum 1.2), Hanover, 1885, 187; id., De Virtutibus Sancti Martini Episcopi, trans. Raymond Van Dam, in: id., Saints and their Miracles in Late Antique Gaul, Princeton 1993, 267.

Italy and France with a flow of the bowels and spots, and beef animals died especially through the aforementioned places".[160] Marius dates the passage to 570, but from the mid-560s he is clearly one year ahead. Much later, in the ninth century, Agnellus of Ravenna, in his *Liber Pontificalis Ecclesiae Ravennatis* (*LPR*), observes that "in the fifth year of Emperor Justin II [570] there was a pestilence of oxen and destruction everywhere".[161]

These accounts of animal mortalities, though overlooked by historians,[162] are encountered in several catalogues of livestock disease and veterinary studies on the rinderpest virus. Discussion in these works has been brief, highly speculative and misguided.[163] The spatial and temporal contours, epizootiological properties and diagnoses of these plagues are far more enigmatic than those already addressed and far less certain than has hitherto been thought. Gregory, Marius and Agnellus appear to illuminate three epizootics – in 569–570, 583–584 and 591 – for which additional evidence is unknown.[164]

160 Marius of Avenches, Chronica, ed. Theodor Mommsen (MGH, Auctores Antiquissimi 11), Berlin 1894, 238. It has long been suggested that Marius refers to two plagues here, one of humans and another of cattle, on account of his use of variola, which many have read as smallpox (Johann Hermann Baas, Outlines of the History of Medicine, New York 1889, 240–41; Jean-Noël Biraben/Jacques Le Goff, The Plague in the Early Middle Ages, in: Robert Forster/Orest Ranum (eds.), Biology and Man in History, Baltimore 1975, 59–60; Donald R. Hopkins, Princes and Peasants. Smallpox in History, Chicago 1983, 24; Devroey, Économie rurale (note 131), 46). There is little reason, however, to identify an outbreak of smallpox here, solely on the basis of this variola (See Dionysios Ch. Stathakopoulos, Famine and Pestilence in the Late Roman and Early Byzantine Empire. A Systematic Survey of Subsistence Crises and Epidemics, Aldershot 2004, 313). Variola did not then designate Variola major or V. minor or necessarily refer to disease in humans.

161 Agnellus of Ravenna, Liber Pontificalis Ecclesiae Ravennatis, ed. Oswald Holder-Egger (MGH, Scriptores rerum Langobardicarum et Italicarum, Hanover 1878, 337; Agnellus of Ravenna, The Book of Pontiffs of the Church of Ravenna, trans. Deborah Mauskopf Deliyannis, Washington 2004, 205.

162 Devroey, Économie rurale (note 131), 26, mentions the 591 plague and Stathakopoulos, Famine (note 160), 313–314, the 569–570 epizootic.

163 Paulet, Recherches historiques (note 3), 73–75, passes over the plague of 569–570, assigns the outbreak Gregory observes in his *De Virtutibus* to 581 and the region of Touraine (a historical province of France located around Tours), seems to think that the plague of 583–584 afflicted equines, and suggests that the 591 plague, which he dates to 592, was zoonotic. Like Paulet, Fleming, Animal Plagues (note 3), 39–41, affixes the outbreak Gregory reports in his *De Virtutibus* to 581, dates the plague of 583–584 to 581, 583 and 584, assigns the plague of 591 to France and Belgium, and, following Wirth, proposes an anthrax diagnosis. Dieckerhoff, Geschichte der Rinderpest (note 3), 25, is confident in a rinderpest diagnosis of the cattle mortalities he dates to 569, 581 and 583. He separates the 569 deaths of people and cattle, suggests that smallpox caused those human losses, and emphasizes that those cattle deaths were not caused by cowpox. Spinage, Cattle Plague (note 2), 88–89, provides a similar account of the epizootics of 569–570 and 591, and suggests that rinderpest did plague Europe in the second half of the sixth century.

164 Neither contemporary writers, such as John of Biclaro or Venatius Forunatus, nor later historians, such as Bede or Paul the Deacon, comment on these animal plagues. The Irish annals, ASC and AC also do not observe a sixth-century epizootic, and the Brut only commences in the early 600s. The vita of Theodore of Sykeon refers to a plague of humans and oxen in Turkey in the region around Ankara, which

The dating of the first and last of these mortalities is clear enough and it is probable that the stock plague Gregory reports in 583 and 584 were one and the same, as Gregory implies in his account of the latter. Gregory notes that the first occurred after a battle between Chilperic I and Guntram, which appears to have taken place in the spring/summer of 583, and in one way or another involved Angers, Bourges, Melun, Nantes, Paris, Poitiers and Tours in central and northwestern France. He reports the second prior to the autumn of 584, and though he does not assign the 584 outbreak any spatial parameters, it is probable, for reasons discussed below, that the disease affected roughly the same region as in 583. Considering the unlikelihood that major diseases of cattle would irrupt near simultaneously in roughly the same area, we may suspect that the 583 and 584 plagues were one, despite Gregory's divided treatment of them. Van Dam suggests that Gregory also refers to this plague in his *De Virtutibus*, as Gregory is thought to have finished the third book of his work on St. Martin, in which this passage is found, in the mid-580s and as Gregory appears to have gathered the miracles encountered in book 3 "as they happened".[165]

If Marius and Agnellus' accounts of the 569–570 die-off are independent of one another, it is quite plausible that they refer to the same mortality, considering again the improbability that multiple large plagues would irrupt contemporarily in roughly the same region (Marius places the outbreak in France and Italy, and in his *LPR* Agnellus primarily addresses events in northern Italy). It is likely that Marius and Agnellus' accounts are independent. They show no verbal parallels and it is unclear whether Agnellus made use of Marius' *Chroncia* at all when writing the *LPR* in the 830s and 840s. Although the extant sources Agnellus is known to have drawn upon do not refer to the plague, he does cite two non-surviving texts, a *Chronicon* by Maximian of Ravenna, which may have been continued into the 570s, and an "annalistic source," which, though unknown, is thought to have extended at least until 573.[166] Agnellus, unlike Marius, assigns no spatial parameters to the plague, fails to mention symptoms, writes of *pestilentia* and *boves*, rather than *morbus* and *animalia bubula*, and neither qualifies the disease as *validus* nor the mortality as *valde*. Still, we must pay heed to Evans' aforementioned caution made in a different context but nonetheless applicable here. As Marius is considered to have written his text shortly after it ends in 580, it is possible that we possess two independent and contemporary or near contemporary references to the 569–570 plague. Of the animal mortalities Gregory documents in his

Stathakopoulos, Famine (note 160), 310, suggests can be dated roughly to the reign of emperor Justin II (565–578). It is possible, though far from certain, that this plague was related to those of 569–570 or 583–584. Stathakopoulos has turned up no additional evidence for livestock plagues in the last four decades of the sixth century in his survey of late antique and early Byzantine texts.

165 Van Dam, Saints (note 159), 142–144, 267, n. 82.

166 Agnellus of Ravenna, Book of Pontiffs, trans. Mauskopf Deliyannis (note 161), 49.

LHX, only that of 591 can be regarded as strictly contemporary, as Gregory appears to have written the majority of this text in the early-590s.[167]

These passages, despite their contemporaneity, clearly furnish us with little knowledge about the symptoms and epizootiology, and thus identity, or impact of these three plagues, the later two in particular. Gregory assigns no spatial parameters to the epizootics he records, nor does Agnellus, and the parameters Marius affixes to the 569–570 mortality are rather general. It is plausible that the 569–570 plague afflicted a wide region, as both Marius and Agnellus claim, particularly if their accounts are independent and corroborate one another. Whether the disease was prevalent across all France and Italy is less certain. Marius tends to focus on Burgundy, the region in which he lived, worked and wrote, and the mortalities he references may be thought to have occurred there and in neighboring northern Italy.[168] Agnellus likely refers to mortalities in roughly the same regions, as he and his sources seem to have been primarily concerned with Ravenna and northern Italy. That Gregory does not report this plague in the *LHX* may signify that it did not reach the regions of France with which he was primarily concerned, those around Tours, where he was bishop from 573, or Clermont-Ferrand, his hometown. It is noteworthy that Gregory limits his discussion of the human epidemics of the mid-550s and early-570s to these regions.[169] Alternatively, the 569–570 epizootic may simply not have been part of Gregory's historical consciousness or, possibly, Gregory may not have had a use for an animal die-off then in his narrative.

We may suspect that at least Tours and Clermont-Ferrand were hit in 583–584 and 591. The connection Gregory draws between the plague of 583 and Chilperic and Guntram's conflict implies strongly that animal deaths then occurred in central and northwestern France. Marius' *Chronica* concludes in 580 and while Agnellus does not refer to epizootics in the mid-580s or early-590s, his text does not, unlike the *LHX*, regularly comment on natural disasters but focuses largely on the activities of Ravenna's bishops. With the evidence available, it would be unwise to strictly limit the 583–584 and 591 plagues to central and northwestern France, or the 569–570 plague to Burgundy and northern Italy, considering the emphasis that Gregory, Marius and Agnellus put on the magnitude of these mortalities and the unlikelihood that diseases capable of causing significant cattle die-offs would be enzootic to the regions in which they occurred, unless, of course, they represent repeated spillovers of a pathogen locally hosted in another animal.

---

167 Alexander C. Murray, Chronology and the Composition of the Histories of Gregory of Tours, in: Journal of Late Antiquity 1 (2008), 157–196.

168 Ian Wood, The Merovingian Kingdoms, 450–751, London 1994, 31, 43. In the sixth century, Burgundy was a large territory centered around Geneva and nearly spanning Arles in the south to Sens in the north, Basle in the east and Bourges in the west.

169 Gregory of Tours, Libri Historiarum X, ed. Krusch (note 156), 148, 16–166.

The temporal parameters and paths of dissemination of the plagues are opaque, and what species were susceptible is somewhat uncertain. That Marius and Agnellus refer explicitly to deaths of cattle strongly suggests, especially if their accounts are independent, that the 569–570 plague primarily afflicted domestic bovines. However, Marius' reference to dead *bubula* appears as an "add on" to his reference to *variola*, which has long been understood as a disease of humans, smallpox specifically – a designation paleogenomics and phylogenetics now complicates. Agnellus' *interitus* may refer to a (pathogenic) destruction of humans. That Gregory only refers to cattle in his two or three passages on the 583–584 plague also signifies that cattle were then principally afflicted. It is not entirely certain, however, that other domesticates were insusceptible. Cattle were, as noted, socio-economically more significant than other stock and their deaths were perhaps more remarkable. Moreover, early medieval authors tend to focus on cattle, of all domesticates, in their works and to only record plagues of cattle. Gregory only documents epizootics that affected cattle, and in his *LHX* he writes more regularly of domestic bovines than any other non-human animal, domesticated or not, with the exception of horses.[170] Cattle were, Gregory reports, the animals primarily susceptible to the 591 plague, though he observes deer and other wild animals died as well. Whether deer were the undomesticated animal chiefly susceptible to the disease is unclear, of course. It is possible that deaths of deer were simply more remarkable for Gregory than deaths of other undomesticates, considering the number of times he refers to deer in the *LHX* (and thereby that deer were not the animal of the forest glades that the plague afflicted most). Gregory rarely mentions wild animals and only feral birds are reported more often than deer. It is also possible that another disease, or the drought Gregory documents, led to the deaths of non-bovine animals in 591, and that Gregory affixed a single cause to unrelated deaths of different animals. That Gregory's plagues were not zoonotic is more certain. Gregory documents disease outbreaks in human populations in 582, 584 and 591,[171] but in each case he clearly differentiates between human and non-human deaths. In fact, he treats the mortalities of people and cows separately.

If the diseases of 569–570, 583–584 and 591 afflicted large regions, as the authors attest, we may suspect that they were capable of high morbidity and neither arthropod- nor soil-borne, but spread between like species. How virulent these plagues were is obscure. Marius emphasizes that the disease of 569–570 was acute and that it gravely afflicted cattle, but he employs similar language in his other accounts of plagues (in 539,

170 See the references in Gregory of Tours, Libri Historiarum X, ed. Krusch (note 156), regarding cattle: 108, 123, 177, 213, 237, 238, 301, 316, 317, 319, 327, 340, 343, 367, 389, 393, 420, 487, 525; horses: 1937:28, 70, 104, 112, 114, 115, 119, 145, 257, 272, 301, 317, 319, 340, 344, 355, 388, 399, 463, 464, 490; wild birds: 59, 104, 116, 132, 390, 431, 522; deer: 83, 86, 183, 525; dogs: 104, 289, 390, 404; fish: 1937:74, 120, 390; wolves: 1937:83, 248, 289; rodents: 1937:40, 419; pigs: 1937:340, 515; rabbits: 1937:200; bear: 1937:419.

171 Ibid., 284, 304, 525.

568 and 570) and often underscores the severity of the disease outbreaks he records.[172] On possibly three occasions Gregory has few cattle surviving the 583–584 plague and he labels the 591 epizootic as severe too. Like Marius, however, Gregory tends to employ the same language in his accounts of plagues and to stress their severity. Indeed, he documents disease outbreaks that occurred in his own lifetime, while he wrote, and long before the sixth century in similar terms. He describes most plagues briefly, often employs the same nouns, adjectives and adverbs, and positions them similarly within the ten books of the *LHX*. Several plagues are titled *morbus*, as are the animal plagues of 583–584 and 591,[173] many, like the animal plague of 591, are attributed the adjective *gravis* or adverb *graviter*,[174] and several others are qualified by *magna*.[175] Many plagues, like the 583–584 and 591 epizootics, are also recorded within a litany of disasters or alongside portents, natural world anomalies, and/or wars.[176] The inclusion of a biblical excerpt or a representative of the Church in the description of an outbreak is likewise characteristic.[177] Of course, that Gregory and Marius appear to have had a method, as rough as it may have been, for reporting disease outbreaks does not in itself signify that the cattle plagues they record were not characterized by high mortality as they assert. As the assessment here of the fourteenth-century panzootic reveals, reports of widespread acute disease in animals encountered in medieval narrative texts should not be disregarded rashly. Gregory may have reported the 591 plague in typical terms, he may have even used it to further the theme of apocalypse and Last Judgment developed in the last book of his histories,[178] but this is not in itself an indication the event was trivial. We simply do not have enough evidence to know.

What precipitated these epizootics is hazy. It does not seem as though extreme weather, a short-term climatic anomaly or food shortage triggered the 569–570 plague, though the shortage Marius observes in northern Italy following the Lombard arrival in 568 may have helped spread the disease.[179] While Gregory reports rain in the winter of 582, the flooding of some rivers in 583, and a drought and poor crops in 584, these phenomena appear neither to have affected wide regions nor produced a food shortage.[180] Any association with the subsistence crisis in the Eastern Mediterranean region *c.*581/82 is unclear.[181] The 591 plague, on the other hand, did take place in a period marked by

172 Marius of Avenches, Chronica, ed. Mommsen (note 160), 236, 238.

173 Gregory of Tours Libri Historiarum X, ed. Krusch (note 156), 245, 326, 428, 441, 485, 517.

174 Ibid., 148, 238, 245, 248, 428, 440, 485, 515, 525.

175 Ibid., 65, 138, 164, 248, 304.

176 Ibid., 230, 238, 248, 304, 477, 515.

177 Ibid., 138, 164–66, 238–39, 326, 442, 517.

178 Martin Heinzelmann, Gregory of Tours. History and Society in the Sixth Century, Cambridge, 2001, 82.

179 Marius of Avenches, Chronica, ed. Mommsen (note 160), 238.

180 Gregory of Tours Libri Historiarum X, ed. Krusch (note 156), 284, 292–293.

181 Stathakopoulos, Famine (note 160), 318.

both extreme weather and food shortage. Gregory observes "strong rains" in 590 and in 591 "ceaseless rain," the flooding of rivers, an "immense drought," a poor harvest and "a strong food shortage" that affected, at the very least, northeastern France.[182] Gregory the Great also documents a shortage of grain and an imminent subsistence crisis in Rome c. 591, and Paul the Deacon a drought and terrible food shortage across Italy.[183] The *ASC*, *AC* and Irish annals provide no insight on possibly relevant environmental phenomena and whether the phenomena that are recorded are relevant is unknown.

Each of the plagues occurred in a period marked to varying degrees by conflict. Gregory reports battles in the early-580s,[184] some of which entailed the looting of cattle, and he first relates the 583–584 animal plague in the context of the war. King Childebert II is also known to have marched into Italy in 584. In 590, Gregory tells us of another Merovingian advance on Lombard Italy, and raiding in the regions of Metz, Nantes, Rennes and Tours.[185] In 568, the Lombards invaded northern Italy from Pannonia (western Hungary) with a large army composed partly of peoples from the Balkans and Germany, and, according to Gregory, Marius and Paul the Deacon, their families and possessions; shortly thereafter some pressed briefly into France.[186] It is possible that the Lombard migration introduced the 569–570 plague to Italy and France, that Merovingian civil wars facilitated the dissemination of disease in 583–584, and that the plague of 591 was tied to extreme weather and food shortage. These are possibilities.

The texts say nothing of the impact of these die-offs, though we may suspect that they had some similar effects on agriculture and human health as later cattle epizootics already surveyed. Yet arable agriculture was less central to diet and economy in these regions in the sixth century than the ninth or tenth, let alone the fourteenth, suggesting that there may have been some important differences. If the sixth-century outbreaks afflicted the same regions their impact may have been cumulative. If restocking was as long and drawn out a process as it was in the fourteenth century, the plague of 583–584 may have cut short efforts to restock following the plague of 569–570, as may have the plague of 591 the plague of 583–584. Still, there is no firm evidence that these die-offs provoked subsistence crises, though the 583–584 and 591 outbreaks may have contributed to the shortages documented in those years.

Definite diagnoses would help us articulate probable impacts. However, the symptoms and epizootiological properties of these plagues, the later two especially, are poorly established, complicating attempts to advance even the most speculative of diagnoses. If

182 Gregory of Tours Libri Historiarum X, ed. Krusch (note 156), 515, 517, 525.

183 Stathakopoulos, Famine (note 160), 322–323.

184 Gregory of Tours Libri Historiarum X, ed. Krusch (note 156), 282–283, 299–302, 314.

185 Ibid., 483–486, 491–494.

186 Ibid., 174, 213; Marius of Avenches, Chronica, ed. Mommsen (note 160), 238; Paul the Deacon, Historia Langobardorum, ed. Ludwig Bethmann/Georg Waitz (MGH, Scriptores rerum Langobardicarum et Italicarum, Hanover 1878), 76–77.

these plagues principally affected cattle, were spatially vast, characterized by high morbidity and mortality, and primarily spread between cattle, RPV and CBPP, of pathogens known to modern science, would again be the best match. Although *variola*, which is encountered for the first time in Marius' text, is not easy to reconcile with RPV or CBPP, Marius' observation of diarrhea certainly suits a RPV diagnosis, as does Gregory's attention to deaths of deer. Rinderpest can cause high mortality in deer, though it appears to spread rather poorly between them.[187] Like most wild ruminants, deer are resistant to CBPP.[188] If the 591 plague was RPV, the other wild animals Gregory refers to may have been wild pigs and wisents, which are susceptible to the virus, as aurochs may have been considering that rinderpest appears to affect most even-toed ungulates belonging to the *Artiodactyla* order.[189] That the Lombards may have introduced the 569–570 plague to Italy and France also fits well with RPV, considering the virus' supposed ancestral homeland. That said, exceptionally little about RPV's early history, as often told over recent generations, is well-founded. If humans died concurrently, as they appear to have, this 569–570 plague, like the 986–988 *scitta*, could evidence a pre-divergence morbillivirus. The *variola*, possibly from the Latin *varius* (changing, varying, different), may refer to the measles-like effect of the RPV ancestor on the appearance of human victims.[190] If the 583–584 and 591 plagues were more circumscribed, and cattle but one of several species affected, anthrax might be suspected. As a virulent soil-borne pathogen, which is most likely to cause marked mortalities in domesticated and undomesticated grazing mammals in periods of drought preceded by heavy rain or flooding,[191] anthrax should be considered alongside rinderpest for the 591 plague. That such epizootiologically dissimilar diseases can be considered for this die-off underscores how little we know about it.

6. Conclusion

This article has teased out six medieval cattle plagues from a wide range of medieval sources, addressed most of the modern scholarship on premodern animal disease, and scrutinized some long-held facts about medieval stock plagues encountered in catalogues of animal disease and in veterinary, virological and policy studies of the rinderpest virus. It has intended to pave the way for a fresh assessment of premodern

187 Paul Rossiter, Rinderpest, in: Elizabeth S. Williams/Ian K. Baker (eds.), Infectious Diseases of Wild Mammals, 3rd ed. Ames 2001, 40; Spinage, Cattle Plague (note 2), 3, 33, 40, 81.

188 Geering/Amanfu, Preparation (note 57), 6.

189 Anderson et al., Manual (note 57), 5.

190 Newfield, Human-Bovine Plagues (note 105), 22–24.

191 Cormack Gates et al., Anthrax, in: Williams/Baker (eds.), Infectious Diseases, 407.

epizootic disease. Four things are clear: the histories of medieval animal plagues encountered in disease catalogues and scientific literature on RPV are fraught with errors, highly assumptive and unreliable, especially for the medieval centuries; the quantity and character of medieval written evidence for livestock disease varies greatly and presents a range of problems and possibilities for interpreting the spatial and temporal parameters, geographical origins, triggers, symptoms, epizootiology, impact and diagnoses of animal plagues; animal plagues, of cattle in particular, were common in premodernity, but enigmatic; and future research on premodern epizootic disease must be collaborative and multi-disciplinary. The contours of numerous plagues, the frequency with which epizootics occurred in particular subperiods and regions, the impacts of animal losses, and the methods employed to absorb mortalities, not to mention the complexities inherent in the practice of retrospective diagnosing, all warrant more consideration. As the forgoing pages have demonstrated. The history of premodern animal plagues is so undeveloped that one can hardly talk about animal plague impacts. Rather, efforts still need to focus on teasing plagues out of the sources, and on establishing their geographies and chronologies.

The firm RPV diagnoses regularly advanced in the scientific literature for the plagues of 569–570, 583–584, 591 and 809–810 need to be re-labeled as speculative. Popular ideas about the vastness of these die-offs, with the exception of the 569–570 and 809–810 plagues, and the devastation they caused need to be treated most gingerly. On account of the survival of manorial accounts and a wide range of textual evidence, the 1314–1325 mortality emerges as sharpest defined cattle plague in Europe before the eighteenth-century panzootics. Yet, its suggested rinderpest identification also must be treated with caution. Although RPV, of pathogens known to modern science, appears to fit several of the plagues addressed here, undeniable proof of the premodern existence of the virus or its ancestor is not found in the fourteenth, tenth, ninth or sixth. Symptoms described by Marius and in the *CC* are rinderpest-like but are not conclusive evidence that RPV or a zoonotic ancestor attacked premodern bovines and people. As disease-causing microorganisms are mutable and retrospective diagnoses assume continuity in disease expressions and epizootiology over considerable periods of time, all diagnoses of premodern stock plagues must remain tentative until they find adequate paleogenomic support. Only then may diagnoses, like those suggested here, be employed to illuminate the extent or impact of past outbreaks, or for that matter be integrated into our understanding of pathogens known to modern science such as RPV. In (re-)assessing the diagnoses of premodern epizootics there is, after all, opportunity to better not only our grasp of premodern plagues but our understanding of the antiquity and evolution of pathogens known to modern science. Evolutionary biologists and palaeogenomicists have much to learn from historians and vice versa. It is noteworthy that analysis elsewhere of the tradition of the great 376–386 panzootic has shown that that plague, as well-known as it may be in some circles, did not even take place, at least not as it has long been said to have.

Our understanding of medieval epizootic disease would benefit from sustained and intensive interdisciplinarity. Paleogenomicists might add weight to speculative diagnoses of past plagues and in doing so further our understanding of their epizootiology, origins, spatial and temporal extent, and impact. Through isotope analyses we might establish the diet and mobility of animal populations affected by disease in centuries and regions, like those discussed in this article, in which livestock trade, diet and transhumance are poorly understood. Attention to mobility could reveal routes by which communicable diseases spread. Paleopathologists can help illuminate the baseline of disease and underlying health conditions of premodern stock, so rarely commented upon in written sources, as well as possible links between epizootic disease, nutrition and chronic sickness. Skeletal evidence may also emerge pertaining to the disposal and butchering of diseased animals, and the impact stock mortalities had on surviving animals in terms of nutrition and exploitation. Before any of this, of course, remains or pits of animals must be unearthed and dated within some reason to documented plagues, a difficult task no doubt for zooarchaeologists. Palaeopathological assessments of human remains dating to shortly after periods of epizootic disease might also inform us of the effects of stock plagues on human health and nutrition, as DeWitte and Slavin's study does.

The palaeoclimatic sciences, as Campbell has shown, are as well of value for the study of epizootic disease. Natural archives of past climate can shine light on the general and specific environmental contexts in which plagues occurred as well as short-term events that may have indirectly contributed to their irruption. At present, the root causes of all the epizootics addressed here, however, are unclear. The relationship with any medieval animal plague to climate, however, remains wholly undetermined. Certainly, no single phenomenon appears to have universally provoked disease outbreaks in cattle and no trigger of any outbreak discussed in these pages is currently known. Extreme weather, short-term climatic anomalies and subsistence crises seem to have been near the root of some significant plagues, including the 1314–1325 panzootic and the 591 outbreak, and conflict and human migration may have been closely associated to some others, such as the 569–570 epizootic, but far from all climatic anomalies, food shortages, wars or human migrations were associated with epizootics. The irruption of the 986–988 and 809–810 plagues cannot be firmly tied to any such phenomena. There are few discernible patterns between these plagues.

The impact of epizootic disease on human populations as well requires further assessment. Medieval textual sources might describe epizootics in the briefest of terms, but, manorial accounts tell us a great deal about the consequences of livestock mortalities on the agrarian economy and, indirectly, human diet and health, though they do so only for England and parts of Wales, and for a limited period of time. While knowledge gleaned from manorial accounts may inform speculation on the impact of epizootics in other regions and periods, it should not be assumed that the English experience with epizootic disease in the thirteenth through fifteenth centuries is wholly applicable to, for instance, then contemporary Scotland, Belgium or Poland, let alone tenth-century

Ireland, ninth-century France or sixth-century Italy. As caution must be exercised when drawing parallels between the eighteenth-century bovine panzootics and earlier cattle plagues, the impact of the 1314–1325 panzootic in England cannot serve as a stand-in for the impact of the earlier plagues addressed here. One might use the English experience of the fourteenth-century as a guide, but to really grasp the consequences of plagues in other regions and periods, consideration will have to be given to human dependence on the afflicted species for agriculture, diet, communication, travel, raw materials and war, as well as to how animals could have been restocked and, thus, livestock production, nutrition and trade. It is certain that the impact of cattle epizootics would not have been altogether similar across Europe throughout the medieval period. While some features may have been near universal, like the contraction of arable, others, like the effect of the die-off on diet, would have varied over time and space, and between cultures and population segments. Of course, the agricultural and economic significance of cattle, and the dietary importance of grain, cow milk and beef, was not constant throughout premodernity.

Much the same can be said about how medieval Europeans attempted to cope with epizootic disease. While some measures adopted in England in the early-1300s to prevent and absorb losses are well documented, it cannot be assumed that panic sales, preemptive culls, the expansion of pasture or the augmenting of unaffected animal cohorts were universal features of the medieval epizootic experience. These phenomena are not universally seen across England in the early-fourteenth century. Herbal remedies and prayers would have been exercised throughout the Middle Ages, though the nature of these too appears to have changed over time, and we can rightly question the efficiency of such measures against diseases like anthrax, CBPP, FMDV and RPV, though histories of these interventions would strengthen our grasp of the experience of these plagues.[192]

Premodern veterinary treatises will give us an idea of how Europeans may have curbed the spread of disease and limited losses. Of course, in using these texts for these purposes we must be careful to differentiate theory from practice. Medieval farmers may have segregated sick from healthy animals, as Columella and Vegetius recommended, but it would be wrong to suppose that quarantining was regularly or effectively practiced, or everywhere and always traditional ecological knowledge. Still, it is clear that premodern Europeans were not completely hopeless in the face of virulent epizootic disease.

192 Lynn L. Remly, Magic, Myth and Medicine. The Veterinary Art in the Middle Ages (9th–15th Centuries), in: Fifteenth Century Studies 2 (1979), 203–209; Briony Aitchison, Holy Cow! The Miraculous Cures of Animals in Late Medieval England, in: European Review of History 16 (2009), 875–92; William Chester Jordan, Charms to Ward Off Sheep and Pig Murrain, in: Miri Rubin (ed.), Medieval Christianity in Practice, Princeton 2009, 67–75.

Before the impact of epizootics, the measures taken by contemporaries to prevent and absorb losses, or the physical remains of plague victims can be assessed, the plagues themselves must be identified. This is a time-consuming enterprise and one not to be overlooked. Sources of all sorts, composed in different regions and different languages, must be combed, and the provenance, contemporaneity and textuality of relevant passages considered. The spatial and temporal proximity of accounts of plagues to the plagues themselves must be addressed, and when few accounts of an epizootic exist the language employed to describe the plague should be read against other accounts of disease in the same text, as was done here for the sixth-century epizootics. In lieu of multiple independent passages, the emphasis given in a single source to the disease's severity or outbreak's scale should be handled carefully. While Gregory's stress on the virulence of the 591 plague should not be rejected, that he employs similar language in descriptions of disease outbreaks throughout his *LHX* and regularly emphasizes the magnitude of plagues, suggests we cannot read too much into his qualifications of individual disease events. The manorial accounts and textual sources for the 1314–1325 panzootic indicate clearly that reports of large animal mortalities in medieval textual sources should not be rashly discounted, but also that medieval writers did on occasion relate incorrect information and borrow imagery and language from earlier authors.

Premodern epizootic disease has long been neglected in the humanities and the histories of ancient, medieval and early modern plagues presented in catalogues of livestock disease, and in veterinary, virological and policy studies of the rinderpest virus, need to be fine-tuned or rewritten. It is hoped that this article, like other recent studies of medieval epizootics, will be but a beginning, and that scholars of different disciplines will come to work together to flesh out histories of premodern epizootics and panzootics. Only then will we begin to come to terms with the parameters, impacts and identities of these animal plagues, which, though largely ignored until now, were potentially of great significance for premodern human populations, no matter how common they were and enigmatic they appear today.

Abstract:

The history of non-human animal plagues in premodernity is very much in its infancy. While our understanding of premodern animal disease has advanced considerably in recent years, specifically in regards to the fourteenth- and eighteenth-century Eurasian bovine panzootics, a great deal remains unknown about the disease outbreaks domesticated and especially undomesticated animals suffered centuries and millennia ago across all world regions. This article seeks to survey the state of our knowledge about animal plagues in western Eurasia, focusing on the European Middle Ages. It employs case studies of animal plagues observed in the sixth, ninth, tenth and fourteenth centuries to probe the limits of what we can glean about premodern animal plagues from written sources alone, to tease out the relevance of recent and ongoing work in the paleo- and phylo-genetic sciences, and to advance a framework for studying animal disease outbreaks in the distant past. There is much work to do and no one discipline can do it alone. To contextual recent histories of epizootic and zoonotic disease, to begin to establish trends in outbreaks over time and space, and to begin to identify triggers of, and risk factors for, animal disease outbreaks, we must advance a new agenda, one that seeks to interdisciplinarily interrogate the diverse evidence we have (or might look to produce) for past animal disease. This article is a step in that direction.

Keywords:
cattle plagues | rinderpest | epizootic | medieval period

Acknowledgments

This volume is the result of an international conference held in Berlin from 30 March to 1 April 2022. The last waves of the Covid-19 pandemic, which inspired us to organise the conference, were still sweeping the globe. Nonetheless, the conference was able to take place in a hybrid format, with some speakers meeting in the technologically sophisticated Akademiesaal in the Henry Ford Building at Freie Universität Berlin, and the other speakers, as well as several discussants from around the world, participating virtually. We would like to thank all those who participated in and contributed to the success of this memorable event, in particular the Fritz Thyssen Stiftung for its financial support; the staff of the FU for their technical assistance; Olivia Mayer for managing the administration; Niklas-Philipp Müller, who helped us with the practical implementation; Eben Kirksey for his inspiring keynote lecture; Jeannette Vaught, who chaired the final discussion; and Maike Riedinger, who wrote the conference report.[1]

We would like to thank the contributors to this volume for substantially revising their papers for publication – and for their exemplary cooperation and patience during the editing process. Madeleine LaRue did a great job of improving the manuscript with her careful editing. Nicole Schraner provided valuable assistance with the formal editing of the texts, and Noemi Fuchs and Simona Baumgartner supported us in creating the index. We are indebted to the Böhlau publishing house, and especially to Dorothee Wunsch and Julia Roßberg for their competent support during the publication process.

Finally, we would like to thank the University of Klagenfurt and the University of Lucerne for making possible the publication of this volume in print and as an open-access publication.

The Editors
Berlin/Kassel/Klagenfurt/Lucerne, June 2023

1 See Maike Riedinger, Animals and Epidemics in Historical Perspective, 30.03.2022–01.04.2022, Berlin und digital, Conference Report in German, in: H-Soz-Kult (6 June 2022), https://www.hsozkult.de/conferencereport/id/fdkn-127993 (6 June 2023).

Index

Animals

People

W

Y

Places

Concepts